MEDICATION A.R.E.A.S. BUNDLE

A Prescription Solution for Value-Based Healthcare

Elizabeth Oyekan
PharmD, FCSHP, CPHQ

Cover design by Victoria V

Published by BookCrafters, Parker, Colorado.
www.bookcrafters.net

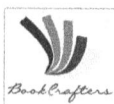

Dedication

This book is dedicated to God, who has showered me with His kindness along with wisdom and understanding. He is also making everything work out according to His purpose.

To my husband, Richard, for his love, incredible support and encouragement, and for this mantra: Good enough never is; therefore, be ever-learning.

To my children, Adedoyin, Oluwasola, and Oluwafemi, for enriching all our lives, supporting me through challenging times, and for doing some of the research in this book.

To my moms (maternal and paternal), dad, sisters, brothers, and family members around the world who have contributed in countless ways.

Acknowledgments

My thanks to Donna Poole, Joe and Jan McDaniel (BookCrafters), Karen Pitcavage, Kimberlee Kiefer, Susan Hindman, Victoria V., and many others for their help in getting this book assembled, typed, fact-checked, verified, designed, edited, and published on a very short time frame. Thank you so much for a job well done.

My gratitude to Carole C., Carole L., Dennis H., June G., Kris K., Ruth D., and my cherished friends near and far for their incredible support, especially during the time I was writing this book.

My indebtedness to my leaders and teachers, management teams, staff members, physician partners, patients, mentors, and sponsors over the years, for the experiences that have contributed to this book.

Table of Contents

Preface

Healthcare delivery systems are undergoing unprecedented change to meet competing priorities that include increased demands for healthcare services; the goal of providing high-quality, affordable care to the general population; and the (unsustainable) rising costs of care and lower reimbursements from payers for services.

In the United States, the passage of the Affordable Care Act (ACA) in 2010 acted as a catalyst to further drive healthcare changes, as well as to promote a focus on healthcare value and the Institute for Healthcare Improvement calls the Triple Aim: improving the patient experience of care (including quality and satisfaction); improving the health of populations; and reducing the per capita cost of healthcare.

While healthcare systems are working to transform the delivery system to improve the quality and affordability of care for millions of people, healthcare in the United States remains unaffordable. The quality of care remains a challenge across the delivery system, especially for the highest utilizers of healthcare: patients with multiple chronic conditions (MCC).

According to the Centers for Disease Control and Prevention (CDC), the number of people in the United States with MCC has risen from 21.8% of the adult population in 2001 to 26% in 2010; this means one out of four Americans has MCC. People with MCC and/or complex conditions are the most frequent users of healthcare, accounting for 96% of drug costs, 91% of all prescriptions filled, 83% of all healthcare spending, 81% of hospital admissions, and 76% of all physician visits.

Let me introduce you to the Smith family who, over time, contributed to my quest to help make the Triple Aim a reality in healthcare, especially for MCC patients. In 2014, Mr. Smith was diagnosed with

1

uncontrolled type 2 diabetes and high cholesterol levels. At the same time, Mrs. Smith was diagnosed with type 2 diabetes, hypertension, and clinical obesity.

The Smiths worked with their physicians, pharmacists, and healthcare team members to develop treatment plans that included diet modifications, physical exercise, and new medications to manage their disease conditions. In October 2014, however, Mr. Smith lost his job. With three children in college, the couple had to rely solely on Mrs. Smith's income, and each family member began hunting for a job.

Because their insurance was through Mr. Smith's job, their healthcare benefits were lost, as well. Mrs. Smith began searching for affordable insurance, but to her dismay, the least expensive full coverage option was the all-too-familiar narrow network plan:

- Monthly premium of $2,000
- Annual family deductible of $10,500
- No maximum limit on out-of-pocket expenses by the family
- Coinsurance of 40%–50% after the deductible for all medical services, depending on the service
- Co-pays of $10 for a 30-day supply of generic medications, and a four-tier co-pay plan for brand and specialty medications

In addition, the family would only be able to receive care from certain doctors, hospitals, labs, pharmacies, and other providers. Visiting out-of-network providers would result in higher out-of-pocket costs.

Their current financial situation made this option impossible, so they explored the health insurance plans and prices on the Marketplace Healthcare Exchange established by the ACA. They found a bronze plan, the cheapest of the four plan levels offered with the following payments:

- Monthly premium of $1,200
- Annual family deductible of $6,500
- Maximum out-of-pocket for medical and drugs of $8,500

- Coinsurance of 40% for all medical services and drugs, regardless of the service

So, in January 2015, the Smith family enrolled in this plan. By September, Mr. Smith was still unemployed, and it was becoming more difficult to pay the premiums. The family was forced to make the very difficult decision to drop their insurance.

Unfortunately, this story is not unique. Situations even more challenging than theirs happen in families every day. They are forced to choose between insurance or paying the mortgage, prescription drugs or college tuition, buying healthy food or the cheapest food that will feed the family. These difficult choices go on and on.

Before the ACA, many families chose to go without insurance, even if they had preexisting conditions, because they could not afford it. And while the ACA has made insurance more affordable, it is still unattainable for many. Uninsured people with complex, preexisting, and/ or chronic conditions chance complications and risk rapid progression of their illnesses, leading to lower quality of health and higher costs to the healthcare system. Yet, even those who have insurance have often been forced into bankruptcy, due to significant out-of-pocket costs, premiums, and catastrophic events.

Under the ACA, the hope was that there would be a more equal proportion of healthy and sick patients in the healthcare pool to help balance the cost of care. However, the reality is that the relatively healthy people are opting out of insurance and choosing to pay the penalties instead. This has left a larger population of sick individuals in the healthcare pool, thus increasing healthcare costs and causing some insurance carriers to drop coverage in some areas.

In my 24-plus years in healthcare, I've known hundreds of providers who have encountered thousands of people like the Smiths, and I know there are millions more like them who do not have access to healthcare for various reasons.

Getting to know the Smith family over a two-year period gave me renewed insight into the challenges that millions of people experience with the current healthcare system. It inspired me to help find a solution that would be meaningful to millions of MCC patients. I spent 18 months extensively researching the challenges and opportunities in healthcare, and hundreds of hours talking with leaders and patients about the challenges in healthcare—and I have come up with a "prescription" to promote healthcare value in this new healthcare environment. This prescription will contribute to optimizing patient health outcomes; lowering the total cost of healthcare to allow more patients to gain access to affordable, high-quality care; and at the same time, improving the performance of organizations and creating a competitive advantage.

I present to you an approach in this book that addresses the above, divided into two sections:

Part I: Challenges in Healthcare and Opportunities to Drive a Value-Based Healthcare System

This section examines the US healthcare system—the good and the challenging aspects of it. Then, it reviews the ACA, its purpose, primary components, successes, challenges, current fate and discusses how the ACA has become a catalyst to promote better care, smarter spending, and healthier communities. Next, it addresses the new Medicare Access and Children's Health Insurance Program Reauthorization Act (MACRA), the Quality Payment Program (QPP), and current programs and measures that are in place to promote healthcare value and accountability (including the transition from fee-for-service to pay for value). Finally, it looks at the organizations involved in supporting the transformation to a value-based healthcare system.

Part II: The Medication A.R.E.A.S. Bundle (MAB) Rx Strategy —A Prescription for Healthcare Value

This section focuses on the prescription solution for healthcare value by condensing and integrating a set of medication practice elements into what I call the Medication A.R.E.A.S. Bundle—Adherence,

Reconciliation, Engagement, Affordability, and Safe Medication Use. I use the acronym MAB or MAB Prescription (Rx) to refer to all of this. Then I took MAB Rx and coupled it with a framework for its implementation, as well as the necessary infrastructures, capabilities, and personnel support needed to ensure its success, scalability, spread, and sustainability. Together, this forms the Medication A.R.E.A.S. Bundle Prescription Strategy, or the MAB Rx strategy. It is my hope that the contents of this book will contribute to the transformative changes of today and improve the health outcomes and quality of life for millions of people; reduce the total cost of healthcare; improve the health and wellbeing of the communities served; and improve the performance outcomes of each organization that adopts the proposed prescription strategy and implements it across the continuum of care for patients with multiple chronic conditions.

When you implement this strategy, please share your successes, challenges, and insights with me. Together, we can make this and other strategies more successful as we work to improve the health of those who have entrusted us with their lives.

My Best to You Always,

Elizabeth Oyekan, PharmD, FCSHP, CPHQ
MABRxStrategy@gmail.com
@MABRxStrategy

Part I:

Challenges in Healthcare and Opportunities to Drive a Value-Based Healthcare System

Chapter 1:
Healthcare in the United States—
The Good and the Challenging

"If you think about how healthcare is delivered, it's on an ad hoc basis. Someone comes into a hospital, someone comes into a pharmacy, someone comes into a doctor. But beyond those touchpoints, the patients are on their own. There's no real continuity of care."
Christopher A. Viehbacher, CEO, Sanofi[1]

Topics Covered:

- An introduction to the US healthcare system: its good and the challenging aspects
- Factors, trends, and drivers contributing to the unsustainable increases in healthcare costs
- US healthcare compared to other countries

The United States has traditionally been perceived to have one of the better healthcare systems in the world, both in terms of technical advances and healthcare quality. In fact, 45% of Americans surveyed in 2008 said that US patients receive better quality of care than do those in other nations and has the world's best healthcare system.[2] With increasing globalization and information sharing, however, it is now evident that, while the US healthcare system has pockets of excellence and has made significant strides to improve over the years, the system as a whole remains challenged. Let's look at the US healthcare system—the good and excellent aspects, as well as the challenging ones, including the drivers of unsustainable cost trends.

The Good

Many Americans, like Jeff Goldsmith, president of Health Futures Inc., believe the US health system's performance has improved. In recounting his experiences in 1979 and 2015, Goldsmith noted significant improvements in surgical procedures such as the total hip replacement for severe arthritis. In 1979, the procedure took about 4½ hours, and the patient stayed in the hospital for approximately three weeks and had about a six-month course of rehabilitation. By 2015, that same procedure took a little over one hour. The patient was walking on the joint within 90 minutes post-op, was discharged home within 24 hours, started physical therapy about 48 hours post-surgery, and, after discharge, had a week of required home health visits to ensure proper pain control and management of any complications such as blood clots or infections. The patient was walking without a limp within two weeks and was driving within one month.[3]

With ongoing refinements of clinical processes, enhanced technology and therapies, education, and patient engagement, the following other improvements have taken place:

- A 25% decline in age-adjusted deaths from cancer from 1990 to 2014, which has resulted in nearly 14.5 million cancer survivors, according to the American Cancer Society[4]
- A 76% drop in deaths from age-adjusted strokes from 1970 to 2014 due to advances in stroke care and public reporting of core stroke measures[5]
- A 67% decline in deaths from heart disease from 1970 to 2014, despite the escalation of cardiac risk created by the obesity epidemic and increased prevalence of diabetes[6]
- Significant improvements in invasive cardiac care due to the introduction of bypass graph surgery and cardiac stents[7]
  These successes have been critical for patients with complex

illnesses. Also, the creation of more effective and consistent care management protocols and the development of consensus standards for successful clinical practices have contributed to the ongoing refinements and improvement in the US healthcare system.[8]

Other good and excellent aspects include:

- *Historic lows in employer health cost growth rates*: Based on the historical cost information for private health insurance tracked by the federal government, healthcare costs have been in a prolonged period of relatively low growth. The average trend from 1984 to 1994 was 10%; from 1994 to 2004, 7.9%; and from 2004 to 2014, just 4.2%.[9]
- *Innovation*: People from around the world come to the United States to get some of the best care available, including cutting-edge medical treatments and techniques. Also, for people with financial means, there are more options for care and doctors.
- *Coverage for the most vulnerable*: The US government provides Medicare insurance for senior citizens and the disabled, Medicaid insurance for low-income people, and the Children's Health Insurance Program (CHIP) for millions of uninsured children. With the ACA, children and young adults are covered under their parents' or guardians' insurance until age 26, and as of 2015, an additional 16 million people who would not have been insured are covered by the ACA.[10]
- *Safety regulations*: The US drug supply chain remains one of the safest in the world. The Food and Drug Administration (FDA) safeguards its integrity and prevents counterfeits, diversion, cargo theft, and importation of unapproved or substandard drugs. Without these safeguards, unsafe, ineffective drugs could enter US distribution and reach consumers.[11]
- *Patient privacy*: With the Health Insurance Portability and Accountability Act of 1996 (HIPAA), all patients receiving care in this country know their health information is secure and protected.[12]

- *Guaranteed emergency care*: The Emergency Medical Treatment and Labor Act (EMTALA) is a federal law that requires anyone coming to an emergency department to be stabilized and treated, regardless of their insurance status or ability to pay. Patients who have nowhere else to go for medical help can seek emergency treatment and not be turned away. This provides some care to the uninsured.[13]
- *The best research*: US university-affiliated hospitals lead the world in research. They develop many of the newest medications, procedures, and technologies that benefit everyone.[14]
- *Increased survival rates*: According to a study in The Lancet, the United States has some of the highest survival rates for heart attacks, strokes, and cancer. American women have a 63% five-year survival rate after a cancer diagnosis, compared to 56% for European women. For American men, the five-year survival rate is 66% compared to 47% for European men. Also, Americans have the highest survival rates for colon, rectal, breast, and prostate cancers compared to 17 European countries. Americans also have one of the highest survival rates for melanoma, ovarian cancer, cervical cancer, and both Hodgkin's and non-Hodgkin's disease lymphoma.[15]
- *Preventive screenings*: The United States has some of the highest percentages of women who get Pap smears and mammography screenings compared to many other countries. It also has the highest rates of cervical cancer screening compared to 23 other developed countries. In addition, more US senior citizens get their flu vaccinations compared to other developed countries.[16]
- *Patient empowerment*: American patients are more likely to seek second opinions, ask questions about their healthcare and medications, and, when necessary, complain and be listened to than patients in health systems in other countries.[17]
- *Pleasing hospital environments*: Many US hospitals are more comfortable and accommodating than hospitals in most other countries around the world. These accommodations include single

or semi-private rooms, gender-separate rooms, food selection choices, and less noise, when possible.

- *Customized convenient services*: Consumerism and market forces have caused organizations to focus on convenience and customized service as a competitive strategy. Examples include: walk-in clinics, online scheduling, transferring of healthcare information electronically, and inclusive one-stop healthcare centers with a lab, pharmacy, other services, and medical offices.[18]
- *Drug development incentives*: The US government offers extended patents and grants to drug companies that are willing to develop medications for patients with rare diseases who have no options.[19]

The Challenges

Unfortunately, the US healthcare system has been spiraling out of control for many years. Some people refer to it as "the healthcare crisis." The challenges have been enabled by the following drivers and trends: high administrative costs; escalation of chronic conditions; fragmentation of the healthcare system; fraud, waste, and abuse; high cost of medications; a lack of focus on prevention and wellness; the fee-for-service reimbursement model; overutilization of services and technology; and the practice of defensive medicine, to name a few. These have led to unsustainable increases in healthcare costs, millions of uninsured people, personal debt and bankruptcies, and patients with poor outcomes in spite of the high costs of healthcare.

The US spends more on healthcare than Japan, Germany, France, China, the United Kingdom, Italy, Canada, Brazil, Spain, and Australia combined. If the US healthcare system were a country, it would have the sixth-largest economy on the planet. Back in 1960, an average of $147 was spent per person on healthcare in this country. By 2009, that number had skyrocketed to $8,086. In 2016, the number is projected to reach $10,345 per capita.[20,21] Let's take a closer look at these challenges and their consequences.

According to the Centers for Medicare and Medicaid Services (CMS), American health spending is about 18% (around $2.6 trillion) of the gross domestic product (GDP) and is projected to reach nearly $5 trillion, or 20% of the GDP by 2021.[22] Other advanced nations are able to provide healthcare services for significantly less: United Kingdom 9.6%, Germany 11.6%, and Japan 9.5% of their respective GDPs.[23]

Despite this high level of healthcare spending, the United States lags behind other countries in many healthcare outcomes and quality measures. This discrepancy illuminates the need to reduce spending while improving care, and the necessity to carefully examine the structural aspects of the healthcare system that contribute to inefficiency and wasteful spending.

Spending on health did not always comprise such a large fraction of the US economic activity. The percentage of our GDP devoted to healthcare spending has doubled over the last 30 years.[24] This rapid growth in health expenditures has created an unsustainable burden on America's economy, with far-reaching consequences.

So, what are the drivers responsible for our high levels of health spending today? Based on many studies—including the Bipartisan Policy Center report titled "What Is Driving U.S. Health Care Spending?"—they include:[25]

- *Administrative costs*: The complex payment and delivery systems have led to increased paperwork and greater administrative burdens on providers, raising their costs.
- *Aging and chronic conditions*: Population aging, rising rates of chronic disease, and comorbidities, as well as lifestyle factors and personal health choices, have had a significant impact on healthcare spending growth.
- *Consolidations*: Changing trends in healthcare market consolidation and competition for providers and insurers have increased the prices of some services.
- *Fragmentation*: Fragmentation in care delivery occurs because providers are paid for volume rather than patient outcomes. This generates little financial incentive to coordinate with others to deliver more efficient care.

- *Fraud and waste*: Experts agree that about 20% to 30% of spending—up to $800 billion a year—goes to care that is wasteful, redundant, or inefficient. In Medicare and Medicaid, fraud, waste, and abuse costs $50 billion to $100 billion or more annually.[26]

- *High cost of medications*: Medication costs escalated by 12.6% in 2014, according to estimates in a new report on trends in healthcare costs by the CMS, and will most likely continue to increase in the upcoming years at a faster pace than other components of healthcare spending.[27] One of the major factors for this significant increase is the FDA's approval of highly effective, but extremely expensive, specialty drugs. This will have an impact on insurance premiums and consumer out-of-pocket spending. Escalating deductibles, co-pays, and medication costs are already adversely impacting what consumers need to stay healthy. For many Americans, medications may become unaffordable. They already pay significantly more for their medications than people elsewhere in the world, something that has not changed in spite of the criticism of the pharmaceutical industry and medical device manufacturers for their role in these increased costs.

- *Insurance benefit design*: People with lower out-of-pocket costs and co-pays tend to use more healthcare services. Access to healthcare services with little cost sharing can encourage increased utilization and lead to more spending.

- *Lack of value*: There is a lack of transparency about cost and quality of services, compounded by limited data to inform consumer choices. Without reliable information that enables a fair comparison of quality and outcomes and the cost associated with these outcomes, patients and clinicians are ill-equipped to utilize the best, most cost-effective treatments.

- *Lack of focus on prevention and wellness*: It is disturbing that such an enormous number of people suffer from chronic diseases, illnesses, and injuries. Even more disheartening is the fact that most of those conditions could likely have been avoided or significantly delayed if people could have changed all of the small but significant daily choices that led to those unintended consequences. Yet, the medical care system in the early 21st century remains focused on treatment and repair, rather than prevention.

- *Regulations and compliance*: Healthcare's legal and regulatory environment, including current medical malpractice and fraud and abuse laws, drives up costs to our healthcare system and prevents transition to more cost-effective systems of care.[28]

- *Reimbursement model*: Fee-for-service reimbursement generates a strong incentive to perform a high volume of tests and services, regardless of whether those services improve quality or contribute to broader efforts to manage care. The new focus on pay for volume versus value will begin addressing the perverse incentives and inefficiencies in the US healthcare system—which spends nearly twice as much on healthcare per person as other advanced countries, but has average-to-poor health outcomes, including a lower life expectancy.[29]

- *Scope of practice*: The short supply of qualified professionals and the way the health profession's workforce is structured—with restrictions to scope of practice, trends in clinical specialization, and conditional access to providers—leads to higher costs and missed opportunities to utilize a lower cost provider.

- *Technology and utilization*: Advances in medical technology have both increased health system efficiency and encouraged unnecessary utilization of expensive treatments in the fee-for-service payment model. Many studies have shown higher US spending is a result of greater utilization of medical technology and higher prices, rather than use of routine services, such as more frequent visits to primary care physicians and providers.

- *Defensive medicine*: Aside from the costs of medical lawsuits and high malpractice insurance premiums, our inefficient medical malpractice system also contributes to high healthcare costs through the practice of "defensive medicine"—meaning, the tests and treatments that physicians prescribe largely in response to the threat of lawsuits. In a 2003 survey of physicians in high-risk specialties, 93% reported they had ordered additional diagnostic procedures, tests, and imaging technology services due to concerns over growing malpractice costs. In total, these defensive medicine costs are estimated to range from $45.6 billion to over $650 billion per year.[30]

Rising healthcare costs adversely impact the United States on multiple fronts. For families and seniors, the higher costs of medical care and insurance mean less money in their pockets and force hard choices about balancing food, rent, and needed care.

For small businesses and Fortune 500 employers alike, the costs make it more expensive to add new employees, more difficult to maintain retiree coverage, and harder to compete in the global economy. For the federal, state, and local governments, rising healthcare costs have led to higher Medicare and Medicaid costs. This has forced cuts to other priority programs such as education, public safety, and infrastructures.[31]

The following are the consequences of all these challenges:

- *Impact on the economy*: Businesses that provide health insurance to their workers are less competitive internationally and have fewer resources to invest in innovation and new technologies. For employees, the increasing cost of employer-provided health insurance contributes to the stagnation of middle-class wages, because salary increases are offset by an employer's healthcare benefit subsidies. Additionally, the growing expense of private health insurance has reduced the resources that consumers would ordinarily have for everything else, ranging from food to housing to savings for their children's education.

  Increased spending on government healthcare programs, primarily Medicare and Medicaid, has consumed a growing portion of federal and state budgets, crowding out other priorities while also increasing public debt and reducing investment in the economy.

- *Impact on the GDP*: Healthcare spending represented 17.0% of our GDP in 2010, and is expected to reach 20% by 2021. Medicare alone accounted for 15% of our federal budget in 2011, and without reform, this share is expected to grow as the baby boomer generation continues to retire. Rising healthcare costs both contribute to our federal deficit and reduce our ability to spend in other important areas, including education, housing, and economic development. In addition, these high costs directly impact businesses and consumers: both the family and employer shares of employer-based coverage doubled between 2001 and 2011.[32]

- *Personal debt*: According to the *American Journal of Medicine*, personal debt and bankruptcies from healthcare costs increased from 46% in 2001 to 62% in 2007. Most of those who filed for bankruptcy were well-educated, middle-class homeowners.[33]

In less developed nations, those in the low-income bracket who are in need of treatment will often avail themselves of whatever help they can get from either the state or nongovernmental organizations without going into debt. In most developed countries, public coverage of healthcare costs are comprehensive, but in the US, even when the patient has insurance coverage, considerable medical costs remain the patient's responsibility.

The rising healthcare costs have made it more difficult for consumers to pay for medical care, and, in some cases, medical debt has become a primary cause of personal bankruptcy, even for those with health insurance. In 2013, an estimated 1.5 million Americans declared bankruptcy. Many people may chalk up that misfortune to overspending or a lavish lifestyle, but a new study suggests that more than 60% of people who declare bankruptcy are actually capsized by medical bills.[34]

US Healthcare Compared to Other Countries

When healthcare experts meet to assess the healthcare system of a certain country, they look at three main dimensions: cost, quality, and access. Cost is basically how much is spent on healthcare in the country. Quality is how the care is provided, and access is whether people can get the care that they need.[35]

The Commonwealth Fund's most recent (2011) national health system scorecard: The Overall Ranking of 11 OECD Countries		
Information from the World Health Organization (WHO) & Organization for Economic Cooperation and Development (OECD)		
	OECD Country with #1 / #2 ranking	U.S. Ranking of the 11 OECD Countries
Overall Ranking (2013)	UK / Switzerland	11
Quality Care	UK / Austria	5
Effective Care	UK / New Zealand	3
Safe Care	UK / France	7
Coordinated Care	UK / New Zealand	6
Patient-Centered Care	UK / Switzerland	4
Access	UK / Germany	9
Cost Related Problem	UK / Switzerland	11
Timeliness of Care	Sweden / Netherlands	5
Efficiency	UK / Sweden	11
Equity	Sweden / UK / Switzerland	11
Healthy Lives	France / Sweden	11
Health Expenditures / Capita 2011	New Zealand ($3,182) / UK ($3,405)	$8,508
http://www.commonwealthfund.org/publications/fund-reports/2014/jun/mirror-mirror		

Figure 1.1 The Commonwealth Fund's most recent (2011) national health system scorecard

According to the Commonwealth Fund's report "Mirror, Mirror on the Wall—How the Performance of the U.S. Health Care System Compares Internationally," the US healthcare system is the most expensive in the world, while underperforming on most dimensions of performance, compared to other countries. Among 11 of the 35 Organization for Economic Cooperation and Development (OECD) nations studied in this report—Australia, Canada, France, Germany, the Netherlands, New Zealand, Norway, Sweden, Switzerland, the United Kingdom, and the United States—the United States ranked last in the following performance categories: overall healthcare ranking, access, cost-related problems, efficiency, equity, and healthy lives.

However, it ranks well in preventive care, patient-centered care, and timeliness of care. The United Kingdom ranks first overall and continues to demonstrate high performance; Switzerland ranks second overall. This report (see Figure 1) also incorporates patients' and physicians' survey results on care experiences and ratings on various dimensions of care.[36]

Key Findings:

- *Quality*: In the following four categories of quality indicators— effective care, safe care, coordinated care, and patient-centered care—the United States did very well on preventive and patient-centered care, but not as well on the other quality indicators compared to 10 other OECD countries.
- *Access*: With the ACA, more people have access to healthcare. However, millions of Americans still do not have access to much needed healthcare, primarily due to cost. And, according to one study, while Americans have more rapid access to specialized care services, they are less likely to have rapid access to primary care services than people in other countries.[37]
- *Efficiency*: Of the 11 OECD countries, the United States ranks last in this category. This is in part due to its poor performance on measures of national health expenditures, administrative costs, administrative hassles, avoidable emergency room use, and duplicative medical testing.
- *Equity*: The United States also ranks last in measures of equity, in part due to Americans with low incomes being more likely to report the following compared to their counterparts in other countries: not visiting a physician when sick; not getting a recommended test, treatment, or follow-up care; or not filling a prescription or skipping doses when needed because of costs. Over one-third of low-income Americans reported going without care due to costs.[38]
- *Healthy lives*: On all indicators of healthy lives, infant mortality,

healthy life expectancy at age 60, and mortality amenable to medical care, the United States ranks last.[39]

Moving forward, the United States hopes to address disparities in access to service by expanding insurance coverage to the uninsured, ensuring Americans have access to primary care and medical home services, providing low- and moderate-income families with financial assistance when they apply for coverage, and continuing to adopt healthcare technology to help providers deliver more effective and efficient care. Also, many US health systems and hospitals are committed to improving healthcare, the quality of care, service, and patient safety, while simultaneously learning from other countries doing well in the areas where the United States needs to improve.[40]

Chapter 2:
The Affordable Care Act—
Its Successes, Challenges, and Fate

"The controversy of healthcare reform continues. Some believe that the Affordable Care Act (ACA or Obamacare) has improved the US healthcare system by reducing the number of uninsured and promoting the focus on value instead of volume. Others believe the ACA will increase our deficit, lead to unsustainable costs, hurt job creators, and reduce innovation. This has led to the newly proposed American Health Care Reform Act (AHCA)."
Elizabeth Oyekan

Topics Covered:

- The components, successes, opportunities, and fate of the ACA
- The role of the ACA in transforming the quality and value of healthcare
- An overview of the National Quality Strategy and the CMS Quality Strategy
- A preliminary comparison of the ACA and AHCA
- Principles worth keeping

On March 23, 2010, President Barack Obama signed into law a federal statute, the Patient Protection and Affordable Care Act (PPACA), also known as the ACA or Obamacare. The ACA, together with the Health Care and Education Reconciliation Act, became the most significant overhaul of the US healthcare system since the passage of Medicare and Medicaid in 1965. The ACA was introduced to address many of the challenges in the healthcare system. Its goals were to help make health insurance more affordable and accessible to lower and middle income Americans and small business employers; improve the quality and value of healthcare provided; implement important new consumer protections; enforce many new rules to help eliminate wasteful spending; bend the cost trends; and initiate reforms to address and transform the healthcare system.[1]

The 8 Primary Components of the ACA

The ACA included several provisions that took effect in 2010. The eight most significant reforms took place from 2010 to 2014:

1. *Early consumer protections and health insurance reforms*: As soon as the ACA became law, reforms to the private health insurance market and consumer protections began. These included preventing most health plans from imposing preexisting condition exclusions on children under 19 years old, prohibiting lifetime limits on coverage, and ending insurance coverage rescissions. The reforms also included improved consumer appeals rights, which enabled people to better understand claim or coverage rejections and appeals, and to obtain independent third-party reviews of insurer's decisions, when needed.

2. *2010–2013 improvements in coverage and affordability*: The law required health plans to cover children up to 26 years old, required free coverage for certain recommended preventive services, began the process of closing the donut hole in Medicare, and required insurers to spend at least 80% of premium dollars on clinical services and quality improvement. The law also focused on the expansion of coverage through Medicaid.

3. *2014 improvements in coverage and affordability*: Some of the most significant and impactful reforms went into place on January 1, 2014. The law prevented discrimination based on preexisting conditions and barred charging women more than men for the same coverage. Most plans had to cover essential healthcare benefits, such as maternity care and prescription drugs. Also, the health insurance marketplaces were created, providing consumers with new types of plans and choices.

4. *Healthcare delivery system improvements*: The ACA included provisions to improve the quality of the healthcare system and the reimbursement infrastructure. This required moving from the fee-for-service model to paying for care delivered. The law also created the National Quality Strategy (NQS) to promote the development of new healthcare quality measures by tying provider reimbursement to quality through value-based payment programs. In addition, the Centers for Medicare and Medicaid Innovation Center (CMMI) was created to test innovative programs and care delivery models that would contribute to improving quality and reducing costs. To further promote this transformation to value-based payment models, the secretary of Health and Human Services (HHS) proposed having 30% of Medicare payments in new advanced alternative payment models (APMs) by the end of 2016, increasing to 50% by the end of 2018 (for more on this, see Chapter 3). HHS has called on state and commercial payers to meet or exceed those goals.[2] To support these efforts, there has been a new focus on data sharing and transparency to make healthcare quality data more available to consumers, providers, and researchers.

5. *Medicaid and Children's Health Insurance Program improvements*: The ACA increased funding for both Medicaid, to cover adults who were previously not eligible, and the Children's Health Insurance Program (CHIP)—making them true safety net programs for low-income Americans. These enhanced programs contain provisions to streamline the application process, improve the quality and effectiveness of the coverage, expand long-term services, enhance coordination between the Medicaid and Medicare programs for the duel eligible populations, and lower the cost of drugs for the Medicaid program.

6. *Medicare program improvements*: The ACA had over 60 provisions to support healthcare system improvements. These provisions: increased access to preventive services; reduced the cost of prescription medications; promoted the adoption of new care delivery models, to optimize care and care coordination; reduced Medicare Advantage plan payments; adjusted Medicare rates to promote effective

value-based care; and altered Medicare payments to hospitals based on their readmission and hospital-acquired infection rates.

7. *Public health, prevention, and capacity expansion*: The ACA's approach to improving health and healthcare expanded into the community to support the reach and sustainability of community-based services, public health programs, and the healthcare workforce. The law has supported the following:

- The investment of funds in a broad range of activities, including community and clinical prevention initiatives, public health research, surveillance, and tracking
- Public health infrastructure, immunizations and screenings, and tobacco prevention
- Workforce training
- The community health center fund, which provides significant support for the operation, expansion, and construction of health centers nationwide
- Healthy eating programs for new mothers, workers, and seniors through standardized menu labels
- Expansion of the National Health Services Corps, which provides scholarships and loan repayment to healthcare providers who work in underserved communities, along with other training programs

8. *Transparency, program integrity, and fiscal responsibility:* The Congressional Budget Office estimated the ACA would reduce the deficit by more than $100 billion during the first 10 years and more than $1 trillion the following 10 years. The ACA also made provisions to aggressively go after fraud, waste, and abuse in the healthcare system, Medicare, and Medicaid. The ACA has promoted accountability and transparency through public reporting in key measures, nursing home safety, changing charitable hospitals' billing practices, and reforming gifting practices from drug and device manufacturers to physicians and teaching hospitals.[3]

ACA: Transforming the Quality and Value of Healthcare

The passage of the ACA has been the catalyst for extensive reform of the US healthcare delivery system. The law established the Health Insurance Marketplace (also known as the exchanges) to extend access to affordable care and provided strong incentives in publicly financed healthcare programs to connect provider payment to quality care and efficiency. The ACA offered better access to coverage for persons with preexisting conditions and young adults, as well as expanding access to preventive services.

The ACA required the HHS to establish an infrastructure to improve healthcare by setting priorities and providing a plan for achieving its goals of better care, affordable care, and healthier people and communities. As a result, the NQS was created—the first overarching strategy and policy designed to lead federal, state, and local efforts to improve the quality of care and align public and private payers in their quality and safety efforts.

Beyond expanding health insurance and access to care, the ACA has numerous other provisions related to improving the quality of care, including:

- The creation of the Center for Quality Improvement and Patient Safety, to conduct and support research on best practices for improving how healthcare is delivered
- The creation of the Patient-Centered Outcomes Research Institute (PCORI), to support the generation of patient-centered evidence that can be used in measure development
- Public reporting on the quality of health insurance plans in the marketplaces
- Data reporting on race, sex, ethnicity, and language
- Health plans that focus on implementing initiatives and activities to reduce healthcare disparities
- Establishment of a mandatory physician quality reporting program and the physician compare website for Medicare beneficiaries

- New payment and care delivery models that would stimulate progress by focusing on value[4]

ACA'S SUCCESSES, CHALLENGES, and FATE

The Successes

Below are the benefits and protections Americans realized between 2010 and 2016, according to the ACA website.

Coverage expansion and its effects

- For the first time in history, nine out of 10 Americans have health insurance, with the nation's uninsured rate falling from over 16% in 2010 to just 9.1% at the end of 2015.
- So far, 35 states and the District of Columbia have expanded Medicaid, giving 4.4 million previously uninsured people access to healthcare and bringing the total number of people covered under Medicaid to about 14 million.
- Over 170 million people now have more transparent access to their coverage information and are able to compare plans, costs, and other ratings.

Improved health and patient care

- About 129 million Americans, including up to 19 million children, with preexisting conditions are now protected from reduced benefits and coverage denials.
- About 2.3 million young Americans gained coverage between 2010 and 2013 because they could stay under their parents' healthcare plans until age 26.
- Preventive care and screening services are now accessible for free for over 137 million Americans (including 55 million women): flu shots, smoking cessation, bone mass measurements, annual check-ups, certain cancer screenings, reproductive counseling, obesity screening, birth control, and behavioral assessment for children.

- The ACA expanded mental health and substance use disorder benefits for 60 million people.
- Over 10 million Medicare prescription drug beneficiaries have saved an average of nearly $2,000 per person due to the phasing out of the "donut hole" coverage gap.

Reduced costs for payers, providers, and patients

- About 105 million Americans have benefited from the annual limits on out-of-pocket spending and the elimination of annual and lifetime limits on coverage. This includes almost 40 million women and 28 million children.
- Close to 8 million Americans have received tax credits, allowing them to purchase healthcare coverage through the insurance marketplaces.
- Between 2011 and 2014, more than $2.4 billion in refunds were paid to consumers—and in 2015, consumers received about $470 million in rebates—from insurers whose spending on health benefits and quality of care, as opposed to advertising and marketing, was too low.
- Medicare Advantage enrollment has grown by about 50% to over 17.1 million, while premiums have dropped by about 10%.

Health and delivery system reform

- Almost 750 accountable care organizations (ACOs) have been created to serve about 23 million people under Medicare, Medicaid, and private insurers (see discussion of ACOs in Chapter 3).
- Medicare Advantage plans have to spend at least 85% of their Medicare revenue on patient care; overpayments to these programs have been phased out.
- Hospitals now receive incentives to reduce hospital-acquired infections and avoidable readmissions (and are penalized if they don't).

Improved structure

- The Partnership with Patients collaborative health-safety learning network now includes over 3,200 hospitals to promote successful and best practices.

- The NQS was created to coordinate and align public and private efforts at the federal, state, and local levels to improve the quality of health and healthcare.[5]

"Because of the Affordable Care Act, more than 100 million Americans have gotten free preventive care like mammograms and contraceptive care with no co-pays, millions of seniors on Medicare have saved hundreds of dollars on their prescription medicine, insurance companies can no longer put lifetime limits on the care your family needs or discriminate against children with preexisting conditions. ... That's a good thing." (Remarks by President Obama on the Affordable Care Act in 2013)[6]

The Challenges

Below are the challenges facing the ACA in 2016.

Reduction in coverage
- In many states, increasing numbers of Americans are losing coverage as insurers are forced to cancel policies due to either standards that do not satisfy the ACA's requirements, financial losses, and/or the costs of the law's mandates and regulations.

Choice limitations
- An increasing number of health plans under the ACA come with narrower networks, which prevents many Americans from keeping the providers they are familiar with and limits the choices of finding new ones.

Cost issues
- Premiums are rising by double digits (an average of 25% in 2017) in the exchange in many parts of the country and will become unaffordable for an increasing number of people. While these increases were predicted at the start of the law, the realities of them have become a challenge for many families and enrollees.[7]
- Insurance companies are backing out of participating in the ACA because fewer healthy Americans than anticipated are signing up;

that in turn raises insurances costs for everyone, which then further drives down participation.[8]

- Premium tax credits do not extend to many middle-income families who need them in order to afford the rising premiums.

Other challenges

- In a 2015 Deloitte survey, only 30% of exchange participants were satisfied with their insurance plan, which was significantly lower than other insured cohorts (42% of enrollees in employer-based coverage, 48% in Medicaid, 58% in Medicare, and 46% of total insured).[9]
- Sixteen of the ACA's 23 healthcare cooperatives have either closed down or announced imminent closing, leaving over 800,000 people looking for new plans and more than $1.7 billion in federal loans that won't be paid back.[10]
- In John Goodman's article "Six Problems with the ACA That Aren't Going Away" in *Health Affairs*, there are at least six major problems that need to be addressed. These include unworkable subsidies, perverse incentives for insurers, perverse incentives for buyers, lack of access to care, the impossible burden for the elderly and the disabled, and the impossible mandate.[11]
- Twenty-one states have chosen not to expand their Medicaid programs—which would give an additional 4 million Americans access to healthcare—due to budget pressures, concerns that the federal government will not pay for the expansion long term, and ideological objections.[12]
- More than 18 million people eligible to buy health insurance still have not done so—especially young people, Hispanics, and those who object to being told to buy insurance. In 2017, the penalty for not having health insurance will be $695 per adult or 2.5% of family income, whichever is greater.[13]

While the ACA has not and will not solve all the healthcare issues and challenges, it has been an important step forward. It has made healthcare coverage more accessible for over 20 million Americans;

promoted the focus on healthcare value over volume; helped ensure consumer protections and health insurance reforms; focused on improvements to the healthcare delivery system, Medicaid and CHIP, and the Medicare program; ensured a renewed focus on public health, wellness, and prevention; promoted ongoing work to reduce healthcare disparities; and promoted increased transparency, program integrity, and fiscal responsibility of our healthcare resources.[14]

The Fate of the ACA: Pros and Cons of Repealing It

As part of his 2016 campaign for president, Donald Trump vowed that on his first day in office, he would ask Congress to repeal the ACA and begin the process of replacing it with reforms that would make healthcare more affordable. In addition, Republicans in both the Senate and the House have pledged to continue their efforts to kill the ACA because they believe that President Obama overstepped his authority when implementing the healthcare law. These efforts would put the insurance coverage for 20 million Americans in jeopardy.

The pros and cons of repealing the ACA have been detailed at the Obamacare Facts website.[15] Below are some of them.

Pros:
- Rules on insurers could be loosened, which could decrease premium growth in the long term.
- Subsidies would be repealed, which would mean less federal spending; but if taxes are cut along with subsidies, it would have much less impact on federal spending.
- Tens of millions of people would receive tax credits, based on age and income, to help lower the cost of their premiums and coverage.
- People would have to make an active decision to renew their plan (there would be no automatic renewals).
- Children under 26 would remain covered for now, but this might change.
- Medicaid expansion would be eliminated, saving taxpayers money.

- With options not to provide benefits, rights, or protections by insurers, this will mean less spending and lower rates.
- There would be no rules for what health insurance must offer or who insurers can sell to, which would mean lower rates for some people.[16]

Cons:

- Since so much of the healthcare reform law has already been implemented, it would be incredibly difficult to make changes without a tremendous amount of disruption to beneficiaries, healthcare organizations, and numerous agencies.
- Many of the benefits, rights, and protections—such as protection of Americans with preexisting conditions—could be eliminated. This would be a major blow to the new consumer rights and protections regarding healthcare, with little to no curbing of federal, state, or personal healthcare spending.[17]
- The estimated cost of repealing the law could be as much as $6.2 trillion over the next 75 years, according to a 2013 report by the Government Accountability Office.[18]
- A June 2015 report from the Congressional Budget Office showed a $137 billion net increase to the deficit over the next decade if the ACA is repealed.[19]
- Millions of women could lose access to free preventive care such as mammograms, contraception, and cancer screenings.
- Millions of Americans would lose access to free preventive services and wellness programs.

There could be a further increase in healthcare disparities for people without access to care.[20]

Bottom line, repealing all of the ACA would most likely result in a net increase to the deficit, lead to tens of millions of people being uninsured and lacking access to more affordable care, and possibly cause major chaos and upheaval.

Preliminary Components of the American Health Care Reform Act and Comparisons to the ACA

On March 6, 2017, House Republicans introduced the American Health Care Reform Act (AHCA) of 2017, a legislative bill to repeal and replace the ACA. According to the Henry J. Kaiser Family Foundation, as of March 20, 2017, the overarching components of the AHCA are:

- *Eliminate/repeal the following*: the ACA mandates, Medicare Hospital Insurance (HI) tax increase, and other ACA revenue provisions; funding for the Prevention and Public Health Fund; the standards for health plan actuarial values; federal Medicaid funding for Planned Parenthood clinics; the enhanced Federal Medicaid Assistant Percentage (FMAP) for Medicaid expansion as of January 1, 2020 (the FMAP is what the federal government uses for Medicaid allocations to the states - some exceptions will apply); and the premium and cost-sharing subsidies
- *New additions and modifications*: encourage the use of Health Savings Accounts by increasing annual tax-free contribution limits and through other changes; imposing a late enrollment penalty for people who do not stay continuously enrolled; in 2020, replacing ACA income-based tax credits with flat tax credits adjusted for age; converting the federal Medicaid funding to a per capita allotment and limiting growth beginning in 2020; and modifying ACA premium tax credits for 2018–2019 to increase the amount for younger adults and reduce it for older adults (also applies to coverage sold outside of exchanges and to catastrophic policies)
- *Establish/provide the following*: new state innovation and stability program grants with federal funding of $100 billion over nine years to help fund high-risk individuals, promote access to preventive services, provide cost sharing subsidies, and for other purposes as well as supplemental funding for community health centers of $422 million for FY 2017
- *Retain the following*: guaranteed issue coverage; prohibition on

discriminatory premiums and preexisting condition exclusions; requirement that the marketplaces provide dependent coverage for children up to age 26; annual open enrollment periods and special enrollment periods; and no changes to Medicare benefit enhancements or provider/Medicare Advantage plan payment savings[21]

Comparing the ACA and the proposed AHCA

On March 21, 2017, three new modifications were made to the AHCA to increase the possibility of passage but no to avail.
1. New Medicaid restrictions:
   - States could no longer expand Medicaid to adults above 133% of the federal poverty line.
   - After March 2017, enhanced funding for states that choose to expand Medicaid would be limited.
   - States would have the option to add a work requirement for nondisabled, nonpregnant, nonelderly enrollees to receive coverage.
   - Block grants would be an option for states in addition to the per capita allotment program.
2. Additional funds for seniors:
   - Age-based tax credits may get additional funds.
   - The Medicaid inflation adjustment for elderly enrollees would be increased to help offset high premium costs.
3. Relief from ACA taxes:
   - Effective in 2017, several of the ACA taxes would be repealed, including the over-the-counter medication tax, the health savings account tax, medical device tax, health insurance tax, and tanning tax.
   - The ACA's Cadillac tax on luxury employer-sponsored health plans would be delayed an extra year, to 2026.[22]

As the negotiations continue to get enough votes to repeal and replace the ACA or Obamacare, the repeal and replace process has been broken down into three overarching phases:

- Adoption of the AHCA which takes full advantage of the budget reconciliation process to avoid a Democratic filibuster
- Administration actions mainly by the HHS to stabilize the health insurance market, increase choices, and lower costs
- Additional legislative policies, such as allowing individuals to purchase coverage across state lines, that by Senate rules cannot be included in a reconciliation bill

Now that the AHCA has collapsed, what will happen next? Will we see another attempt to repeal and replace the ACA (Obamacare) or will our leaders work together to come up with legislation that will promote a better healthcare system - focusing on lowering costs and improving quality while expanding coverage to those who need it? Only time will tell. However, below are key principles worth keeping on behalf of all.

PRINCIPLES WORTH KEEPING

According to Jim Collins, co-author of Built to Last, "In this era of dramatic change, we're hit from all sides with lopsided perspectives that urge us to hold nothing sacred, to 'reengineer' and dynamite everything, to fight chaos with chaos, to battle a crazy world with total, unfettered craziness. Everybody knows that the transformations facing us—social, political, technological, economic—render obsolete the lessons of the past. Well, I submit that 'everybody' is wrong. The real question is, What is the proper response to change? We certainly need new and improved business practices and organizational forms, but in a turbulent era like ours, attention to timeless fundamentals is even more important than it is in stable times."[23]

Many healthcare leaders, policy makers, analysts, and citizens believe that we should not just throw out everything that is associated with the ACA and replace it with something else, which appears to be the belief of some of the alternative ACA plans. While there are components of the ACA that need to be changed, deleted, updated, and improved to stimulate progress, there are fundamental aspects of it that should be preserved and are core to basic healthcare coverage for all Americans. Below are some of the core principles that the ACA was built on and the provisions it offers that must be preserved moving forward:

Better Care
- Affordable prescription medications
- Incentives and penalties for hospitals and health systems to reduce the most common causes of preventable admissions and readmissions (such as hospital-acquired infections)
- Increased focus on mental health and substance use disorders
- Maintenance of the NQS
- Free preventive care and screening services
- Prohibition of sudden cancellations of health insurance due to changes in health conditions
- Protection from coverage denials for people with preexisting conditions
- Provisions to recruit and train qualified healthcare providers to address the new challenges in this era of value-based healthcare

Smarter Spending
- Provide ways for Americans to purchase healthcare (for example, subsides, tax credits)
- Establish partnerships to promote and spread successful, best practices
- Find ways to encourage younger and healthier people to enroll in the system to balance the risk pool and lower overall costs
- Have organizations continuously look for ways to reduce the cost of care and pass savings on to individual and group purchasers (for example, preventing the unnecessary use of the most expensive facilities like emergency rooms and urgent cares for basic healthcare needs – venue management)
- Reform medical liability to reduce frivolous lawsuits and the practice of defensive medicine

- Make access to coverage information transparent so that plan costs and other ratings can be compared
- Promote innovations, research, and best practices in clinical practice, care delivery, and the healthcare systems (for example, the creation of alternative payment models) that make the Triple Aim a reality
- Don't charge women more for healthcare than men

Healthier Communities

- Have annual limits on out-of-pocket spending on essential healthcare benefits and the elimination of annual and lifetime limits on insurance coverage
- Retain coverage for young Americans under their parents' healthcare plans until a predetermined age
- Ensure effective safety net programs (such as Medicare and Medicaid) that will help improve care and reduce costs for our most vulnerable populations
- Make healthcare available and affordable for all Americans
- Reduce healthcare disparities and inequities
- Support wellness programs and create incentives for people to make healthy choices and adopt healthy behaviors

According to Bob Galvin, former CEO of Motorola, "Change unto itself is essential. But, taken alone: it is limited. Yes, renewal is change. It calls for 'do differently.' It is willing to replace and redo. But it also cherishes the proven basics."[24]

ACA	AHCA (SUBJECT TO CHANGES)
Date Introduced: March 23, 2010	Date Introduced: March 6, 2017
• Require most U.S. citizens and legal residents to have health insurance. • Create state-based health insurance exchanges through which individuals and small businesses can compare plans, apply for financial assistance, and purchase coverage. • Provide refundable premium tax credits, based on income and cost of coverage, for individuals/families with income between 100% and 400% of the federal poverty level. • Impose new insurance market regulations, including requiring guaranteed issue of all non-group health plans during annual open enrollment and special enrollment periods; limiting rating variation to 4 factors: age, geographic rating area, family composition, and tobacco use; prohibiting preexisting condition exclusion periods; prohibiting lifetime and annual limits on • coverage; and extending dependent coverage to age 26. • Require 10 essential health benefits be covered by all individual and small group health insurance • Require plans to provide no-cost preventive benefits and limit annual cost-sharing.	• Repeal ACA mandates (2016), standards for health plan actuarial values (2020), and premium and cost-sharing subsidies (2020). • Modify ACA premium tax credits for 2018–2019 to increase amount for younger adults and reduce for older adults, also to apply to coverage sold outside of exchanges and to catastrophic policies. • Retain private market rules, including requirement to guarantee issue coverage, prohibition on discriminatory premiums and preexisting condition exclusions, and requirement to extend dependent coverage to age 26. • Retain health insurance marketplaces, annual open enrollment periods, and special enrollment periods. • Impose late enrollment penalty for people who don't stay continuously covered. • Establish State Innovation Grants and Stability Program with federal funding of $100 billion over nine years.

ACA	AHCA (SUBJECT TO CHANGES)
Date Introduced: March 23, 2010	Date Introduced: March 6, 2017
<ul><li>Expand Medicaid to 138% of the federal poverty level at state option and require a single, streamlined application for tax credits, Medicaid, and CHIP.</li><li>Extend CHIP funding to 2015 and increase the match rate by 23 percentage points up to 100%.</li><li>Close the Medicare Part D doughnut hole and enhance coverage of preventive benefits in Medicare.</li><li>Reduce Medicare spending by reducing payments for Medicare Advantage plans, hospitals, and other providers.</li><li>Establish the Independent Payment Advisory Board and the Center for Medicare and Medicaid Innovation (CMMI).</li></ul>	<ul><li>Repeal funding for Prevention and Public Health Fund at the end of Fiscal Year 2018 and rescind any unobligated funds remaining at the end of FY2018. Provide supplemental funding for community health centers of $422 million for FY 2017.</li><li>Encourage use of Health Savings Accounts by increasing annual tax-free contribution limit and through other changes.</li><li>Eliminate enhanced FMAP for Medicaid expansion as of January 1, 2020 (some exceptions apply)</li><li>Convert federal Medicaid funding to a per capita allotment and limit growth beginning in 2020.</li><li>No change to Medicare benefit enhancements or Provider/ Medicare Advantage plan payment savings.</li><li>Repeal Medicare Hospital Insurance tax increase and other ACA revenue provisions.</li><li>Prohibit federal Medicaid funding for Planned Parenthood clinics.</li></ul>

Figure 2: Comparing the Affordable Care Act and the proposed American Health Care Act.
Source: Kaiser Family Foundation,
http://kff.org/interactive/proposals-to-replace-the-affordable-care-act/

Chapter 3:
MACRA's Quality Payment Program—
Supporting the Transition from
Volume to Value

"The MACRA legislation Congress passed ... was a milestone in our efforts to advance a health care system that rewards better care, smarter spending, and healthier people. We have more work to do, but we are committed to implementing this important legislation and creating a health care system that works better for doctors, patients, and taxpayers alike. We look forward to listening and learning from the public on our proposal for how to advance that goal."
HHS Secretary Sylvia M. Burwell[1]

Topics Covered:

- An introduction to QPP and MACRA, and key concepts to prepare clinicians and organizations for both
- An overview of merit-based incentive payment systems
- An overview of alternative payment models, examples of them, and a framework for private-sector payers

In April 2015, a bipartisan majority in Congress passed the Medicare Access and CHIP Reauthorization Act of 2015 (MACRA) to make comprehensive changes to how Medicare pays for physician services. While built on the principles set by the ACA, MACRA will most likely remain regardless of what happens to the ACA. MACRA's focus is supporting the ongoing transformation of healthcare delivery by tying Medicare reimbursements to quality of care through merit-based incentive payment systems and alternative payment programs to support the NQS aims of better care, smarter spending, and healthier people. It also moves closer to the new CMS strategy of addressing the care delivery system and promoting information sharing.

The passage of MACRA terminated the sustainable growth rate, the long-standing formula for determining Medicare payments to physicians and other eligible health professionals, and combined the existing provider payment programs—the Physician Quality Reporting System, the Value Modifier program, and the Medicare Electronic Health Record (EHR) Incentive Program—into one overarching program.[2]

In 2016, the HHS and CMS developed the Quality Payment Program (QPP) framework to operationalize MACRA with the following strategic goals:

- Modernizing and aligning Medicare payments with the cost and quality of patient care for eligible clinicians
- Moving toward reimbursement systems that are based on performance incentives or APMs
- Rewarding eligible clinicians for value over volume
- Streamlining other existing quality reporting programs into one new system
- Furthering the development of delivery models for physicians and other clinicians
- Improving Medicare beneficiaries' outcomes
- Improving data and information sharing

The QPP policy will reform Medicare payments to more than 600,000 US clinicians and will be a major step in improving care across the entire healthcare delivery system.[3]

QPP offers the following two paths (see Figure 3.1) to help clinicians transition from payments based on volume (fee-for-service) to payments based on value (fee-for-value):

- Merit-Based Incentive Payment System (MIPS)
- Advanced APMs (AAPMs)

The Medicare Access & <u>CHIP</u> Reauthorization Act of 2015 (MACRA) / Quality Payment Program (QPP) to reform Medicare payment by:

1. Implementing a new payment framework to reimburse for VALUE instead of VOLUME

2. Ending the Sustainable Growth Rate (SGR) formula for health care providers' services

3. Combining components of the Quality Reporting Programs into one new system

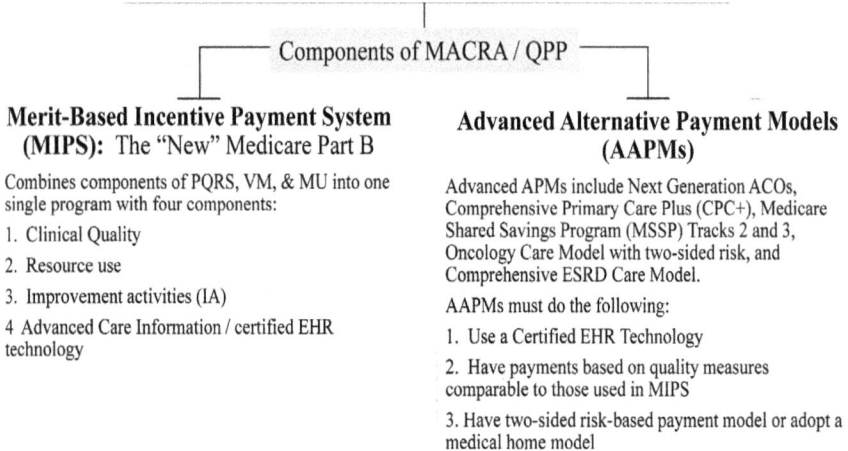

Components of MACRA / QPP

Merit-Based Incentive Payment System (MIPS): The "New" Medicare Part B

Combines components of PQRS, VM, & MU into one single program with four components:

1. Clinical Quality

2. Resource use

3. Improvement activities (IA)

4 Advanced Care Information / certified EHR technology

Advanced Alternative Payment Models (AAPMs)

Advanced APMs include Next Generation ACOs, Comprehensive Primary Care Plus (CPC+), Medicare Shared Savings Program (MSSP) Tracks 2 and 3, Oncology Care Model with two-sided risk, and Comprehensive ESRD Care Model.

AAPMs must do the following:

1. Use a Certified EHR Technology

2. Have payments based on quality measures comparable to those used in MIPS

3. Have two-sided risk-based payment model or adopt a medical home model

Figure 3.1: The two tracks of MACRA's Quality Payment Program

New HHS and CMS Goals for Value-Based Payments

In January 2015, HHS and CMS set goals for value-based payments within the Medicare fee-for-service (FFS) system (see Figure 3.2) and invited private-sector payers to match or exceed the following two goals:

- 85% of all Medicare FFS payments would be tied to quality measures and value, such as value-based purchasing, the Hospital Readmissions Reduction Program, and others by the end of 2016, increasing to 90% by the end of 2018.

- 30% of Medicare payments would be tied to quality or value through alternative payment models (APMs) by the end of 2016, increasing to 50% by the end of 2018.

Medicare Payment Changes 2011-2018

CMS aims to link 90% of Medicare payments to quality programs and 50% to alternative payment models by 2018.

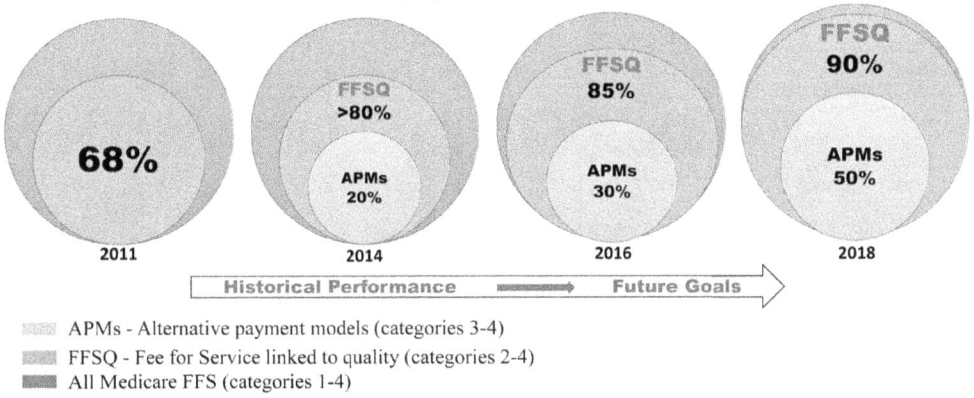

2011   2014   2016   2018

Historical Performance ➡ Future Goals

APMs - Alternative payment models (categories 3-4)
FFSQ - Fee for Service linked to quality (categories 2-4)
All Medicare FFS (categories 1-4)

Figure 3.2: Medicare payment changes from 2011 to 2018

This was the first time HHS and the Medicare program set explicit goals for APMs and value-based payments with the goal to move the Medicare program and the healthcare system at large toward paying providers based on quality rather than quantity of care provided. To make these goals scalable beyond Medicare, the HHS secretary also announced the creation of a Health Care Payment Learning and Action Network. Through this network, HHS will work with private payers, employers, consumers, providers, states and state Medicaid programs, and other partners to expand APMs into their programs.[4] (See more about payments options for MIPS and AAPMs in Appendix A.)

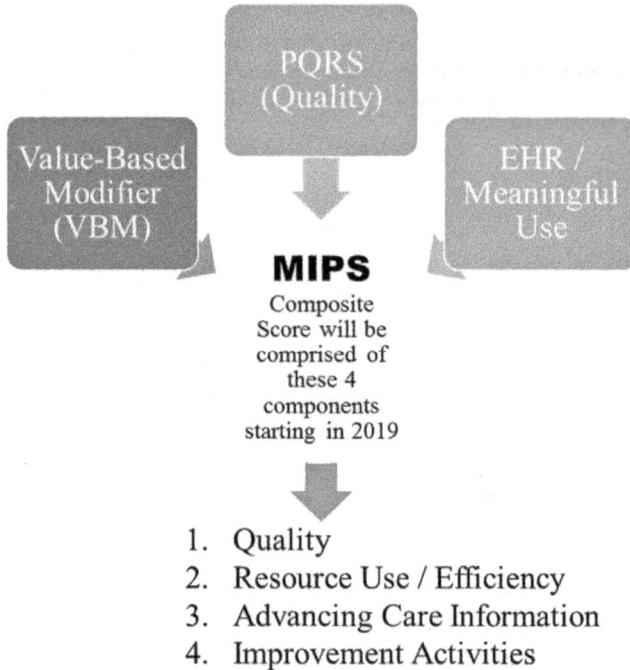

Figure 3.3: The combination of three programs into one single payment program—MIPS

MERIT-BASED INCENTIVE PAYMENT SYSTEM (MIPS)

MIPS combines the current Physician Quality Reporting System (PQRS), Value-Based Payment Modifier, and EHR incentive programs into a single payment system (see Figure 3.3). These three existing clinician-level quality programs will sunset at the end of 2018. Under the MIPS program, each eligible clinician and groups of eligible clinicians under Medicare Part B will be moved into a performance-based payment system that will give them the flexibility to choose activities and measures that will be most meaningful to their practices from the following four categories: quality, resource use, improvement activities, and Advancing Care Information (ACI, replacing the Meaningful Use program for Medicare clinicians). Each provider will be assigned a composite performance score (from 0 to 100) based on the four categories, and their payments will then be adjusted based on a comparison of their composite scores to a performance threshold and their level of participation.[5]

When Does MIPS Begin and How Will It Work?

Performance: MIPS begins in 2017. The first performance period opened January 1, 2017, and closes December 31, 2017. During the year, clinicians will need to record quality data and their use of technology to support their practices. Practices that are Advanced APMs can provide care during the year through that model.

Send in performance data: To potentially earn a positive payment adjustment, clinicians will need to send in data as described in Appendix A to MIPS by March 31, 2018. Advanced APMs will send in their quality data to earn the 5% incentive payment for participating in an Advanced APM.

Feedback: Once the data has been submitted, Medicare will provide feedback about their performance to clinicians and practices between April and December 2018.

Payment: Clinicians may earn a positive MIPS payment adjustment beginning January 1, 2019,[6] if they submitted their 2017 data in time. The positive adjustments will be based on the performance data submitted, not the amount of information or length of time submitted. Clinicians who submit their 2017 Advanced APM data may earn a 5% incentive payment in 2019. The timeline for MIPS is outlined in Appendix B.

MIPS: Provider Eligibility, Scoring, Weighting, and Payment Adjustments

- *Provider/clinician eligibility*

  Eligible clinicians (ECs) for MIPS in the first two years (2019 and 2020) include physicians, physician assistants, nurse practitioners, clinical nurse specialists, nurse anesthetists, and groups including such clinicians (see Figure 3.4). To be eligible for the QPP, a clinician must bill more than $30,000 and see more than 100 Medicare beneficiaries.

In the third year and beyond, ECs will include occupational therapists, speech-language pathologists, audiologists, nurse midwives, clinical social workers, clinical psychologists, and dieticians/nutrition professionals. Medicare Part B providers who are exempt from MIPS will be ECs participating in APMs, first-time Medicare clinicians, and clinicians with low patient volume threshold (they charge Medicare less than or equal to $30,000 a year or see 100 or fewer Medicare Part B patients a year).[7]

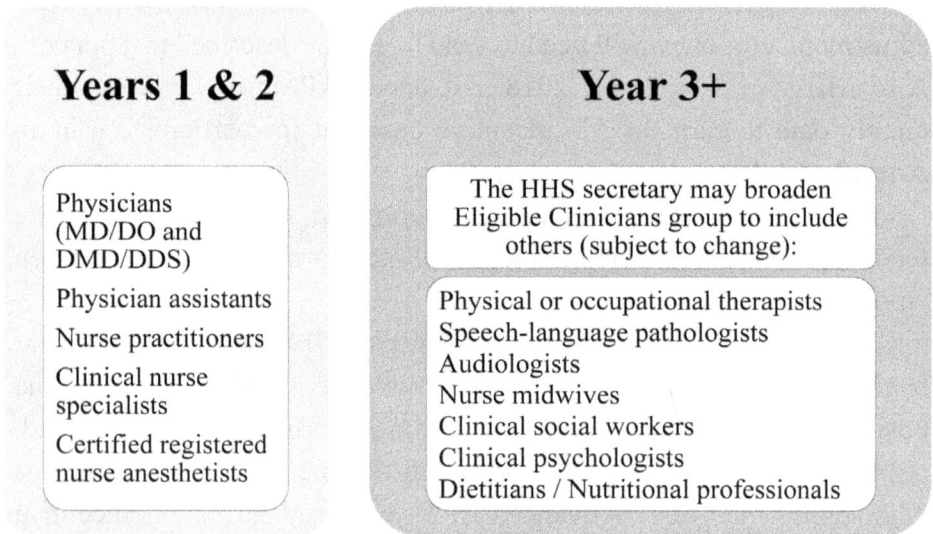

Years 1 & 2

Physicians
(MD/DO and
DMD/DDS)

Physician assistants

Nurse practitioners

Clinical nurse
specialists

Certified registered
nurse anesthetists

Year 3+

The HHS secretary may broaden
Eligible Clinicians group to include
others (subject to change):

Physical or occupational therapists
Speech-language pathologists
Audiologists
Nurse midwives
Clinical social workers
Clinical psychologists
Dietitians / Nutritional professionals

Figure 3.4: MIPS eligible clinicians (ECs) that will participate in MIPS. The types of Medicare Part B eligible clinicians affected by MIPS may expand in future years.

- *Weighting*

    Eligible clinicians' MIPS performance is based on the four categories, which contribute to the MIPS composite performance score of up to 100 points (see Figure 3.5). In year one (2017 performance year aligned with the 2019 payment year), the proposed category weightings are quality (60%), ACI (25%), improvement activities (15%), and resource use (0%).

MIPS Performance Category Weights - Year 1

Final MIPS Performance Category Weights - in 2021 (subject to change)

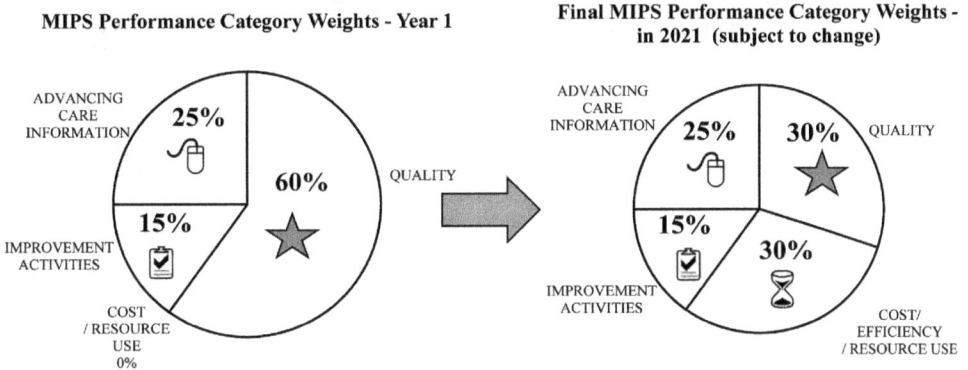

Figure 3.5: The MIPS performance categories and weights

By the 2019 performance year aligned with the 2021 payment year, it is proposed that the quality and resource use/cost categories will change from 60% and 0%, respectively, to 30% each (subject to change). Under certain circumstances where the eligible clinician's performance cannot be determined for a given category, MIPS will set that category to 0% and redistribute the weight to the quality category, but this may change in the future.[8]

- *Scoring*
  Each performance category is scored independently as a percentage of the maximum possible points in that category. Then the scores from each category will be weighted based on the weight for that category (see Figure 3.6).

  Details of calculating the scores for each section and calculating the final score under MIPS can be found at https://www.cms.gov/Medicare/Quality-Initiatives-Patient-Assessment-Instruments/Value-Based-Programs/MACRA-MIPS-and-APMs/Quality-Payment-Program-Long-Version-Executive-Deck.pdf, pages 35–45.

Summary of MIPS Performance Categories	Maximum Possible Points per Performance Category	Percentage of Overall MIPS Score (Performance Year 1, 2017)
Quality: Clinicians choose six measures to report to CMS that best reflect their practice. One of these measures must be an outcome measure or a high-priority measure, and one must be a cross-cutting measure. Clinicians may also choose to report a specialty measure set. This replaces the Physician Quality Reporting System (PQRS).	Clinicians receive 3 to 10 points on each quality measure based on performance against benchmarks	60%
Advancing Care Information: Clinicians will report key measures of interoperability and information exchange. Clinicians are rewarded for their performance on measures that matter most to them. This replaces the Medicare EHR Incentive Program also known as Meaningful Use.	Capped at 100 points	25%
Improvement activities: Clinicians may choose the activities best suited for their practice; the rule proposes over 90 activities from which to choose. Clinicians participating in a patient-centered medical home, medical home model, or similar specialty practice will earn "full credit" in this category, and those participating in APMs will earn at least half credit. This is a new category.	Activity Weights -Medium = 10 points -High = 20 points	15%
Resource use: CMS will calculate these measures based on claims and availability of sufficient volume. Clinicians do not need to report anything. This category replaces the Value-Based Payment Modifier.	Maximum of 10 points per episode cost measure	0% (in 2017)

Figure 3.6: MIPS—Proposed Performance Category Scoring (subject to change)[9,10]

- *Payment adjustments: Provider bonuses and penalties (subject to change)*

  Payment adjustments are determined by the combined weighted score of quality, resource use, meaningful use, and improvement activities. According to CMS, the law requires MIPS to be budget neutral.[11] Therefore, clinicians' MIPS scores would be used to compute a positive, negative, or neutral adjustment to their Medicare Part B payments (see Figure 3.7). Baseline payment adjustments for the following years include:

- Payment adjustment of up to +/- 4% in 2019
- Payment adjustment of up to +/- 5% in 2020
- Payment adjustment of up to +/- 7% in 2021
- Payment adjustment of up to +/- 9% in 2022 and beyond
- 2026 (and beyond): 0.25% annual baseline payment update

Also, between 2019 and 2024, exceptional performers may be eligible for an additional positive payment adjustment.

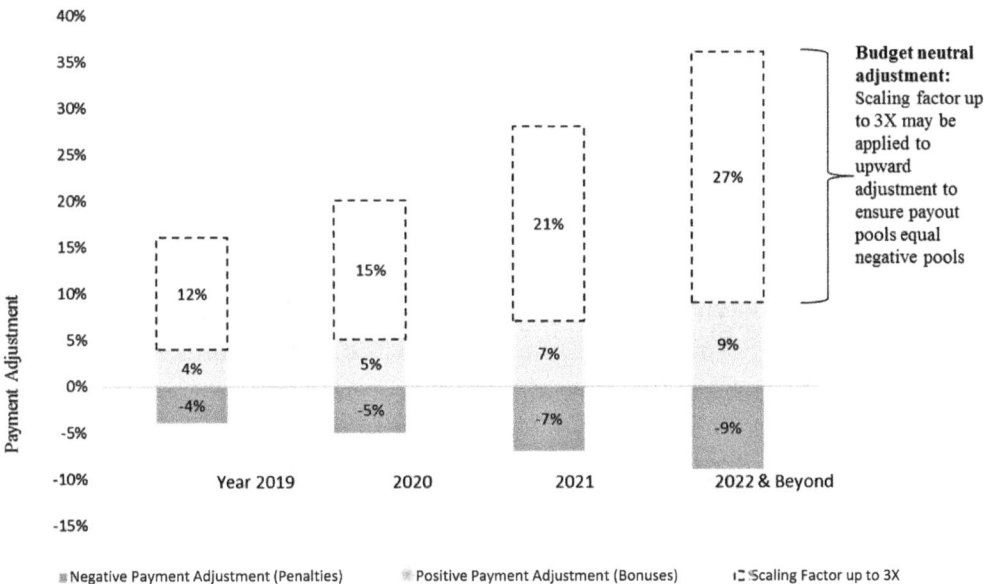

Figure 3.7: Provider payment adjustments—bonuses and penalties

In the first five payment years of the program, the law allows for $500 million in an additional performance bonus that is exempt from budget neutrality for exceptional performance.[12] For more information, go to the CMS website: https://www.cms.gov/Medicare/Quality-Initiatives-Patient-Assessment-Instruments/Value-Based-Programs/MACRA-MIPS-and-APMs/MACRA-MIPS-and-APMs.html.

ALTERNATIVE PAYMENT MODELS (APMs) AND ADVANCED APMs (AAPMs)

What Are They?

In addition to establishing MIPS, MACRA provides incentives to clinicians to participate in APMs that meet criteria specified in the law. APMs are not just incentive models; they fundamentally change how we deliver care and pay for healthcare in this country. They have the potential to change the value we receive from the healthcare system. APMs include:

- Medicare Shared Savings Program (MSSP)
- Accountable care organizations (ACOs)
- Patient-centered medical homes
- Medicare Advantage
- Bundled Payments for Care Improvement (BPCI) initiative
- The Comprehensive Care for Joint Replacement (CJR) model
- All the CMS Innovation Center initiatives except Health Care Innovation Awards and certain demonstration programs

Most clinicians who participate in APMs will also be subject to MIPS, but will receive favorable scoring with correspondingly higher reimbursement rates. They may be eligible for the following:

- Annual 5% lump-sum bonus payments from 2019 through 2024
- Beginning in 2026, higher annual premiums (for some participating providers)
- Increased flexibility through physician-focused payment models

Advanced APMs (AAPMs), also known as "eligible" APMs, are a subset of APMs. These AAPMs must meet the following criteria according to the MACRA law:

- Must be in a risk-based payment model such as:
  - Next Generation ACOs
  - Comprehensive Primary Care Plus (CPC+)
  - Medicare Shared Savings Program (MSSP) Tracks 2 and 3
  - Oncology Care Models (OCMs) with two-sided risk
  - Comprehensive End-Stage Renal Disease (ESRD) care programs
- Base payment on quality measures must be comparable to those in MIPS
- Will require use of certified EHR technology[13]

Currently, about 95% of APM ACOs are participating in Track 1 of the MSSP, which does not qualify them for the eligible Advanced APM category; therefore, they will be scored under MIPS. For Advanced APMs, a bonus payment will be made to clinicians who operate under the Advanced APMs. In addition, they will also receive the regular APM rewards.

CMS is estimating less than 5% of participating physicians will get paid under the APM track. In 2019, clinicians could qualify for incentive payments based, in part, on participation in Advanced APMs developed by non-Medicare payers, such as private insurers or state Medicaid programs.[14] As CMS continues to develop and evaluate APMs, the identification and integration of lessons learned, best practices, and viable measures are essential for the transition to Advanced APMs.

Another important consideration for CMS and MACRA-funded measure developers is to understand the variation and diversity of payment models when identifying clinical quality measures for development. MACRA requires that performance and participation information under MIPS and APMs be made available for public reporting on the Physician Compare website, which will help Medicare consumers make informed healthcare decisions and choices.[15]

Examples of APMs:

Accountable Care Organizations (ACOs)

Accountable care organizations consist of healthcare providers and organizations such as doctors, hospitals, and other providers who come together to coordinate and provide high-quality care to their Medicare patients.[16] The goal of an ACO is to deliver seamless, high-quality care for Medicare beneficiaries, instead of the fragmented care that often results from an FFS payment system, in which different providers receive different, disconnected payments. When an ACO is successful in providing high-quality care and reduces the cost of care by spending and using resources more effectively, the ACO shares in the savings it achieves for the Medicare program.

There are a number of ACO programs such as the MSSP, which was established by section 3022 of the ACA. The program is a key component of the Medicare delivery system reform initiatives included in the ACA and is a new approach to the delivery of healthcare. The MSSP was designed to facilitate coordination and cooperation among providers to improve the quality of care for FFS beneficiaries and reduce the rate of growth in healthcare costs. Eligible clinicians, hospitals, and suppliers may participate in the MSSP by creating or participating in an ACO—and when ACOs meet the program requirements and quality performance standards, they are eligible to share in savings, if earned. ACOs will be responsible for maintaining a patient-centered focus and developing processes to promote evidence-based medicine, promote patient engagement, internally and publicly report on quality and cost, and coordinate care.[17] Other ACO programs include the ACO Investment Model, Comprehensive ESRD Care Model, Medicare Health Care Quality Demonstration, Next Generation ACO Model, Nursing Home Value-Based Purchasing Demonstration, and Pioneer ACO Model. For more information, go to https://innovation.cms.gov/initiatives/index.html#views=models.

Primary Care Medical Home (PCMH) Models

The medical home is best described as a model or philosophy of primary care that is patient-centered, comprehensive, team-based, coordinated, accessible, and focused on quality and safety. It has become a widely accepted model for how primary care should be organized and delivered throughout the healthcare system, and is a philosophy of healthcare delivery that encourages clinicians and care teams to meet patients where they are, from the simplest to the most complex conditions. It is a place where patients are treated with respect, dignity, and compassion, and it enables strong and trusting relationships with clinicians and staff. Above all, the medical home is not a final destination; instead, it is a model for achieving primary care excellence so care is received in the right place, at the right time, and in the manner that best suits a patient's needs.[18]

Bundled Payment Models

Bundled payment is defined as the reimbursement of healthcare clinicians (such as hospitals and physicians) on the basis of expected costs for clinically defined episodes of care. Bundle payment models are also known as episode-based payment, episode payment, episode-of-care payment, case rate, evidence-based case rate, global bundled payment, global payment, package pricing, and packaged pricing.[19]

A bundled payment is a single payment that comprehensively covers the cost of care delivered by two or more providers during one episode of care and/or some specified period of time, and is a hybrid between FFS reimbursement and capitation to reduce healthcare costs. For example, if a patient has total joint replacement surgery, rather than making one payment to the hospital, a second payment to the surgeon, and a third payment to the anesthesiologist, the payer would combine these payments for the specific episode of care.

CMS has developed the BPCI initiative that is composed of four broadly defined models of care, which link payments for the multiple services that beneficiaries receive during an episode of care. Under the initiative, organizations enter into payment arrangements that include financial and performance accountability for episodes of care. These four models include the following:

- *Model 1*: Inpatient stays in acute care setting providing prospective payments using the inpatient prospective system for organizations and to clinicians using the physician fee schedule
- *Model 2*: Acute care hospital inpatient stays plus post-acute care and any services incurred up to 90 days after discharge
- *Model 3*: Initiated at the start of post-acute care services in either a skilled nursing facility, inpatient rehab facility, long-term care hospital, or home health agency
- *Model 4*: A single prospective payment made to an organization encompassing all services during the entire inpatient stay for that episode of care[20]

Figure 3.8 is a diagram that shows the differences between the bundle payment model and the traditional fee-for-service payment model.

Integrated Care and Care Management Models
There are ongoing demonstration projects at the CMMI that are focused on developing integrated care and care management models for dually eligible Medicare and Medicaid beneficiaries. These models include oncology care and other specialty care services where clinicians are paid for care coordination services.[21]

Physician-Focused Payment Models (PFPM)
Due to the large number of medical specialties, there cannot be one single approach to APMs that will work for all physicians and patients. Therefore, a menu of physician-focused APMs has been developed. Below are seven types of APMs that can be used to address the most common types of opportunities and barriers that physicians face. For more information, go to http://www.chqpr.org/downloads/Physician-FocusedAlternativePaymentModels.pdf.

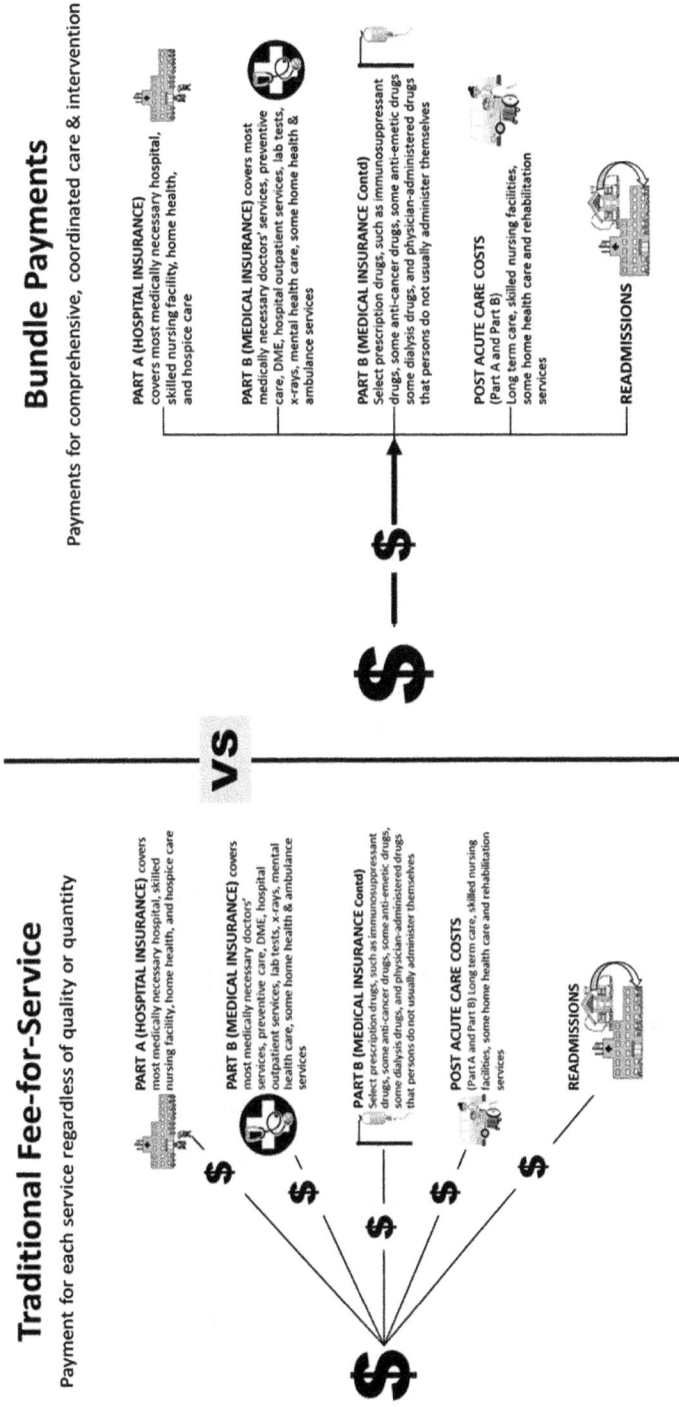

Bundle Payments

Payments for comprehensive, coordinated care & intervention

PART A (HOSPITAL INSURANCE) covers most medically necessary hospital, skilled nursing facility, home health, and hospice care

PART B (MEDICAL INSURANCE) covers most medically necessary doctors' services, preventive care, DME, hospital outpatient services, lab tests, x-rays, mental health care, some home health & ambulance services

PART B (MEDICAL INSURANCE Contd) Select prescription drugs, such as immunosuppressant drugs, some anti-cancer drugs, some anti-emetic drugs some dialysis drugs, and physician-administered drugs that persons do not usually administer themselves

POST ACUTE CARE COSTS (Part A and Part B) Long term care, skilled nursing facilities, some home health care and rehabilitation services

READMISSIONS

VS

Traditional Fee-for-Service

Payment for each service regardless of quality or quantity

PART A (HOSPITAL INSURANCE) covers most medically necessary hospital, skilled nursing facility, home health, and hospice care

PART B (MEDICAL INSURANCE) covers most medically necessary doctors' services, preventive care, DME, hospital outpatient services, lab tests, x-rays, mental health care, some home health & ambulance services

PART B (MEDICAL INSURANCE Contd) Select prescription drugs, such as immunosuppressant drugs, some anti-cancer drugs, some anti-emetic drugs, some dialysis drugs, and physician-administered drugs that persons do not usually administer themselves

POST ACUTE CARE COSTS (Part A and Part B) Long term care, skilled nursing facilities, some home health care and rehabilitation services

READMISSIONS

Figure 3.8: The differences between the traditional FFS and bundle payments

55

- APM #1: Payment for a High-Value Service
- APM #2: Condition-Based Payment for Physician Services
- APM #3: Multi-Physician Bundled Payment
- APM #4: Physician-Facility Procedure Bundle
- APM #5: Warrantied Payment for Physician Services
- APM #6: Episode Payment for a Procedure
- APM #7: Condition-Based Payment [22]

Examples of Advanced APMs (AAPMs)

Next Generation ACO Model

The Next Generation ACOs have been built on the experiences garnered from the Pioneer ACO Model and the MSSP. The goal of the Next Generation ACO Model is to test whether strong financial incentives, along with tools to support better patient engagement and care management, can improve health outcomes and lower expenditures for original Medicare FFS beneficiaries. The Next Generation ACOs will have predictable financial targets, will give clinicians and beneficiaries a greater opportunity to coordinate care, will provide strong patient protections to ensure access to high-quality care, and will aim to attain the highest quality standards of care.

These ACOs will be assuming higher levels of financial risk and rewards than the prior ACOs. These models will be evaluated based on their ability to deliver better care for individuals, better health for populations, and lower growth in expenditures in accordance with the NQS's "better, smarter, healthier" approach to improving our nation's healthcare. In addition, CMS will publicly report on its website the performance of the Next Generation ACOs, focusing on quality metrics and patient experience ratings.[23]

Comprehensive Primary Care Plus (CPC+)

CPC+ is a new APM that will test a different way to reimburse primary care physicians. In January 2017, CMS launched the CPC+ five-year care model program, which will provide preventive services and 24/7 access to care. CMS will pay incentives up-front to all participating practices, but providers will have to return the payments if their performance falls short of certain quality and utilization metrics. The CPC+ model will allow medical groups and physician practices more flexibility to redesign care delivery by doing the following:

- CPC+ may enable primary care practices to provide more services that are not currently billable (for example, conversations with caregivers) or services that don't contribute much to their margins (for example, telehealth and behavioral health)—aligning physician practice incentives with patient health incentives.
- CPC+ will allow practices to offer patients concurrent services that have historically not been billable on the same day. For instance, if a physician sees a patient for a wellness visit and finds that the patient also has unmet psychosocial care needs, the physician cannot, in many cases, bill for physical health and behavioral services on the same day. CPC+ tries to solve that with a care management fee that can support delivering multiple services.
- The care management fees will give providers options for how to utilize the rest of the healthcare team more effectively, because these fees will help pay for services performed by advanced practitioners, pharmacists, care managers, and nurse navigators.

MSSP Tracks 2 and 3 ACO Programs

The MSSP was intended to encourage providers of hospitals and healthcare services to create a new type of healthcare entity, an ACO, that would be accountable for improving the health and experience of care for the FFS patients assigned to the ACO, while reducing the rate of growth in healthcare spending.[24]

CMS implemented a one-sided model (sharing of savings only for the term of an ACO's first agreement) known as Track 1 and a two-sided model (sharing of savings and losses for the term of an ACO's agreement) known as Track 2. Track 1 provided organizations that had little experience with risk models an entry point into the ACO model before transitioning to a risk-based model (Track 2 or 3). Tracks 2 and 3 were established to give more experienced ACOs (ones that were ready to share in losses) the opportunity to enter into a sharing arrangement that provided a greater share of savings, but at the risk of repaying Medicare a portion of any losses.

To provide a greater incentive for ACOs to become accountable for shared losses, Track 2 and Track 3 ACOs have a maximum sharing rate of 60% and 70%, respectively. Also, Track 2 has a performance payment limit that is 15% of the ACO's updated benchmark, and Track 3's limit is 20% of ACO's updated benchmark.[25]

Oncology Care Models with Two-Way Risk
In 2016, CMMI formally launched the Oncology Care Model (OCM) at the Cancer Moonshot Summit. In June of that year, the OCM was a five-year voluntary pilot project intended to improve the quality of cancer treatment and to lower Medicare spending by coordinating care. The OCM is a multi-payer initiative, with 17 private payers and 196 physician practices in 31 participating states. HHS has forecasted that more than 3,200 oncologists will be included in the OCM that will cover approximately 155,000 Medicare beneficiaries. The two-sided risk arrangement will take place after the second year of being in the program. With this arrangement, participants can elect to change to a symmetric two-sided risk model. Only the two-sided risk arrangements will be considered an eligible Advanced APM under the new QPP.[26]

Comprehensive End-Stage Renal Disease (ESRD) Care Programs
CMMI developed the Comprehensive ESRD Care model to reduce expenses while optimizing the quality of care. This was the first ACO with a disease-specific focus intended to improve the coordination and healthcare outcomes of Medicare patients living with end-stage renal disease; this ACO also reduces Medicare costs. The ESRD Seamless Care Organization (ESCO) is an ACO consisting of providers and suppliers who voluntarily united to form a legal entity that offers coordinated care to ESRD patients through the care model.

An ESCO is required to have at least one nephrologist or nephrology group practice as participant owners and must include at least one dialysis facility. Only the care models that take on a two-sided payment arrangement are considered an Advanced APM under the new QPP. ESCOs that contain dialysis facilities from a large dialysis organization are required to be in the two-sided risk track, while ESCOs that do not have a dialysis facility, have the option of choosing the one-sided or two-sided payment tracks.[27]

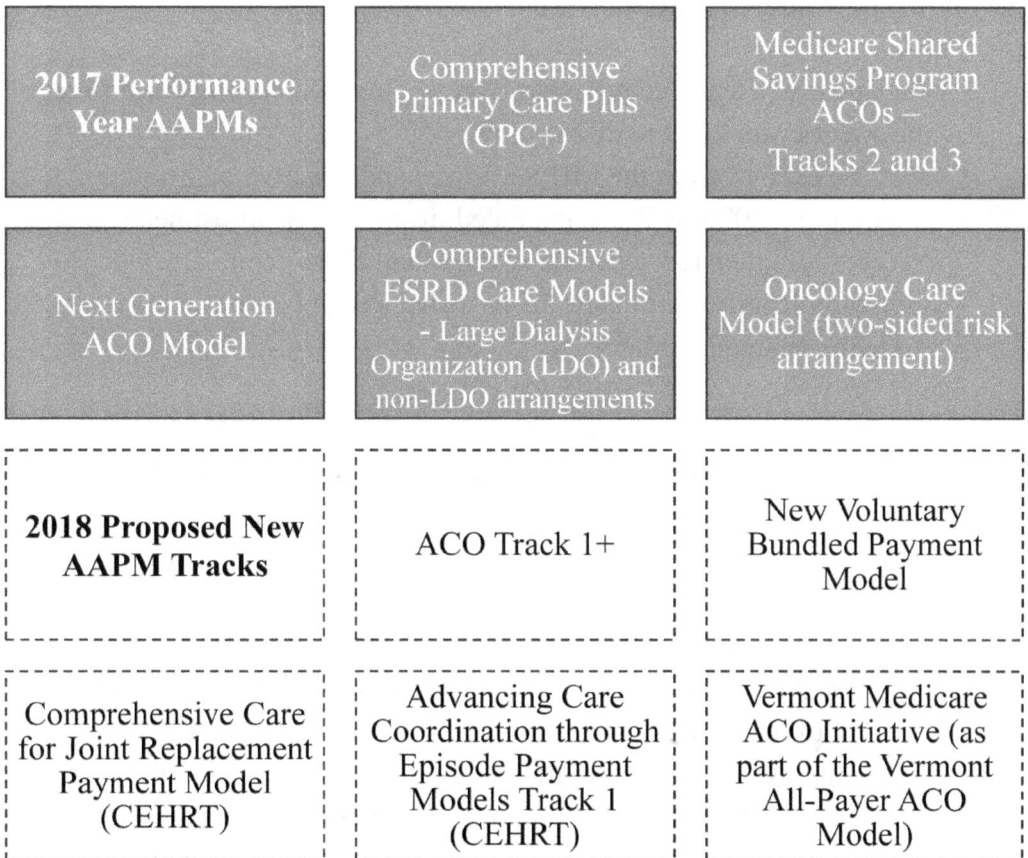

2017 Performance Year AAPMs	Comprehensive Primary Care Plus (CPC+)	Medicare Shared Savings Program ACOs – Tracks 2 and 3
Next Generation ACO Model	Comprehensive ESRD Care Models - Large Dialysis Organization (LDO) and non-LDO arrangements	Oncology Care Model (two-sided risk arrangement)
2018 Proposed New AAPM Tracks	ACO Track 1+	New Voluntary Bundled Payment Model
Comprehensive Care for Joint Replacement Payment Model (CEHRT)	Advancing Care Coordination through Episode Payment Models Track 1 (CEHRT)	Vermont Medicare ACO Initiative (as part of the Vermont All-Payer ACO Model)

Figure 3.9: 2017 performance year AAPMs and proposed 2018 AAPMs

In the 2018 performance year, CMS anticipates reopening applications for new practices and payers in CPC+ and new participants in the Next Generation ACO model. Also, see Figure 3.9 for the additional models that will be considered for the AAPM track. A final 2018 performance year Advanced APM Model list will be published before January 1, 2018.[28]

AAPMs Payment Adjustments—Incentives and Penalties

Clinicians and organizations that qualify to be an APM will be eligible for the following incentives:

- Will receive a 5% Medicare Part B annual lump-sum bonus/incentive payment From 2019 to 2024
- Will be exempt from the MIPS positive and negative adjustments
- Starting in 2026 will be excluded from MIPS adjustments and receive a higher fee schedule update than those clinicians who do not significantly participate in an Advanced APM (0.75% annual baseline payment update)

In 2019 and 2020, the participation requirements for Advanced APMs are only for Medicare payments or patients; but starting in 2021, the participation requirements for Advanced APMs may include non-Medicare payers and patients.[29]

Who Will Participate in AAPMs?

Qualifying APM participants are clinicians who have a certain percentage of their Part B payments for professional services furnished through an Advanced APM entity. Beginning in 2021, this threshold percentage may be reached through a combination of Medicare and other non-Medicare payer arrangements, such as private payers and Medicaid.[30]

Summary of MIPS, APMs, and Advanced APMs

	MIPS	APMs	Advanced APMs
PURPOSE	MIPS streamlines current Medicare value and quality program measures into one program. Clinicians will receive a MIPS score to assess payment adjustment.		Qualifying APMs go further than MIPS to deliver high-quality, efficient care, requiring clinicians to take on more risk. Only advanced alternative payment models (Advanced APMs) qualify for APM bonus payments.
PARTICIPATION	All clinicians should plan on receiving a payment adjustment through MIPS for the first performance year. Clinicians who do not meet APM criteria will be given a MIPS score instead.		All clinicians should plan on receiving a payment adjustment through MIPS for the first performance year. CMS will inform clinicians at the end of the first performance year if they qualified for an APM bonus payment.
PAYMENT	MIPS adjustments and penalties	APM-specific rewards + MIPS adjustments	Advanced APM-specific rewards + 5% lump sum bonus CMS estimates that less than 5% of participating physicians will get paid under the APM track.

Figure 3.10: A summary of MIPS, APMs, and Advanced APMs [32]

APMs' Framework for the Private-Sector Payers

HHS and CMS are now partnering with the private, public, and nonprofit sectors of healthcare to transform the healthcare system by focusing on value over volume to help achieve better care, smarter spending, and healthier people and communities. To further these efforts, HHS has developed the Health Care Payment Learning and Action Network with these partners to align the APM measures with those in the private sector and to advance the work being done across sectors to increase the adoption of value-based payments and APMs beyond the Medicare and Medicaid arena.[31]

Key Concepts to Prepare Clinicians and Organizations for MACRA and QPP

> *"An organization's ability to learn, and translate that learning into action rapidly, is the ultimate competitive advantage."*
> Jack Welch[33]

MACRA was signed into law in April 2015 and finalized by the HHS and CMS in October 2016. The Deloitte Center for Health Solutions surveyed 600 physicians in April 2016 on their level of awareness, thoughts, and perceptions about this new law and its impact on them. The survey found the following:

Awareness and thoughts:
- 50% of non-pediatric physicians had never heard of MACRA, and 32% recognized it by name but were not familiar with its requirements
- 21% of self-employed physicians and those in independently owned medical practices reported they were "somewhat familiar" with MACRA, compared to 9% of employed physicians (employed by hospital or health systems)
- Eight out of 10 providers preferred traditional fee-for-service or salary-based compensation versus value-based payment models

- 74% of surveyed physicians believed that performance reporting is burdensome
- 79% did not support tying compensation to quality, both requirements under MACRA[34]

Perceptions about the outcome of MACRA implementation:
- 87% of solo practitioners expected their reimbursement to fall
- 70% of physicians in groups of two to nine expected their reimbursements to fall
- 55% of physicians in groups of 25 to 99 expected to see their reimbursement rise
- 81% of physicians in groups of more than 100 anticipated getting a reimbursement boost from MACRA
- 80% of physicians believed that MACRA will prompt physicians to join larger organizations or networks
- 58% of respondents said they would join a larger organization (i.e., hospital groups, a larger physician group, clinically integrated networks) to diminish their financial risks and gain access to the information technology and data needed to prove quality under the new reimbursement models[35]

Preparing for MACRA

To significantly improve awareness and reduce pessimism about MACRA, many clinicians, integrated delivery networks, and health systems have now started to:

- Become familiar with the requirements of this law
- Create a sense of purpose, importance, awareness, and criticality around MACRA and QPP, and put together stakeholder groups or coalitions to lead the change
- Do a SWOT (strengths, weaknesses, opportunities, and threats) assessment to determine what needs to be strengthened, stopped or changed

- Conduct a participation readiness assessment to cross walk current reporting processes and measures with those included in MIPS
- Explore strategies and opportunities to score better through performance improvement efforts, preferred reporting mechanisms, clinical practice transformation, and alternate care delivery model exploration
- Build/acquire/optimize data, tools, and infrastructures to support transformation and outcomes
- Create a culture with the behaviors and leadership to successfully navigate through these changes

There are many resources and websites that can help educate organizations and providers about MACRA and how to implement it, including training and advocacy (see Appendix C). There are also many consulting groups and firms that can support these efforts and can be found on the CMS website and Google. These and other resources can help organizations prepare for MACRA. Equipped with information and the support of consultants (if necessary), organizations can develop new value-based strategies for their future that align with their values, mission, and vision.

Organizations that successfully do this will have a business advantage, as they:

- Build strong foundations to operationalize the new infrastructures
- Identify and develop new leaders who will successfully navigate the new environmental changes
- Find ways to continuously improve and leverage new opportunities
- Support the organization in spreading its successful practices across the continuum and eventually to other organizations
- Expand the organization's geographical reach
- Foster a culture that focuses on value for all

Chapter 4:
Measurements Matter
When Transforming Healthcare

"Quality is everyone's responsibility and Transformation
is not automatic, it must be learned; it must be led."
W. Edwards Deming[1]

"Measurement is the first step that leads to control and eventually to
improvement. If you can't measure something, you can't understand it.
If you can't understand it, you can't control it.
If you can't control it, you can't improve it."
H. James Harrington[2]

Topics Covered:

* Understanding the National Quality Strategy and the CMS Quality Strategy
* Introduction to the types of quality measures, how they are used, and the challenges with current quality measures
* The collaborative approach for developing, endorsing, and aligning/consolidating quality measures—and information about the organizations and programs that are doing this

The ACA required the establishment of the National Quality Strategy (NQS), which was developed and then published in 2011. Federal agencies, healthcare payers, purchasers, providers, consumers, and other partners provided input, and the document now serves as a framework for aligning stakeholders across the private and public sectors at the federal, state, and local levels. It serves as a compass for a nationwide focus on quality improvement efforts and on approaches to measuring quality.

The NQS is guided by three aims to provide better, more affordable care for individuals and the community and is supported by six priorities to address the range of quality concerns that affect most Americans. The NQS's three aims closely resemble the Institute for Healthcare Improvement's (IHI) Triple Aim and builds on the work that the IHI has done by giving additional consideration to the health of communities at different levels and by addressing affordability for multiple groups.

The NQS has aligned the nation toward three shared aims:

- *Better care*: Improve the overall quality of care by making healthcare more person-centered, reliable, accessible, and safe.
- *Smarter spending/affordable care*: Reduce the cost of quality healthcare for individuals, families, employers, government, and communities.
- *Healthier people, healthier communities*: Improve the health of Americans by supporting proven interventions to address behavioral, social, and environmental determinants of health, and deliver higher-quality care.[3]

These aims are being advanced through the following six priorities:

- Making care safer by reducing harm caused in the delivery of care
- Ensuring each patient and family member is engaged as a partner in his or her care
- Promoting effective communication and coordination of care
- Promoting the most effective prevention and treatment practices for the leading causes of mortality, starting with cardiovascular disease
- Working with communities to promote wide use of best practices to enable healthy living

- Making quality care more affordable for individuals, families, employers, and governments by developing and spreading new healthcare delivery models.[4]

These six priorities will be achieved with the active involvement and engagement of patients, providers, organizations, and communities. The path to achievement however, may be different due to the different resources and needs states and communities have, but the NQS will help ensure efforts are aligned and consistent with the shared aims and priorities. For more details on the goals of the priorities, see Appendix D.

NQS's Focus to Reduce Variation in Quality Measures and Increase Alignment

At the national level, HHS continues to help coordinate quality measurement efforts that address the NQS's six priorities, while at the same time addressing the abundance of clinical quality measures currently used in national programs. In 2012, the HHS Measurement Policy Council (MPC), composed of key stakeholders from major agencies and programs, convened to focus on measurement alignment and discussed the following:

- Proliferation of measures used by HHS agencies for numerous programs and initiatives
- Redundancies and overlaps leading to provider/data collector burden, conflicting results, inefficient use of HHS resources, and lost opportunities to drive improvement through reinforcing program use of key measures
- The need to develop a process to align, coordinate, approve development, implement, and retire measures across HHS programs
- Take into account the precedent work done by Million Hearts, Partnership for Patients, the internal CMS Quality Measures Task Force, and Meaningful Use Stage 2[5]

The MPC's short-term goals focused on alignment and prioritization of measures in six major areas: hypertension, depression, smoking cessation, hospital-acquired conditions, care coordination (closing the referral loop), and patient experience of care. The MPC's long-term goals concentrated on the development of a process to review and make recommendations on the following major functions: measure alignment, new measure development and implementation, and measurement policy/management.

So far, the MPC had reviewed nine topics: hypertension control, hospital-acquired conditions/patient safety, Hospital Consumer Assessment of Healthcare Providers and Systems (HCAHPS), smoking cessation, depression screening, care coordination, HIV/AIDS, perinatal, and obesity/BMI. While these measures are used for federal programs, the MPC supports state and private-sector efforts to adopt core measure sets for further harmonization and alignment across the health and healthcare community.[6]

The other areas of focus for MPC include:

- Ensure ongoing connection with the work of the Measure Applications Partnership (MAP)—a multi-stakeholder partnership that guides HHS on the selection of performance measures for federal health programs.
- Develop consensus on decision rules for categorization of measures in partnership with the National Quality Forum (NQF).
- Continue retrospective and prospective alignment of measures.
- Review quarterly the agency "action plans" for measure alignment.
- Oversee the work of the MCG to coordinate measure development.
- Promote transparency of measure development pipeline.
- Be the vehicle for early engagement of federal stakeholders in the pre-rulemaking process.
- Understand how to leverage relevant population surveys, surveillance systems, and other data collection systems to promote alignment.

The CMS Quality Strategy

The CMS Quality Strategy is built on the foundation of the CMS strategy and aligns with the NQS.[7] The six priorities of the NQS have become the goals in the CMS Quality Strategy as listed in Figure 4.1. To guide these six goals, CMS has established four foundational principles: eliminating racial and ethnic disparities, strengthening infrastructure and data systems across all settings of care, enabling local innovations, and fostering learning organizations.

The successful implementation of the NQS and the CMS Quality Strategy will contribute to ensuring healthcare is person-centered, provides incentives for the right outcomes, is sustainable, emphasizes coordinated care and shared decision making, and relies on transparency of quality and cost information. These strategies will also promote APMs, including ACOs, bundle payment models and episode-based payment models, integrated care, and patient-centered medical and health home models.[8]

Quality and Value Measurements

As previously mentioned, quality measures are used to evaluate the performance of health plans and healthcare providers on many different levels and against many recognized national quality standards. They can take many forms and can be used to evaluate care across the full range of healthcare settings, from doctors' offices to imaging facilities to hospital systems.

In many parts of the US, the quality of care is below average, with only about 55% of patients receiving proper diagnosis and care. There are also variations in care, healthcare quality, access, patient outcomes, and misuse of services resulting from the fragmented, overly complex, and uncoordinated healthcare system. This leads to serious harm or even death.[9]

Quality measurements are used to make these issues transparent and to improve health and healthcare across the continuum of care. Other common uses of quality measurements include public reporting, provider incentive programs, and accreditation and/or certification of providers and health plans.

National Quality Strategy (NQS) Priorities	CMS Quality Strategy Goals and Objectives	The Proposed Strategic Results
Making care safer by reducing the harm caused in the delivery of care	**Goal 1:** Make care safer by reducing harm caused in the delivery of care Objectives: • Improve support for a culture of safety • Reduce inappropriate and unnecessary care • Prevent or minimize harm in all settings	Healthcare-related harms are reduced.
Ensuring patients and their families are engaged as partners in their care	**Goal 2:** Strengthen person and family engagement as partners in their care Objectives: • Ensure all care delivery incorporates patient and caregiver preferences • Improve experience of care for patients, caregivers, and families • Promote patient self-management	Persons and families are engaged as informed, empowered partners in care.
Promoting effective communication and coordination of care	**Goal 3:** Promote effective communication and coordination of care Objectives: • Reduce admissions and readmissions • Embed best practices to manage transitions to all practice settings • Enable effective healthcare system navigation	Communication, care coordination, and satisfaction with care are improved.
Promoting the most effective prevention and treatment practices for the leading causes of mortality, starting with cardiovascular disease	**Goal 4:** Promote effective prevention and treatment of chronic disease Objectives: • Increase appropriate use of screening and prevention services • Strengthen interventions to prevent heart attacks and strokes • Improve quality of care for patients with multiple chronic conditions • Improve behavioral health access and quality care • Improve perinatal outcomes	Leading causes of mortality are reduced and prevented.
Working with communities to promote wide use of best practices to enable healthy living	**Goal 5:** Work with communities to promote best practices of healthy living Objectives: • Partner with and support federal, state, and local public health improvement efforts • Improve access within communities to best practices of healthy living • Promote evidence-based community interventions to prevent and treat chronic disease • Increase use of community-based social services support	Best practices are promoted, disseminated, and used in communities.
Making quality care affordable for individuals, families, employers, and governments by developing and spreading new healthcare delivery models (affordable care)	**Goal 6:** Make care affordable Objectives: • Develop and implement payment systems that reward value over volume • Use cost analysis data to inform payment policies	Quality care is affordable for individuals, families, employers, and governments

Figure 4.1: NQS and CMS priorities, goals, objectives, and proposed results

Types of Measures: What Are the Types of Quality Measures?

Quality measures are used to assess the care provided in all practice settings in the healthcare delivery system, from the level of individual physicians to health insurance plans and organizations. Quality measures fall in to five broad categories: structure, process, outcomes, patient experience, and balanced measures. A combination of these type of measures are what organizations use to get a picture of the quality of care that is been provided and received by patients.

1. *Structure Measures*

Structure measures evaluate the infrastructure of healthcare settings like hospitals or doctor offices and how well those healthcare settings deliver care. These measures are used by payers and regulators to determine if a provider or organization has the capacities needed to deliver high-quality care (for example, EHRs to order labs or medications electronically). They also determine the certification and accreditation of health plans and providers.

Two key reasons for using structure measures are that characteristics of healthcare settings can significantly affect the quality of care, and care settings that meet certain standards have an advantage when it comes to providing high-quality care. However, structure measures do not capture whether or not what has been measured actually occurs. For example, some forms of provider accreditation and certification require providers to use electronic health records; the provider could buy an electronic health record system but continue to rely on paper records and still meet this structural requirement.[10]

To address structure measures, organizations might ask the following:

- Does a pharmacy program have an antibiotic stewardship program to reduce antibiotic-resistant superbugs?
- Does the surgical department have the Surgical Care Improvement Program (SCIP) in place?
- Does a physician's office use EHRs for prescription data entry?

2. *Process Measures*

Process measures determine the extent to which providers regularly give patients specific services that are consistent with recommended guidelines and evidence-based care. They are generally linked to treatments or procedures that will improve the health outcomes of patients and minimize complications. Process measures are useful in providing organizations and clinicians with clear, actionable feedback to improve performance; however, they are just another piece in the puzzle of the true picture of what is happening with a patient. Also, process measures are not available for all areas of care, and, in some cases, do not capture the true quality of care provided.[11]

Questions organizations might ask to determine process measures include:

- Is a qualified healthcare team member consistently performing eye exams in diabetic patients?
- Do providers ensure their patients receive recommended colorectal cancer screenings?
- Are physicians prescribing the appropriate drugs to their cardiovascular disease patients?

3. *Outcome Measures*

Outcome measures evaluate the patient's health after the care provided. These measures examine the impact the care made on the patient's health, and whether or not the goals of care were met. Outcome measures include survival rates and incidences of disease, but are not able to fully assess the extent of a patient's experience.

One of the challenges with outcome measures include their difficulty to obtain them. Gathering enough data can be challenging, and differences in patient populations can make it difficult to achieve.[12]

Examples of questions to ask include:

- What was the quality of pain relief for patients who had hip surgery?

- What was the rate of blindness in patients with diabetes?
- What is the five-year survival rate for patients who have had breast cancer?

4. *Patient Experience Measures*

Patient experience measures provide feedback based on a patient's experience with the care provided, ranging from the clarity and accessibility of information providers give patients, to whether providers tell patients about test results, to how quickly patients are able to get appointments for a surgical procedure. Studies have shown patients are more engaged in their care when they have better care experiences.[13] Experts are increasingly advocating for the inclusion of patient experience as a key measure of quality in healthcare. NQS includes measures of patient experience as part of its key priorities.[14]

Organizations might ask:

- How long did patients have to wait in the exam room before they were seen?
- Do patients report that their provider explains their treatment options in easy-to-understand ways?
- Did a patient receive an email or text from the provider's office with lab test results?

5. *Balancing Measures*

Balancing measures focus on examining the system from a different point of view to make sure the changes being made to one part of the system are not causing problems in another part of the system.[15] For example:

- To increase compliance with regular visits for preventive care or required testing, make sure not to exceed the scheduling capacity.
- To reduce time patients spend on a ventilator after surgery, make sure reintubation rates are not increasing.

- For reducing patients' length of stay in the hospital, make sure readmission rates are not increasing.[16]

Current Challenges with Quality Measures

As knowledge about the many factors that shape individual and population health has advanced, the scope of health measurement has broadened to include a large number of process and outcome measures relevant to health and healthcare. This, however, has unleashed a multitude of uncoordinated, inconsistent, and often duplicative measurement and reporting initiatives from multiple agencies and organizations. Federal agencies, states, payers, independent organizations, and employers have their own programs, approaches, and initiatives, usually focusing on different measures or on the same things measured differently. These quality measures are still taken very seriously by health systems and organizations because they are used for accreditation, monitoring the effectiveness of these entities, monitoring the population health status and patient experiences, payment, and transparent public reporting and benchmarking.

The current quality measurement systems and programs have led to inefficiencies in the healthcare systems, a rise in healthcare costs, and too many redundant measures that have not necessarily helped patients and populations make better healthcare choices. And it has placed a significant burden on providers who have to report these requirements to the multiple sources. Also, in spite of the hundreds of quality measures in existence, there are still many gaps:

- Too few measures that are patient centered or outcome focused
- Measures not compatible or consistent from one program to another
- Coverage gaps
- Variations in data quality and availability
- Measurement gaps in our understanding about what works in care coordination, quality healthcare, cost control, patient safety, and patient engagement

This has led to a renewed focus on consolidating existing measures and identifying new ones to close the above gaps and challenges. In the meantime, physicians and other providers participate in these various programs and initiatives to demonstrate the quality of care they provide to their patients, for reimbursement and payment purposes, and to help consumers make informed choices about their care. They also report multiple quality measures to different sources—a major burden and challenge. Figure 4.2 shows the confusion and complexity that results when measure requirements are not aligned among payers, agencies, and organizations.[17]

Government Agencies	Private-Sector Organizations	Independent Organizations
• Centers for Medicare & Medicaid Services • Agency for Health Care Research & Quality	• Anthem, BCBS, Aetna, Humana, Kaiser, United, Cigna, and others • Consultants and others	• National Committee for Quality Assurance • National Quality Forum • The Joint Commission • U.S. Preventive Services Task Force • American Diabetes Association, et. al. • Specialty societies
Government Measures • PQRS – 29 • Meaningful Use – 33 • ACO – 33 • Medicare Advantage Varied	**Private-Sector Measures** • Clinical • Service – e.g., access • Patient satisfaction • Productivity • Health status	**Independent Organizations Measures / accreditation** • PCMH, HEDIS, CAHPS, others • Efficiency measures • Disparate measures • Condition focused

Figure 4.2: Examples of the multiple sources of quality measures for primary care

This complexity and the challenges of data collection and monitoring are further complicated when agencies, states, payers, and employers set requirements for providers and organizations to meet in different practice settings, such as hospitals, clinics, ACOs, nursing homes, and others. Figure 4.3 lists common quality reporting programs that providers, health systems, and organizations participate in and report to.

The full benefits of investments in these programs and measurements are being diminished, due in part to minor variations in measure methodologies that lead to multiple different reporting requirements for the same target. These variations have led to significant inefficiencies, redundancies, unnecessary costs, and waste, because the results ascertained cannot usually be compared across geographic areas, institutions, or populations.[18]

Value-Based and Quality Reporting Programs

Hospital Reporting Programs	Physician and Certain Eligible Provider Reporting Programs	Health Plans Reporting Programs
• Hospital Inpatient Quality Reporting Program (Hospital IQR Program) • Hospital Value-Based Purchasing Program (Hospital VBP Program) • Hospital Readmissions Reduction Program (HRRP) • Hospital-Acquired Condition Reduction Program (HAC) • Reduction Program Medicare and Medicaid Electronic Health Record (EHR) Incentive Program for Eligible Hospitals and Critical Access Hospitals (EHR EH) • Hospital Outpatient Quality Reporting Program Hospital (OQR Program) • Ambulatory Surgical Center Quality Reporting Program (ASCQR Program) • Inpatient Psychiatric Facility Quality Reporting Program (IPFQR Program) • Prospective Payment System-Exempt Cancer Hospitals Quality Reporting Program (PCHQR Program)	• Physician Quality Reporting System (PQRS) • Medicare Electronic Prescribing Incentive Program (eRx Incentive Program) • Medicare and Medicaid Electronic Health Record (EHR) Incentive Program for Eligible Professionals (EHR EP) • Physician Compare Physician Compare Medicare Part C (Display or Star Ratings) Part C • Medicare Part D (Display or Star Ratings) Part D	• NCQA accreditation - Healthcare Effectiveness Data and Information Set • eValue8 • Medicare Part C (Display or Star Ratings) Part C • Medicare Part D (Display or Star Ratings) Part D • Patient Experience of Care (HCAHPS / CAHPS Survey)
		Medicare ACOs
		• Medicare Shared Savings Program (MSSP) • Other Contracts

Figure 4.3: Value-Based and Quality Reporting Program

Development, Endorsement, Alignment, and Consolidation of Quality Measures

There are a number of organizations and programs contributing to the transformation of health and healthcare quality by leading, developing, evaluating, and/or consolidating critical value measures (quality, care, and cost). These measures, as well as the strategies and initiatives being created, are used by virtually all healthcare delivery systems, payers, providers, and health plans to do the following:

- Reflect on how well they are taking care of their patients (improving patient outcomes)
- Determine how effective they are compared to other providers, organizations, and plans
- Evaluate their performance by recognized, national quality standards
- Hold health insurance plans and healthcare providers accountable for ensuring high-quality care
- Identify what works in healthcare and what doesn't
- Measure and address disparities in how care is delivered and health outcomes
- Monitor progress as leaders work to transform their organizations (new value goals)
- Optimize reimbursements opportunities (while minimizing penalties)
- Prevent the overuse, underuse, and misuse of healthcare, promote patient safety, drive healthcare improvement, and increase accountability for providing the best care
- Help consumers make informed choices about their care[19]

Understanding these challenges and gaps, the following list highlights some of the private and government organizations, agencies, and programs that are collaborating to develop, evaluate, endorse, consolidate, and align existing quality measures where possible, and create new measures where necessary to meet the NQS goals of better care, smarter spending, healthier people, and communities.

Key Players

Over the last 10–20 years, quality improvement initiatives, task forces, and reports have been implemented and published. Today, there are federal and state organizations, private entities, trade associations, nonprofits, and private for-profit organizations that have developed and continue to develop quality measures. The following are key players:

Private Nonprofits

1. *National Quality Forum (NQF)*: NQF was formed in response to a presidential commission's recommendation to develop a forum on healthcare quality measurement and reporting. The organization's mission includes building consensus on national priorities and goals for performance improvement, and working in partnership with the public and private sectors. The mission also includes ensuring and maintaining best-in-class standards for measuring and publicly reporting on healthcare performance quality, attaining national healthcare improvement goals, and using standardized measures through education and outreach programs.[20]

2. *National Committee for Quality Assurance (NCQA)*: NCQA's mission is to transform healthcare quality through measurement, transparency, and accountability. It represents the first broad-based attempt at value-based purchasing. NCQA oversees the Healthcare Effectiveness Data and Information Set (HEDIS), which consists of approximately 81 measures in five domains, and it is used by more than 90% of health plans to measure performance. It also offers accreditation programs (for example, for ACOs), certification programs (for example, for disease management), physician recognition programs (for example, for patient-centered medical homes), and health plan report cards.[21]

3. *Institute for Healthcare Improvement (IHI)*: IHI's mission is to improve health and healthcare worldwide. Its vision is for everyone to receive the best care and have the best health possible. IHI works closely with health systems to drive down costs and enhance sustainability in both clinical and operational settings by

identifying proven and evidence-based strategies that demonstrate efficiency through the removal of waste, harm, and variation. It has also developed a number of measures for use by the organizations within its sphere of activities, accelerated improvement through its partnerships, and formulated the Triple Aim concept of better care, lower cost, and better health, which has become a standard reference point for many health improvement efforts.[22]

4. *The Joint Commission (TJC) on Accreditation of Healthcare Organizations*: TJC's mission is to continuously improve healthcare for the public, in collaboration with other stakeholders, by evaluating healthcare organizations and inspiring them to excel in providing safe and effective care of the highest quality and value. TJC also plays an important role in the assessment of care quality by administering on-site surveys to thousands of healthcare systems across the nation and makes each healthcare organization's accreditation public to ensure transparency for all interested stakeholders and the community at large. In many states, TJC accreditation fulfills state regulatory requirements for healthcare providers, as well as Medicare and Medicaid certification.[23]

5. *International Consortium for Health Outcome Measurement (ICHOM)*: ICHOM is a nonprofit organization founded by three institutions. Its purpose is to transform healthcare systems worldwide by measuring and reporting patient outcomes in a standardized way. ICHOM's mission is to unlock the potential of value-based healthcare by defining global standard sets of outcome measures that really matter to patients with the most relevant medical conditions. It drives adoption and worldwide reporting of these measures. ICHOM believes outcomes are the ultimate measure of success in healthcare and is working toward publishing 50 standard sets by 2017 to cover more than 50% of the global disease burden.[24]

6. *The Patient-Centered Outcomes Research Institute (PCORI)*: PCORI, an independent nonprofit, nongovernmental organization, was authorized by Congress in 2010. Its goal is to determine which

of the many healthcare options available to patients and those who care for them works best in particular circumstances. This is done by taking an approach to clinical effectiveness research called Patient-Centered Outcomes Research, or PCOR. This research addresses the questions and concerns most relevant to patients and involves patients, caregivers, clinicians, other healthcare stakeholders, and researchers throughout the process. The PCORI vision is for patients and the public to have information they can use to make decisions that reflect their desired health outcomes.[25]

7. *The Leapfrog Group*: Founded in 2000 by large employers and other purchasers, The Leapfrog Group is a national nonprofit organization driving a movement for giant leaps forward in the quality and safety of American healthcare. The Leapfrog Hospital Survey collects and transparently reports hospital performance, and its hospital Safety Score initiative assigns letter grades to hospitals based on their record of patient safety. This helps consumers protect themselves and their families from errors, injuries, accidents, and infections. So far, about 1,800 hospitals complete this survey annually.[26]

8. *World Health Organization (WHO)*: WHO's goal is to build a better, healthier future for people worldwide. Working through offices in more than 150 countries, WHO's staff works side by side with governments and other partners to ensure the highest attainable level of health for all people. WHO strives to combat diseases, especially infectious diseases like influenza and HIV and non-communicable ones like cancer and heart disease. It also helps to ensure the safety of air quality, food, water, and medicines and vaccines.[27]

9. *International Society of Quality in Healthcare (ISQua)*: ISQua's mission is to inspire and drive improvement in the quality and safety of healthcare worldwide. It does this through education and knowledge sharing, external evaluation, supporting health systems, and connecting people through global networks. ISQua achieves this through a network that spans 100 countries and five out of six continents.[28]

10. *Pharmacy Quality Alliance (PQA)*: PQA's mission is to improve the quality of medication management and use across healthcare settings. Its goal is improving patients' health through a collaborative process to develop and implement performance measures and recognize examples of exceptional pharmacy quality. PQA develops medication-use measures in areas such as medication safety, medication adherence, and appropriateness. It does so by identifying the high-priority areas for healthcare and identifying gaps in existing performance measure sets. It focuses on the priorities identified through the National Priorities Partnership and aligns its activities with the NQS.[29]

11. *URAC (originally known as Utilization Review Accreditation Commission)*: URAC is an independent, nonprofit organization whose mission includes improving quality and accountability of health care organizations using utilization-review services (i.e., where organizations determine if health care is medically necessary for a patient). URAC also accredits many types of health care organizations such as health plans, preferred provider organizations, and ACOs.

Government Organizations

HHS is the US government's principal agency for protecting the health of all Americans and providing essential human services, especially for those who are least able to help themselves. HHS manages programs that cover a vast spectrum of activities that impact health, public health, and human services outcomes throughout the population's lifespan. The mission of the HHS is to enhance and protect the health and wellbeing of all Americans by providing for effective health and human services and by fostering advances in medicine, public health, and social services.[30]

The HHS accomplishes its mission through the following agencies and programs:

1. *Agency for Healthcare Research and Quality (AHRQ)*: AHRQ has undertaken a number of projects aimed at improving measurement

of healthcare performance. These include assessments of national healthcare performance through the National Healthcare Quality Report and the National Healthcare Disparities Report, both of which describe the current status and trends in care effectiveness, patient safety, access, timeliness, and patient-centeredness.

AHRQ has also developed a number of indicators for gauging healthcare quality, including the Prevention Quality Indicators, Inpatient Quality Indicators, Pediatric Quality Indicators, and Patient Safety Indicators. It has supported and overseen the Consumer Assessment of Healthcare Providers and Systems (CAHPS) program and stores evidence-based measures and measure sets in the National Quality Measures Clearinghouse and compiles measures used by HHS in the HHS Measure Inventory.[31]

2. *Centers for Disease Control and Prevention (CDC)*: The CDC operates a number of categorical clinical preventive service programs (for example, immunization and cancer screening) with elements aimed at improving the quality of those services, in part through measurement. CDC's Immunization Grant Program provides aid to underinsured and low-income families for whom vaccinations impose a significant cost challenge.[32]

3. *The CMS Overall Hospital Quality Star Rating*: This rating has been designed to help individuals, their family members, and caregivers compare hospitals in an easily understandable way and, at the same time, encourage hospitals to improve the quality of care they provide. This new rating summarizes data from existing quality measures publicly reported on CMS's Hospital Compare website into a single star rating for each hospital, making it easier for consumers to compare hospitals and interpret complex quality information.

The ratings are a composite metric of one to five stars, with five being the best. They intend to convey the overall quality of nearly 4,000 US hospitals and are posted to the Hospital Compare site.[33] For grading hospitals on their overall quality, the CMS uses 64 measures across the following seven domains: mortality, safety of care, readmissions, patient experience, effectiveness of care, timeliness of care, and efficient use of medical imaging. Details of the 64 measures can be found at: https://www.medicare.gov/hospitalcompare/Data/Data-Updated.html#.

Details about comparing hospitals can be found at: https://www.medicare.gov/hospitalcompare/search.html.

4. *Centers for Medicare and Medicaid Services (CMS)*: CMS has perhaps the greatest impact in the quality measurement arena, leveraging measures for multiple purposes in Medicare, Medicaid, and CHIP. It has applied measures to its payment programs including:

- MSSP (ACOs), Medicaid health homes, and Innovation Center projects
- Public reporting programs, such as Hospital Compare Physician Compare, and Medicare Advantage Star Rating
- Quality tracking, such as Medicaid Adult Health Care Quality measures and Medicaid/CHIP Children's Health Care Quality measures

Moreover, CMS provides technical assistance on measurement through the Quality Improvement Organization program and coordinates with a variety of measurement organizations on measure development and accreditation. CMS is also working with the Office of the National Coordinator for Health Information Technology (ONC) within HHS to spearhead the implementation and application of EHRs and the exchange of health information across the system. To further encourage the adoption of health information technology, two HHS programs—the Medicare EHR Incentive program and Medicaid EHR Incentive program—provide financial incentives for providers and hospitals to use EHRs meaningfully. The capture and reporting of quality measures are required for meaningful use.

CMS administers several comparative programs, including accountability systems such as CMS Medicare Hospital Compare and Physician Compare that provide information for the public, and programs that report data on Medicare and Medicaid performance in terms of geographic variation and healthcare expenditures. CMS also operates a variety of systems that collect monitoring and compliance data to ensure that high-quality care is delivered to Medicare and Medicaid beneficiaries.[34]

5. *CMS Quality Measurement Development Plan (MDP)*: Under the MACRA legislation from the ACA, HHS and CMS were tasked to coordinate, consolidate, align, and identify the quality measures that will be used by MIPS and certain Medicare APMs. These quality measures were to be aligned with the NQS and the CMS Quality Strategy. To meet these MACRA requirements, CMS created the MDP to serve as a strategic framework for the future of clinician quality measure development to support MIPS and advanced APMs. The MDP will align the resultant quality measures with the following six CMS quality domains for use in MIPS: clinical care, safety, care coordination, patient and caregiver experience, population health and prevention, and efficiency and cost reduction.

These domains align with the NQS priority areas and CMS Quality Strategy goals. The measures assigned to these domains will be used to address gaps, drive quality improvement, and ensure the CMS Quality Strategy goals are achieved. The final MDP was posted on the CMS. gov website May 1, 2016. Updates to the MDP, which will be released annually or otherwise as appropriate, will prioritize the development of additional quality measures to address identified gaps and other priority areas using MACRA funding.[35]

The evolution and success of this plan will depend on partnering with patients, caregivers, frontline clinicians, professional societies, payers and other stakeholders, and across federal agencies, to shift the focus of our national healthcare system to paying clinicians and other providers based on value rather than volume.[36]

Other Public- and Private-Sector Entities

Professional societies such as the American Heart Association, American College of Surgeons and American College of Cardiology, various health plans, and payers are also developing, testing, and submitting measures for evaluation by the NQF. Other organizations such as Healthgrades are developing measures that are being used to "grade" healthcare providers. Some states, such as Minnesota, have established a standardized set of quality measures to encourage provider accountability, and many other organizations are leveraging existing measures to ensure quality without creating new reporting.[37]

After quality measures are developed, they are often evaluated and endorsed by professional societies and/or consumer groups. The endorsement process is consensus-based and allows stakeholders to evaluate the proposed measure(s). Organizations such as the NQF and the AHRQ convene stakeholders to rigorously review potential quality measures and endorse those that meet preestablished standards. These stakeholders include healthcare professionals, consumers, payers (such as insurance companies), employers, hospitals, and health plans.

Reducing the Burden of Data Reporting

ONC has launched the Health eDecisions Standards and Interoperability Initiative, with significant private-sector participation, to standardize and enable the sharing of clinical decision support interventions and tools.

In 2014, CMS achieved unprecedented alignment across its data reporting programs, leading to some reductions in burden on providers, while still fostering accountability for quality outcomes. Also, CMS and other federal agencies have identified opportunities to align reporting requirements. For example:

- Eligible professionals participating in the Shared Savings Program received credit for the PQRS program for certain measures that were satisfactorily reported by their accountable care organization.
- Providers can report once to receive credit for both PQRS and the EHR Incentive Programs.

- Alignment of measures and reporting mechanisms across these programs reduce the burden on healthcare providers and allow them to focus on the measures that matter.
- The Hospital Value-Based Purchasing program uses a subset of the Hospital Inpatient Quality Reporting (IQR) program posted on Hospital Compare. The hospital IQR measure data can also be used to determine if a hospital has met its Hospital Value-Based Purchasing measure data reporting requirements.
- In 2012, CMS launched the process for using electronic health records to directly report the quality data required by other hospital programs. This process also allowed hospitals using certified EHR technology to use the same data (and often in the same format) to report on quality measurement and deliver clinical care.
- In 2012, the Health Resources and Services Administration (HRSA) established the Measures Management Review Board to promote the use of nationally recognized measures used in the CMS EHR Incentive Programs and PQRS and measures endorsed by the National Quality Forum.[38]

The organizations and entities that have the most difficult task in this process are the ones below, assigned to the consolidation and alignment of the quality measures to reduce administrative burdens and increase value. They have had to review hundreds of measures and measure requirements to address issues of necessity, relevance, redundancy, and overlaps.

- ***Measurement Policy Council (MPC)***: One of the outcomes of the ACA was the formation of the National Quality Strategy (NQS) under the HHS umbrella to provide a forum for addressing the plethora of clinical quality measures currently used in national programs. The goal of the NQS is to get to measures that matter and minimize provider burden. In 2012, HHS established the MPC to work on the alignment of measures across agencies and programs.
- ***MAP***: The Measure Applications Partnership, or MAP, is a public-private multi-stakeholder partnership convened by the NQF to

guide HHS for providing input (for its pre-rulemaking process) on selecting performance measures for public reporting, performance-based payment, other programs, and the selection of performance measures for federal health programs. The goal of this partnership is essentially to streamline performance metrics—examining which metrics are relevant for various federal applications, providing input to HHS, and encouraging alignment of public- and private-sector measurement initiatives. MAP is set up to encourage alignment across federal programs and implicitly encourages public-private alignment.[39]

- *America's Health Insurance Plans (AHIP)*: AHIP, CMS, and NQF have collaborated to align measures across public and private programs in hopes of creating consistency in the quality measures being used in government programs and by private insurers. The goal of this collaboration (in partnership with both public and private payers, physician specialty organizations, employers, and consumers) is to offer consumers useful information for healthcare decision making and to reduce the burden on providers of reporting quality measures. AHIP has been working with patients and provider groups to develop consensus around core sets of measures in particular areas, including primary care, liver disease, gastroenterology, medical oncology, and cardiology.[40]

- *Specifications Manual for National Hospital Inpatient Quality Measures (IQM)*: Collaboration between the CMS and the Joint Commission to work to align these common measures resulted in the creation of the IQM common set of measures, which is used by both organizations.[41]

- *The Institute of Medicine's Committee*: The Institute of Medicine's Committee on Core Metrics for Better Health at Lower Cost is an ad hoc committee exploring measurement of individual and population health outcomes and costs, identifying weaknesses and gaps in healthcare systems, and considering approaches and priorities for developing the measures necessary for continuously learning and improving the health system. In its report from 2015, the committee proposed a basic, minimum slate of core metrics for use with respect to people's engagement and experience in healthcare, quality, cost, and health.[42]

- **The IMPACT Act**: The Improving Medicare Post-Acute Care Transformation Act of 2014 (IMPACT Act) provides new and streamlined quality measures across nursing homes, home health agencies, and other post-acute care providers participating in Medicare. The act also requires more frequent surveys of hospice providers—a measure the hospice community and the National Hospice and Palliative Care Organization has championed for more than a decade.[43]

- **NQF**: In December 2016, the NQF published a report titled "Variation in Measure Specifications—Sources and Mitigation Strategies." This report identified key reasons for the variation in measure specifications and the impact of such variation, and provided guidance on ways to mitigate or prevent variation. According to Dr. Helen Burstin, chief scientific officer with NQF, "We have an urgent need to focus on the measures that really matter for quality improvement. To make care better for patients, in addition to reducing variations in measures, it's also important that we eliminate measures that are duplicative, ineffective or that have reached the limits of their usefulness."[44]

These groups and organizations will have to further consolidate over time to continuously address overlapping, redundancy, and the additional administrative burdens put on providers with monetary and time costs, but with little to no added value.

Most, if not all key stakeholders (plans, providers, employers, and consumers) are embracing the vision of a core, consolidated set of outcomes-based quality measures that can be used across payers—because the measures and complexity of the current systems are not achieving their potential in improving quality of care. However, achieving the vision has proved incredibly challenging, because individual stakeholders have generally failed to achieve consensus around which measures should be prioritized and how they should be used.

While these individual stakeholders' concerns about particular measures are often valid, the objections have undermined their broader consensus about what is needed to achieve their goal of a much more workable and actionable approach. In part, the failure to reach consensus is a disagreement on the purpose of the measures and whether the measurement actually achieves its purpose.

While there will never be a perfect set of measures with a universal consensus, today's healthcare delivery models are moving forward at an unprecedented rate. And the current patchwork of measures is also moving forward toward meeting the goal of transitioning from volume to value.[45]

PART II:

The Medication A.R.E.A.S. Bundle (MAB) Rx Strategy— A Prescription for Healthcare Value

Chapter 5:
An Introduction to the Medication
A.R.E.A.S. Bundle Prescription (MAB Rx)

*"Increasing the effectiveness of adherence interventions may
have a far greater impact on the health of the population than
any improvement in specific medical treatments."*
WHO[1]

*"Synergy is the interaction of two or more entities to produce a
combined effect greater than the sum of their separate effects –
Medication Adherence, Reconciliation, Engagement and Education,
Affordability, and Safe Medication Use (A.R.E.A.S.) are the elements
that when 'prescribed' and leveraged together in patients with
multiple chronic conditions, will produce a combined outcome
far greater than the sum of their separate components"*
Elizabeth Oyekan

Topics Covered:

- The purpose of the Medication A.R.E.A.S. Bundle Prescription
- The importance of MAB Rx for patients with multiple chronic
  conditions
- Key facts and important consequences when each MAB
  component is not optimized
- The MAB Rx strategy for implementation

The national focus on creating a value-based healthcare system to
ensure better care, smarter spending, and healthier communities

has become a driving force to transform the US healthcare system. One key aspect is the transformation of the healthcare payment structure from a focus on volume to a focus on value, by linking healthcare payments to quality and outcomes in the new QPP. This commitment to healthcare value and the QPP has led organizations and provider practices to begin transforming their current delivery systems by:

- Adopting new, alternative care delivery models and evidence-based practices, such as care coordination and population management
- Focusing on standardizing and automating processes to improve quality and reduce costs
- Using technology and analytics to augment provider practices; provide critical insights into issues, patterns, and trends; and identify populations for personalized interventions
- Identifying talent and leaders with the skills and potential to maneuver the new healthcare landscape and successfully leverage these new practices, tools, and infrastructures to expand their geographic reach

These are some of the critical infrastructures that organizations are putting in place to ensure success and a business advantage in the new value-based healthcare system. Organizations are also looking for new strategies that will leverage these infrastructures to support the positive outcomes of their populations, reduce costs, and significantly improve their performance.

Patients with multiple chronic conditions (MCC) are one group of patients who, when successfully identified and strategically managed in this new healthcare environment, will result in better care and patient health outcomes, lower total healthcare costs, and better organizational performance.

Driven by factors such as aging, increased obesity, and cardiovascular diseases, the number of people with MCC has risen significantly. According to the CDC, the prevalence of MCC has increased from

21.8% of the adult population in 2001 to 26% in 2010—one out of four Americans. Consider the following:

- Chronic diseases are responsible for seven out of every 10 deaths in this country, killing more than 1.7 million Americans every year.
- Approximately 27% of Americans with MCC account for 66% of the nation's health expenditures.[2]
- Chronic diseases can be disabling and reduce a person's quality of life, especially if left undiagnosed or untreated.
- People with chronic and/or complex conditions are the most frequent users of healthcare. They account for the following:

  - 96% of drug costs[3]
  - 91% of all prescriptions filled
  - 83% of all healthcare spending
  - 81% of hospital admissions
  - 76% of all physician visits[4]

According to 2010 Medco Data, for 88% of the population with MCC, prescription medications are a first choice for intervention. When medications are used optimally, there are better patient care experiences and improved health outcomes, a reduction in total healthcare costs, and improvement in the health of the communities and of organizational performance in the areas of quality, affordability, service, and other critical measures.[5]

Although medications are effective in improving the health and lives of patients with MCC, the full benefits are often not realized because of the following challenges:

- Approximately 50% of patients do not take their medications as prescribed.
- Patients are unable to afford their co-pays or the cost of the medications.
- Patients experience side effects that prevent the continuation of the therapy.

- Patients are not engaged and/or do not understand the benefits of the therapies.
- Medication errors occur in different healthcare settings.
- Sometimes, unique aspects of patients are not taken into account, such as the elderly and pediatric populations.

These challenges have led to the following adverse outcomes:
- Medication errors that result in 7,000 medication-related deaths per year in many hospitals and approximately 1.3 million injuries annually
- Increased progression of diseases and complications, poor health outcomes, additional illnesses, and even premature death
- Avoidable hospital admissions and readmissions
- A $290 billion burden on the healthcare system from unnecessary healthcare spending annually[6]

Over the last two to three decades, international, national, and local organizations and team members have worked independently and interdependently to understand the barriers that contribute to poor medication use and identify the evidence-based interventions that have been shown to effectively optimize appropriate medication use in patients with MCC. Based on the ample evidence, research, and studies on appropriate medication use and management, a set of medication practice elements has been identified. There is general acceptance that these practice elements will optimize patient care and health outcomes in a consistent manner across the continuum of care. They are expected to reduce the total cost of healthcare, improve the health and wellbeing of the communities served, and improve organizational performance in quality, affordability, service, access, and other critical measures.

These elements have been condensed and integrated into a bundle known as the Medication A.R.E.A.S. (adherence, reconciliation, engagement, affordability, and safe medication use) Bundle Prescription, or MAB Rx.

MAB Rx for Patients with MCC

MAB Rx is a set of practices and interventions for MCC patients on chronic medications that will result in better patient outcomes when implemented together than when implemented individually, regardless of the disease condition. The following are the components of MAB:

- *Adherence*: MCC patients taking their medications at least 80% of the time (higher for certain drugs and disease conditions) as measured using PDC or MPR
- *Reconciliation*: Medication reconciliation of patient medication lists upon admission, transfer between units, at discharge, and when medication therapies or doses change (regardless of the practice setting)
- *Engagement*: Engaging and educating patients and caregivers about their medications
- *Affordability*: Addressing drug costs at every point of contact and minimizing prescription waste
- *Safe medication use*: Promoted from the prescribing process, through the transcription process, to the dispensing and administration processes

These elements of the MAB Rx are not specific to a particular diagnosis but instead have been designed to help physicians, clinicians, and team members reliably and consistently address core medication-related challenges in patients with MCC. Many organizations have strategies, initiatives, and teams in place—such as medication adherence teams, medication safety teams, drug use management teams, and others—to address the challenges associated with each element of MAB Rx and to develop initiatives to improve each. These initiatives and strategies are used to improve core performance and quality measures (discussed in more detail in Chapter 8), while at the same time addressing a multitude of measurements and reporting requests from internal stakeholders and external organizations/ agencies. However, because many of these teams and strategies are separate and not always coordinated, they sometimes fail to leverage their interdependencies.

This has led to duplicative and redundant use of resources and efforts, silo efforts, competing priorities, and waste (in terms of time and resources for duplicate work). While each element can contribute to the improvement of appropriate medication use in MCC patients, it is the combination of all the elements working together interdependently that will reliably produce the optimal outcome results desired.

It is important to understand that this bundle does not represent the comprehensive care for the treatment of chronic conditions. Rather, it is a core set of accepted elements that when implemented and successfully integrated into the clinical practice to manage MCC patients—and supported by the right infrastructures, initiatives and teams—will result in:

- High levels of reliable and sustained performance not seen when working with each individual element[7]
- Better health and quality outcomes for the population, especially the MCC population
- Better care and medication use experience for each individual patient
- The creation of healthier people and communities
- Lowering the total cost of healthcare
- Improving organizational performance and value reflected in Medicare Stars, HEDIS, QPP, ACO quality measures, APMs quality measures, and other national and local Triple Aim measures

Before focusing on the implementation and integration of MAB Rx into clinical practice, it is crucial to define each element of MAB; provide key facts; and examine the impact, challenges, and consequences when each element is not optimized.

Key MAB Facts—And the Consequences of NOT Optimizing Them

ADHERENCE

According to WHO, adherence is generally defined as the extent to which a person's behavior—taking medication, following a diet, or making healthy lifestyle changes—corresponds with agreed-upon recommendations from a healthcare provider.[8] Medication adherence is generally defined as the patient's conformance with the provider's recommendation with respect to timing, dosage, and frequency of medication taken during the prescribed length of time.[9] Patients are generally considered adherent to their medication if their proportion of days covered (PDC) is equal to or greater than 0.8 (or 80%). Eighty percent is the goal for patients on most classes of chronic medications (antiretrovirals for HIV/AIDS and some cancer oral therapies have an approximately 0.95, or 95%, threshold).[10] To calculate the PDC, visit: http://www.pqaalliance.org/images/uploads/files/PQA%20PDC%20 vs%20%20MPR.pdf.

Key Facts

Incidence of medication nonadherence

- Approximately 187 million Americans take one or more prescription drugs, and up to 50% of them do not take their medications as prescribed.[11]
- A study in the *Annals of Internal Medicine* found that more than 31% of all first-time drug prescriptions were not filled within nine months.[12]
- For disease conditions where there are minimal to no symptoms, such as high cholesterol and high blood pressure, over 50% of people stop taking their medications after 12 months (and sometimes much sooner).[13]
- One out of eight heart attack patients stops taking lifesaving drugs after just one month.[14]

- One out of two prescriptions are not taken as directed. In 2005, over 3.8 billion prescriptions were dispensed, but 1.9 billion prescriptions were not taken as directed.[15]

Most common causes of medication nonadherence along the medication use continuum

Before examining the most common causes and reasons for medication nonadherence, it is essential to understand the medication use continuum. When a patient has been diagnosed with a condition, prescriptions are ordered via either a paper prescription or ePrescribing. From there, the prescription is filled in the pharmacy, the patient is consulted about the prescription, and then the patient takes it home for consumption. If the prescription has refills (or if it is a medication for chronic use), the patient will order the refills in time to prevent a break in use. This is called the medication use continuum. At each point in the continuum, medication adherence can break down (see Figure 5.1).

According to the American Heart Association, in patients with cardiovascular disease, if 100 patients receive a prescription from their provider, about 12 of them will not fill it; 88 will go to the pharmacy to get their prescription filled, but of the 88, about 12 will decide not to take it. Primary nonadherence occurs when a patient does not get the prescription filled or does not take it upon receiving it from the pharmacy.

Of the patients who end up taking their prescriptions, within six months, about another 29 stop or reduce the frequency of use (without their provider's permission). When a patient starts the therapy but stops or reduces the dosage frequency, this is known as secondary nonadherence. So, of the 100 patients who received prescriptions, about half of them are not taking the medication as prescribed within six months.[16]

Research has shown that over 250 barriers have been identified as to why patients do not take their medications as prescribed—ranging from patient abilities, beliefs, and involvement to practical difficulties, medication-related problems, support systems, and patient-provider

The Medication Use Continuum:
Breaking medication adherence down into manageable components

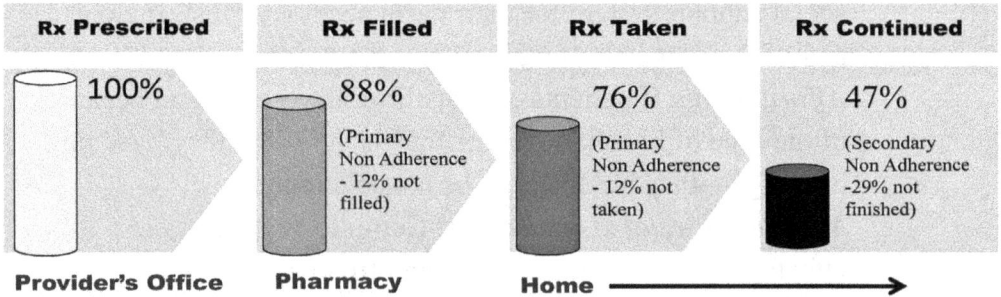

Rx Prescribed	Rx Filled	Rx Taken	Rx Continued
100%	88%	76%	47%
	(Primary Non Adherence - 12% not filled)	(Primary Non Adherence - 12% not taken)	(Secondary Non Adherence -29% not finished)
Provider's Office	**Pharmacy**	**Home** ⟶	

Figure 5.1: Understanding where medication adherence breaks down along the continuum[17]

relationships (see Figure 5.2).[18] Because patients usually have multiple reasons for not taking their medications as prescribed, the interventions have to be multifaceted. Addressing every possible barrier in each patient would not be realistic, and trying to find one solution that will address adherence in all patients rarely works.

Research on medication adherence barriers has indicated there are two sets of barriers that generally impact the majority of patients taking medications. One set generally leads to primary nonadherence, and the second set leads to secondary nonadherence.

- The set of barriers that increase primary nonadherence is identified by the acronym BREAM.
  - *Beliefs and motivation*: Patients will question the necessity of prescribed medication for maintaining health, and express concerns about potential or real negative effects related to the medication, beliefs about illness, religious beliefs, and cultural beliefs.
  - *Relationships*: Poor provider-patient relationship will result in poor adherence, as well as a lack of communication and coordination of prescriptions between providers, which can result in adverse outcomes and nonadherence.

- □ *Experiences*: Has the patient had positive or negative experiences with medications in the past? Have they known others who had positive or negative outcomes? Do they lack a social support system for their basic needs? A "yes" answer to any of these questions may cause a patient to be nonadherent.
- □ *Affordability*: If patients cannot afford the medication because of the type of benefit coverage they have—or if they have no coverage—they are likely to be nonadherent.
- □ *Medication-related challenges*: Complex regimens, side effects, number of medications, and frequency of taking medications can cause patients to be nonadherent.

- The set of barriers that increase secondary nonadherence is known as FRAMME (some descriptions are the same as above):
  - □ *Forgetfulness*: forgetting to take medications as scheduled due to other priorities or conflicts
  - □ *Relationships*
  - □ *Affordability*
  - □ *Motivation*: unable to sustain a new habit of taking medications over an extended period of time
  - □ *Medication-related challenges*
  - □ *Experiences*

Pareto's Principle - 80/20 Rule:
Most common barriers at each point of contact

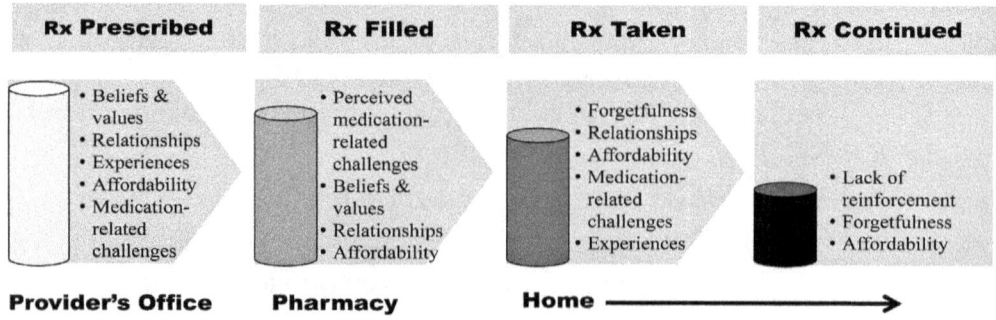

Rx Prescribed	Rx Filled	Rx Taken	Rx Continued
• Beliefs & values • Relationships • Experiences • Affordability • Medication-related challenges	• Perceived medication-related challenges • Beliefs & values • Relationships • Affordability	• Forgetfulness • Relationships • Affordability • Medication-related challenges • Experiences	• Lack of reinforcement • Forgetfulness • Affordability
Provider's Office	**Pharmacy**	**Home** ⟶	

Figure 5.2: Understanding the most common barriers at each point of contact

Impact and Consequences When Medication Adherence Is Not Optimized

Medication nonadherence impacts these major constituents: patients, providers, the healthcare system, health plans and insurers, employers, and pharmaceutical manufacturers. Patients have a reduced quality of life, increased mortality and morbidity, more complications, and higher long-term health costs. In the new value-based healthcare system, providers are at higher risk of revenue loss and penalties for quality measures, many of which are directly or indirectly linked to medication adherence. The entire healthcare system is burdened by increased costs, increased hospitalization rates, and potential penalties for poor quality outcomes due to medication nonadherence. Employers lose productive employees and productivity due to employees missing work. Health plans, insurers, and pharmaceutical companies forego potential revenues worth millions (even billions) of dollars, especially for medications used in chronic conditions.

Overall, the consequences of medication nonadherence include increased hospitalizations and nursing home admits, decrease in population health, increased mortality, increased total healthcare costs, and many other economic impacts. Below are specific examples of these consequences.

Increased Hospitalizations and Nursing Home Admits

- Ten percent of hospital admissions and 23% of nursing home admissions are due to medication nonadherence.[19]
- More than 10% of older adult hospital admissions may be due to medication nonadherence.[20]
- The risk of hospitalization, rehospitalization, and premature death among nonadherent hypertension patients is more than five times higher, compared to hypertension patients who take their medicine.[21]
- Patients with high cholesterol who do not adhere to their medications have a 26% greater likelihood of a cardiovascular-

related hospitalization, compared to patients who adhere to their prescriptions.[22]

- Poor adherence to heart failure drugs is associated with an increased number of cardiovascular-related emergency department visits.[23]

Decrease in Population Health

- Patients with low adherence have shorter times between recurrence, increased medical costs, and diminished quality of life.[24]
- Poor adherence to hypertensive medications leads to increased progression of heart disease, kidney disease, and other complications.
- In the β-Blocker Heart Attack Trial, patients who were nonadherent to propranolol hydrochloride were 2.6 times more likely to die within a year, compared to adherent patients.[25]
- Problems with medication adherence were cited as a contributing factor in more than 20% of cases of preventable, adverse drug events among older persons in the ambulatory setting.[26]
- Data from a study of 1,341 patients, published in *Psychiatry Research*, showed 23.6% were nonadherent over the course of 21 months. The nonadherent patients had a decreased likelihood of achieving remission and recovery, and an increased risk of relapse, recurrence, hospitalization, and suicide attempts. In addition, costs incurred by nonadherent patients during the study period were significantly higher than those of adherent patients (£10231 verses £7379, p<0.05), mainly from inpatient costs.[27]

Increased Mortality

- Nonadherence to prescribed medications causes approximately 125,000 deaths annually in the United States.[28]

- Among older adults, the consequences of medication nonadherence may be more serious, less easily detected, and less easily resolved than in younger age groups.[29]
- A 2008 study showed patients who didn't take any of their prescribed cardiac medication after a first heart attack were 80% more likely to die within a year than those who took all their prescribed drugs.[30]
- If 70% of patients with hypertension get the treatment they need, 46,000 deaths could be avoided each year.[31]

Increased Total Healthcare Costs
- Nonadherence contributes $100 billion to $300 billion annually to avoidable healthcare costs, representing 3% to 10% of total US healthcare costs.[32]
- Indirect costs exceed $1.5 billion annually in lost patient earnings and $50 billion in lost productivity.
- Among Medicaid beneficiaries with congestive heart failure, total healthcare costs for adherent patients were 23% lower than those of nonadherent patients (see Figure 5.3).[33]

Healthcare Spending by Level of Adherence among Medicaid Beneficiaries with Congestive Heart Failure

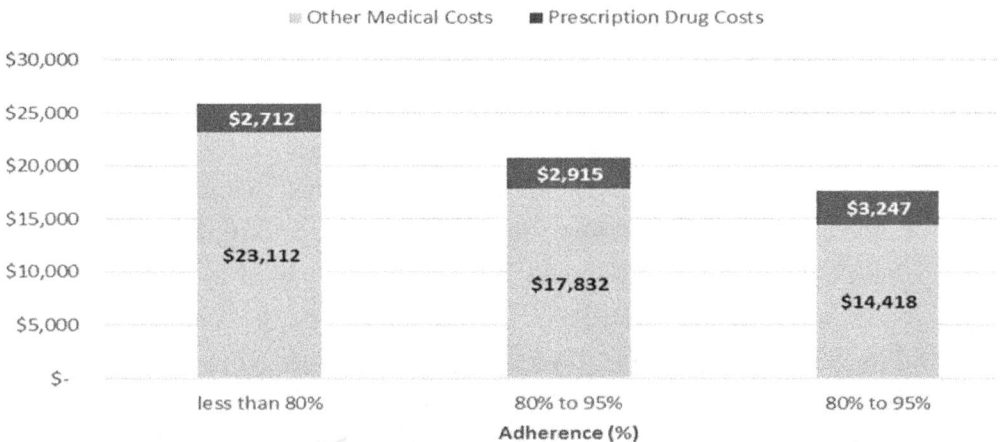

▒ Other Medical Costs   ■ Prescription Drug Costs

Adherence (%)	Prescription Drug Costs	Other Medical Costs
less than 80%	$2,712	$23,112
80% to 95%	$2,915	$17,832
80% to 95%	$3,247	$14,418

Figure 5.3: Healthcare spending by level of adherence in Medicaid beneficiaries with heart failure[34]

Other Economic Impacts

- According to the benefits consulting firm Watson Wyatt Worldwide, some corporate health insurance premiums have seen annual double-digit growth rates, and 20% to 25% of employers' healthcare expenses are direct and indirect consequences of nonadherence to medications.[35]
- Pharmaceutical manufacturers potentially lose billions of dollars in revenue, especially for chronic diseases such as hypertension, hyperlipidemia, osteoporosis, and mental disorders due to patients not filling their prescriptions. It is estimated that pharmacies lose nearly $8 billion yearly from non-refilled prescriptions.[36]

Improving Adherence with Medication Regimens Can Make a Positive Difference

- In the HOPE (Heart Outcomes Prevention Evaluation) Study, patients at high risk of cardiovascular events who were adherent to the study medications had significantly less episodes of myocardial infarction, stroke, and cardiovascular death compared to patients not on the medications, resulting in improved morbidity and mortality.[37]
- Diabetic patients with coronary heart disease in the Scandinavian Simvastatin Survival Study (4S) who were adherent to their cholesterol-lowering Simvastatin medication showed improved prognosis compared to nonadherent patients.[38]
- A 2005-2008 CVS Caremark integrated pharmacy study looked at the impact of medication adherence in chronic vascular disease on health services spending for patients age 65 and older. It found that the annual per person healthcare savings totaled $7,893 for congestive heart failure, $5,824 for hypertension, $5,170 for diabetes, and $1,847 for dyslipidemia. The average benefit-cost ratios from adherence for this group were 8.6:1 for congestive heart failure, 13.5:1 for hypertension, 8.6:1 for diabetes, and 3.8:1 for dyslipidemia.[39]

- In a study that looked at preventing myocardial infarction MI) and stroke with a simplified bundle of cardioprotective medications, patients who were adherent to their statin and ACEI/ARB medications showed a reduction of the risk by up to 60% in hospitalization for MI and stroke.[40]
- The Sokol study titled "Impact of Medication Adherence on Hospitalization Risk and Healthcare Cost" found that for a number of chronic medical conditions (diabetes, hypercholesterolemia, hypertension, and heart failure), as adherence improved, hospitalization decreased.[41]

RECONCILIATION

Medication reconciliation is the process of identifying errors and acting on discrepancies in patients' medication histories by obtaining and maintaining accurate and complete medication information for a patient and using this information to ensure safe and effective use.[42] Medication reconciliation is a key aspect of patient safety as it engages providers and patients in the process of verifying the patient's medication list at key transition points to identify which ones have been added, discontinued, or changed over time.

According to WHO, medication reconciliation is the formal process in which healthcare professionals partner with patients to ensure accurate and complete medication information transfer at interfaces of care.[43] TJC defines the medication reconciliation process as the identification of the most accurate and up-to-date list of all medications a patient is taking, at the time of admission, transfer, and discharge within the healthcare environment, using the following five-step process to prevent or reduce medication (errors):

1. Develop a list of current medications including the medication's name, dosage, frequency, and route of administration.
2. Develop a list of medications to be prescribed.
3. Compare the medications on the two lists.

4. Make clinical decisions based on the comparison.
5. Communicate the new list to appropriate caregivers and to the patient.[44]

Key Facts

Medication Errors Resulting from Medication Reconciliation Failures
A medication error is defined as any preventable event that may cause or lead to inappropriate use or patient harm while the medication is in the control of the healthcare professional, patient, or consumer.[45] The main types of medication errors that can be eliminated or significantly reduced with an effective medication reconciliation include:

- Drug **interactions**: when one medication, such as an over-the-counter medications, supplements, or herbals, affects the activity of another medication when both are administered together
- Drug **duplications**: the prescribing of multiple medications for the same indication without a clear distinction of when one agent should be administered over another
- Errors of **commission**: dispensing the wrong drug or dose, administering a drug incorrectly, prescribing the wrong dose, and/or entering the drug incorrectly into the computer system
- Errors of **omission**: failing to administer a drug that was prescribed, not administering a drug in a timely manner, failing to counsel the patient, or omitting important medication information on the label

Medication reconciliation should be done at every transition of care when new medications are ordered or existing orders are rewritten, to prevent the interaction, duplication, commission, and omission (IDCO) errors. For medication reconciliation to become more than a paperwork exercise, TJC has added the following to step 3 of the five-step process: compare the medications on the two lists "with the patient and/or caregiver." This is known as participatory reconciliation, which goes beyond the traditional patient-centered reconciliation process.[46]

Incidence of Medication Errors Resulting from Medication Reconciliation Failures

In three randomized controlled trials, readmissions and emergency department visits were significantly reduced by up to 23% when medication reconciliation was combined with other interventions specifically aimed at reducing readmissions.[47] Based on the United States Pharmacopeia (USP) MEDMARX reporting program that captures errors involving medication reconciliation failures, between September 2004 and July 2005 there were 2,022 reports of medication reconciliation errors. Sixty-six percent occurred during the patient's transition or transfer to another level of care, 22% occurred during the patient's admission to the facility, and 12% occurred at the time of discharge. Of the types of medication reconciliation errors reported to MEDMARX, the majority involved improper dose/quantity, followed by omission error and prescribing error. The other less frequently reported types of errors included wrong drug, wrong time, extra dose, wrong patient, mislabeling, wrong administration technique, and wrong dosage form.[48]

Impact and Consequences When Medication Reconciliation Is Not Optimized

The Hospital Readmissions Reduction Program (HRRP) was implemented in 2012 by CMS to address the unacceptable rate of patients readmitted to hospitals. Hospitals face steep financial penalties if they are unable to align readmission rates with the new quality standards.

In the program's first year, about 66% of the 3,400 hospitals failed under HRRP and were penalized, totaling $280 million in losses. These penalties are expected to increase over time. Studies have shown that adverse drug events resulting from medication misuse and IDCO errors have significantly contributed to the increase in readmissions.

Erroneous medication histories can lead to discontinuity of therapy, recommencement of discontinued medicines, inappropriate therapy, and failure to detect a drug-related problem. Up to 27% of hospital prescribing errors can be attributed to inaccurate or incomplete medication histories on admission to a hospital, with the omission of a regular medicine being the most common error. Older patients (≥ 65 years) and those taking multiple medicines experience a higher incidence of errors.[49] In fact, studies show that inconsistent knowledge and record keeping about medications directly threatens patient safety, causing up to 50% of all medication errors in the hospital and up to 20% of adverse drug events.[50] These errors and adverse outcomes can be reduced or prevented through an effective medication reconciliation process and education.[51]

ENGAGEMENT

Patient and family engagement strategies have shown such promise that they have been incorporated into the majority of recent efforts to improve healthcare quality. CMS describes patients and their families as "essential partners in the effort to improve the quality and safety of health care."[52]

The American Institutes for Research (AIR) defines patient and family engagement as patients, families, caregivers, and health providers working in active partnerships at various levels across the healthcare system to improve health and healthcare.[53] AHRQ defines patient engagement as "the involvement in their own care by individuals (and others they designate to engage on their behalf), with the goal that they make competent, well-informed decisions about their health and health care and take action to support those decisions."[54]

With the focus on healthcare value, patient engagement and education have gained prominence and are recognized as crucial components of high-quality healthcare services and better patient outcomes. And when patients are engaged, they are more likely to understand what they are being taught about their medications and to ask questions when they do not.[55]

Other organizations have different definitions of patient and family engagement; however, the key concepts are similar, and all emphasize that specific actions must be taken by patients, providers, and others in healthcare systems to create collaborative partnerships to improve both the individual's health and the healthcare system. Patient engagement is now a key quality component in value-based and alternative payment incentive models, such as ACOs and PCMHs, and is key to new federal initiatives that explore ways to help patients better understand medical treatment options and share in healthcare decision making. It is important to note that, to be most effective, patient engagement should not be considered a one-time event, but rather part of an ongoing conversation.

Key Facts

Incidence of Non-Engagement
A Deloitte report showed the following:

- One in three healthcare consumers is currently disengaged, reporting less need for care, preventive action, interest in resources, and financial preparation.
- There is an increase in the number of "passive" healthcare consumers.
- One in two healthcare consumers follows a "passive patient" approach, relying on doctors for decisions, preferring standard care, and adhering to treatment. Another cause for concern is that the number of "active" healthcare consumers is in decline. Two in five healthcare consumers are classified as more "active" in managing their health and navigating the healthcare system. However, this segment has experienced a decrease, from 51% in 2008 to 44% in 2012.[56]

According to a study in the *Annals of Internal Medicine*, patients who are engaged and have a clear understanding of their after-hospital care instructions, including how to take their medicines and when to make follow-up appointments, are 30% less likely to be readmitted or visit the emergency department than patients who lack this information.[57]

Factors for Patient Non-Engagement

There are many factors that contribute to lower levels of engagement, including the recession, which caused many families to have fewer resources to spend on healthcare. Although the economy has recovered in many parts of the country, many families are still experiencing economic hardship. Some families have to choose between food, shelter, medical costs, and medications; therefore, getting medications often drops to the bottom of their priority list.

In addition to socioeconomic factors, there are also cultural barriers to patient engagement. These include racial and ethnic cultures that have a history of mistrusting medicine and healthcare and also have practices of traditional healing, prayer, meditation, or herbal supplements that they feel their providers will not support.[58] Patient and family engagement can be viewed as a means of health equity, where providers and systems focus on patient-centered care, and patients and families partner in a way they choose.

Research shows that patients and providers support engagement and believe that increased involvement in healthcare by patients and families can lead to improved experiences and outcomes.[59] In 2012, 63% of healthcare consumers were dissatisfied with the US healthcare system, giving it a report card grade of C, D, or F. Healthcare organizations interested in boosting their scores should consider the benefits of patient and family engagement. One study found that patients who were highly engaged were 10 times more likely to report high patient satisfaction scores when compared to patients who were not engaged.[60] Increasing levels of patient and family engagement may lead to increases in patient satisfaction and experience of care scores.

In addition to becoming more involved in their own care and well-being, patients and families can also be involved in the governance and oversight of healthcare organizations and systems. Healthcare systems implementing patient engagement efforts have seen reductions in medical errors, hospital-acquired infections, and other serious safety events.[61]

Despite initial awareness of the importance of patient engagement, the number of disengaged patients has grown. A report by the Deloitte Center for Health Solutions found the number of disengaged patients increased from 23% in 2008 to 34% in 2012, with disengagement defined as "reporting less need for care, preventive action, interest in resources and financial preparation." The report found that patients in this group "are simply not engaged because they don't see the need." At the same time, the report found that many healthcare consumers are, in fact, motivated to engage more fully based on individual circumstances, including experience with a new medical problem or disruption in employer-sponsored coverage. The report suggests that the trend toward greater patient engagement will increase along with these circumstances.[62]

AFFORDABILITY

Prescription drugs play a critical role in helping to prevent, manage, and cure disease, yet they are a key factor in rising healthcare costs. While the rate of growth of health spending in the United States continues to increase (5.3% in 2014, up from 2.9% in 2013), the rate of prescription drug spending has far outpaced that.[63] According to the IMS Institute for Healthcare Informatics, Americans filled 4.3 billion prescriptions and spent nearly $374 billion on medications in 2014. The rate of prescription drug spending accelerated by 12.2% in 2014, compared to 2.4% growth in 2013. This rapid growth in 2014 was primarily due to increased spending for new medications, especially specialty drugs used to treat complicated conditions like hepatitis C, cancer, and rheumatoid arthritis.[64]

In 2015, prescription drug spending totaled about $457 billion, nearly 17% of total health spending.[65] These double-digit trend increases are also due to increased utilization (due to more people being insured and gaining prescription drug coverage as a result of the ACA), no significant new generics, increased costs of brand and generic medications, and more patients requiring medications for chronic conditions. There are three types of prescription drugs: generic, brand, and specialty:

- Generic medications are defined as drug products that are comparable to a brand drug product in dosage form, strength, route of administration, quality and performance characteristics, and intended use.[66]
- Brand medications are defined as medications that have a trade name and are protected by a patent (and can be produced and sold only by the company holding the patent).[67]
- Specialty drugs are generally defined as high-cost prescription medications that treat complex conditions, are bioengineered using a living source, and require special handling and administration.[68]

Figure 5.4 below shows the percent of prescription volume breakdown of brand, generic, and specialty drugs compared to the percent contribution each has to the total prescription drug spending.

This rapid growth in prescription medication prices over the last few years has become a national issue and the subject of a number of congressional hearings and probes.

CVS Caremark analysis presentation[69]	% of prescription volume of the total prescription drug spend	% of cost of the total prescription drug spend
Brand	14.5%	36%
Generics	84%	33%
Specialty	1.5%	31%

Figure 5.4: Brand, generic, and specialty drug volume
vs. cost of the total prescription drug spend

Key Facts

In 2013, the United States spent $329.2 billion on prescription drugs—eight times more than the $40.3 billion spent in 1990.[70] Although prescription drugs have historically accounted for a small proportion of national healthcare spending, compared to hospital and physician services, in recent years, it has grown rapidly. Between 2009 and 2014, there was a fundamental shift in spending trends in the US market toward high-priced medicines used to treat substantially smaller patient populations.

According to an analysis of the top 100 selling drugs, a new report known as the "Budget-Busters: The Shift to High-Priced Innovator Drugs in the USA" revealed that:

- The median price of the top 100 drugs increased from $1,260 in 2010 to $9,400 in 2014, representing a sevenfold increase.
- The median patient population size served by a top 100 drug in 2014 is 146,000, down from 690,000 in 2010.
- There are now seven treatments priced in excess of $100,000 per patient per year in 2014, versus four in 2010.[71]

Generic Drugs

While the cost of generics is increasing due to fewer generic drug manufacturers (from consolidation), shortages of active ingredients, and fewer blockbusters going generic in the next three to five years, generics are still a good option compared to brand name alternatives. In addition, for every 1% increase in generic medication mix as a total percentage of one's brand-generic-specialty mix, a health plan can see from $500,000 to $1 million in savings (depending on total population in the health plan).

Specialty Drugs

Specialty pharmacy is the fastest growing sector of pharmacy spending today, with spending trends of 18.3% in 2012 and 15.6% in 2013.[72] Much of the spending on specialty pharmaceuticals is concentrated in just four therapy classes: inflammatory conditions, multiple sclerosis (MS), cancer, and HIV. Drugs to treat these four conditions account for almost 70% of the total per member per year (PMPY) spending on specialty pharmaceuticals.[73] In addition:

- Over the last 20 years, the number of specialty pharmaceuticals increased from 10 to more than 900.[74]

- Although less than 1% of the US population uses specialty drugs, they account for more than 25% of total pharmacy spending.[75]
- Specialty drugs are generally very expensive compared to traditional medications, costing tens of thousands of dollars per treatment.[76]

Given these facts, it is understandable why the health insurance industry is campaigning against the high prices of specialty drugs. For its part, the brand-name pharmaceutical industry insists that health insurers often put these specialty drugs on the most expensive tier of their formularies, requiring patients to pay high out-of-pocket costs.[77] However, any government policy forcing insurers to cover a higher share of the price of a specialty drug will not reduce the cost of medications; instead, they will shift the cost to patients' premiums, further burdening the consumer.[78]

Impact and Consequence When Affordability Is Not Optimized

Based on a recent survey by *Consumer Reports*, 33% of Americans are paying an average of $39 more out of pocket for their regular prescription medications, and 10% are paying as much as an extra $100 per month. Among the drugs that have seen the highest increases are medications for asthma, high blood pressure, and diabetes, which went up by more than 10% in 2014. For low-income and many fixed-income Americans, paying the rising cost of prescription drugs means cutting back on daily expenses like groceries and rent payments.[79] According to the survey:

- One out of four people who had an increase in their prescription drug costs were unable to pay their medication bills.
- Seven percent said they missed a mortgage payment.
- One in four people stopped getting their prescriptions filled.
- One out of five skipped scheduled doses.[80]

This is hardly a prescription for good health. These price increases also affect employers and insurers, who are transferring some of these costs to consumers; state Medicaid programs for the poor; and Medicare programs. So, despite the number of people who have health insurance or qualify for government-assisted programs for medical care, an increasing number of people are unable to pay for the medications they need.[81]

Based on a Bloomberg survey conducted in 2014, 73 of the top branded drugs had price increases of 75% or more from late 2007 to early 2014. Generic drugs are also increasing at alarming rates. As insurers and employers pass on costs to patients in the form of higher co-pays and out-of-pocket payments, more and more people are unable to afford medical care and their medications, leading to a public health crisis.[82]

US drug prices compared to other countries according to the International Federation of Health Plans (IFHP) 2013 Comparative price report					
Drug (cost per month)	Canada	UK	Spain	Netherlands	US
Enbrel (autoimmune)	$1,646	$1,117	$1,386	$1,509	$3,000
Celebrex (pain)	$51	$112	$164	$112	$330
Copaxone (MS)	$1,400	$862	$1,191	$1,190	$3,900
Cymbalta (depression)	$110	$46	$71	$52	$240
Gleevec (leukemia)	$1,141	$2,697	$3,348	$3,321	$8,500
Humira (arthritis)	$1,950	$1,102	$1,498	$1,498	$3,049
Nexium (acid reflux)	$30	$42	$58	$23	$305

Figure 5.5: US drug prices compared to other countries in 2013

Many Americans have turned to importing medications from other countries. Research has shown that importation from legitimate, verified, international online pharmacies can be a safe and affordable option for

Americans. Medications from these pharmacies cost an average of 50% less than identical products in American pharmacies. Figure 5.5 shows US drug prices compared to other countries, according to the International Federation of Health Plans (IFHP) 2013 Comparative Price Report.[83] It is now estimated that over 5 million Americans each year rely on importation to access the medications they need at prices they can afford. The Pharmaceutical Research and Manufacturers of America (PhRMA) believes the international comparisons are misleading because list prices do not take into account discounts available to US insurers. While these discounts do drive down the actual price paid by US insurance companies, similar confidential discounts are also offered to big European buyers such as Britain's National Health Service.[84]

SAFE MEDICATION USE

The 1999 Institute of Medicine (IOM) report "To Err Is Human: Building a Safer Health System" found that medication-related errors were a significant cause of morbidity and mortality in the United States, accounting for at least 1.5 million medication-related events or preventable medication-related injuries that occur yearly. Medication errors have been estimated to account for 1.9 million hospital stays, increased length of hospital stays, the most common causes of inpatient complications, and about $3.5 billion in hospital costs.[85] In outpatient/ambulatory settings, medication errors are the most common post-discharge complication, resulting in 3.5 million office/ambulatory visits, and 1 million emergency department visits.

Medication errors also account for one out of every 131 outpatient deaths, and one out of 854 inpatient deaths, totaling more than 7,000 deaths annually.[86] Based on these and other findings, the IOM issued a report in 2007 on medication safety called "Preventing Medication Errors." This report focused on issues such as the importance of reducing medication errors, providing clinicians with information and decision-support tools, and processes to reduce medication errors and adverse outcomes.[87]

Medication-related errors are not just a problem in the United States. Several studies from various countries have reported that 3.7–16.6% of total hospital admissions were associated with adverse events, a substantial proportion of which were attributed to medication use.[88] With the increased reliance on medication therapy as the primary intervention for chronic and acute conditions, patients are exposed to the benefits as well as the potential harm of the medications. Also, as people age, they are more likely to develop one or more chronic illnesses, which will be treated with medications. While appropriate medication can help people live longer, more active lives, these benefits have also been accompanied by increased risks of adverse events, side effects, and errors along the medication process and use continuum.[89]

Key Facts

The Stages of the Medication Use Process Where Medication Errors Can Occur
There are a number of discrete stages along the medication use process continuum where medication errors can occur. Six of the key stages include prescribing, transcribing, preparing, dispensing, administering, and monitoring.[90]

- *Prescribing*: This is when a prescribing healthcare provider chooses the most appropriate medication for a patient's given clinical situation, taking individual factors into account. The provider also selects the most appropriate administration route, dose, time, and regimen.
- *Transcribing*: This is the transfer of information from the provider's orders to the nursing documentation form or to the pharmacy system.
- *Preparation*: After getting the prescription from the provider, the pharmacist reviews it for accuracy, appropriateness, and any errors before picking and preparing (counting, calculating, mixing, or labeling) the drug.

- *Dispensing*: This occurs when the pharmacist delivers the prepared medication to the patient or the ward/unit where the prescription was ordered.
- *Administering*: Administering a medication involves giving it to the intended user or to the caregiver for administration to the patient. Administering always includes the need to check for allergies and to make sure that the correct dose of the right medicine is given to the right patient via the right route at the correct time.
- *Monitoring*: This involves observing the patient to determine whether the medication is working, being used correctly, and not causing harm.[91]

Incidence of Errors Along the Medication Process Stages

Soon after the IOM's report was released, the US Department of Defense (DoD) focused on standardizing its medication error event reporting. The DoD created a reporting system using MEDMARX, an Internet-based commercial reporting application, and captured inpatient and outpatient events between October 2002 and September 2003; that information was compared to the 2002 MEDMARX national database (see Figure 5.6).[92]

The percentage of inpatient and outpatient events, stratified by the medication use stages from the DoD patient safety center registry, Oct. 2002 to Sept. 2003, compared to the 2002 MEDMARX national database				
	Inpatient		Outpatient	
Medication Use Stages	DoD	National	DoD	National
Prescribing	525 (13%)	26,703 (21%)	4,136 (28%)	3,683 (27%)
Dispensing	1,058 (26%)	23,573 (19%)	8,942 (61%)	6,962 (51%)
Documenting / Transcribing	793 (19%)	30,124 (24%)	1,226 (8%)	1,124 (8%)
Administering	1,710 (41%)	43,488 (35%)	381 (3%)	1,832 (13%)
Monitoring	40 (1%)	1,399 (1%)	48 (1%)	113 (1%)

Figure 5.6: The percentage of inpatient and outpatient events.

The data reported to the DoD showed the largest percentage of inpatient events occurred in the administering stage (41%), followed by the dispensing stage (26%) and then the documenting/transcribing stages (19%). In the outpatient setting, the largest percentage of events occurred in the dispensing stage (61%), followed by the prescribing stage (28%) and the documenting/transcribing stages (8%).

The national data showed that the largest percentage of inpatient events occurred in the administering stage (35%), followed by the documenting/transcribing stages (24%) and the prescribing stage (21%). In the outpatient setting, the largest percentage of events occurred in the dispensing stage (51%), followed by the prescribing stage (27%) and the administering stage (13%). While the national and DoD datasets do contain differences, the error distributions compare closely.

The implementation of the MEDMARX electronic reporting system enhanced the DoD's ability to collect and analyze these events and will have significant long-term benefits for the DoD patients.[93]

Dr. Grace Kuo conducted a 20-week study on medication errors that involved 42 family physicians at 42 practices, combined with a 10-week period involving 401 clinicians and staff from 10 diverse family medicine offices. The study showed that a significant number of medication errors were prescribing errors, with more than half reaching the patients. A total of 1,265 medical errors were reported, and 194 reports had errors in medication. Of the 194 reports, 70% involved prescribing errors, 10% administering errors, 10% documenting errors, 7% dispensing errors, and 3% monitoring errors. Of the 194 reports, 41% of the errors were prevented and did not reach patients, while 59% did reach patients. The pharmacists in this study were the most likely to prevent the errors from reaching the patients (40%), while physicians and patients were almost equally likely to intercept the medication error (19% and 17%, respectively). The researchers believe that more widespread use of healthcare information technology, such as electronic medical records or computer physician order entry systems, could have prevented up to 57% of the medication errors.[94]

Conditions and Failures That Contribute to Errors and Potential Patient Harm

There are a number of defenses and safeguards along the medication use process that help prevent errors from occurring. These range from systems approaches (for example, computer alerts when there are drug interactions or duplications, or automated hard stops for potentially dangerous prescribing) to personal expertise to policy and administrative controls.

The Medication Process Stages: The Defenses and the Holes

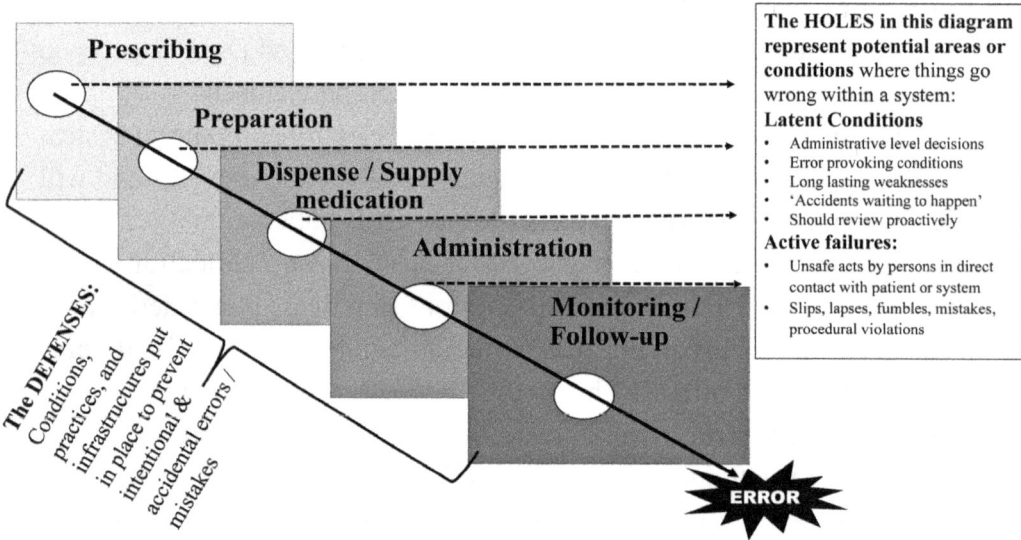

Figure 5.7: The defenses and holes along the medication process stages

According to a study by James Reason, professor of psychology at the University of Manchester, each of these defense and safeguard layers will have systematic processes in place to prevent errors from occurring.[95] In reality, however, these layers are more like slices of Swiss cheese, with holes in each slice. The presence of a hole in one layer (or stage) does not usually necessitate a bad outcome.[96] Errors occur when the "holes" in all layers line up to permit a trajectory of accident opportunity, causing potential harm to the patient.

The holes in the medication process stage defenses arise for two reasons: active failures and latent conditions (see Figure 5.7). Nearly all adverse events and medication errors involve a combination of these two sets of factors.

- *Active failures*: "These are the unsafe acts committed by people who are in direct contact with the patient or system. They take a variety of forms: slips, lapses, fumbles, mistakes, and procedural violations," according to Reason.[97]
- *Latent conditions*: These are the inevitable "resident pathogens" within the system that arise from decisions made by people in the system and top level management. Latent conditions have two kinds of adverse effects: (1) They can translate into error-provoking conditions within the workplace (time pressure, understaffing, inadequate equipment, fatigue, inexperience); and (2) they can create long-lasting holes or weaknesses in the defenses (alarms and indicators that go off constantly, complex or unworkable procedures, design deficiencies). Latent conditions can lie dormant within the system for months to years before they combine with an active failure or trigger, creating an accident opportunity.[98]

Impact and Consequences of Unsafe Medication Use and ADEs

The concern raised in "To Err Is Human" about the prevalence and impact of ADEs (two out of every 100 hospitalized patients) was just the beginning of our understanding of the potential magnitude of the rates of medication errors.[99] IOM's 2007 report ("Preventing Medication Errors") stated that "a hospital patient is subject to at least one medication error per day, with considerable variation in error rates across facilities."[100] In a case-control analysis of ADEs in hospitalized patients during a three-year period, the impact of medication errors on morbidity and mortality were assessed. The investigators found significant increases in the following:

- Cost of hospitalization due to increased length of stay (ranging from $677 to $9,022)
- Patient mortality (odds ratio = 1.88 with a 95% confidence interval)
- Post-discharge disability

There are three areas of focus that demonstrate the impact of unsafe medication use and adverse outcomes: the opioid, diabetic, anticoagulation, and antibiotic drug classes (ODAA), which account for a significant number of adverse outcomes; inappropriate medication use in the elderly; and inappropriate medication use in the pediatric population.[101]

1. *ODAA Drug Classes*

In 2011, ADEs accounted for over 3.5 million physician office visits and an estimated 1 million emergency department visits. Also, almost one in three of all adverse events that occurred while patients were in the hospital were the result of ADEs, affecting nearly 2 million hospital stays annually. Of these nearly 2 million, approximately 66% were related to the prescribing, dispensing, and/or administering of anticoagulants (bleeding adverse events), insulin/oral hypoglycemic agents (hypoglycemia adverse events), and opioids (accidental overdoses, over-sedation, respiratory depression adverse events).[102] Also, according to the CDC, an estimated 700,000 people around the world die every year from antimicrobial-resistant infections, with more than 23,000 deaths and 2 million illnesses occurring within the United States.[103] Other classes of medications that most frequently result in harm include antineoplastics and corticosteroids.[104]

- *Opioid Adverse Events*

In recent years, opioid drug abuse has become a serious public health issue in this country, with drug overdose deaths now the leading cause of injury deaths. According to the CDC, every day an average of 44 people die from overdose of prescription drugs. Overprescribing and illegally obtaining prescription opioid drugs are a large part of the overdose problem. In 2014, more people died from drug overdoses than in any other year on record—more than 28,000 people, a 14% increase from 2013, which was the highest year on record.[105] The rate of overdose deaths involving opioids (both prescription opioid pain relievers like oxycodone, hydrocodone, and methadone, as well as heroin) nearly quadrupled between 1999 and 2014.[106] Despite this increase, there has not been an overall change in the amount of pain that Americans report.[107] In addition, in 2012 there were an estimated 2.1 million people suffering from substance use disorders related to prescription opioid pain relievers and an estimated 467,000 people were addicted to heroin.[108]

The abuse of and addiction to opioids such as heroin, morphine, and prescription pain relievers is not just a serious problem in this country; it is a global problem that affects the health, social, and economic welfare of all societies. It is estimated that between 26.4 million and 36 million people worldwide abuse opioids.

The consequences of this abuse have been devastating. Approximately 75% of heroin users started on the road to addiction with prescription drugs, validating the growing evidence suggesting a relationship between increased non-medical use of opioid analgesics and heroin abuse in the US.[109] To address the complex problem of prescription opioid and heroin abuse in this country, providers are going to have to strike the right balance between prescribing, administering, and monitoring the use of opioids to maximize pain relief while minimizing associated risks and adverse effects.[110]

- *Diabetic Medications Adverse Events*
  Hypoglycemia (low blood sugar) is one of the most common and potentially most dangerous complications of diabetes therapy. Event rates for severe hypoglycemia in patients with type 1 diabetes range from 115 to 320 per 100 patient-years, while in patients with type 2 diabetes, the event rate was about 35 to 70 per 100 patient-years. However, because type 2 diabetes is much more prevalent than type 1, most episodes of

hypoglycemia, including severe hypoglycemia, occur in patients with type 2. Also, due to the longer life expectancy of patients with diabetes, and the focus on having patients work to obtain tight glycemic control (to reduce complications), there has been an increase in the number of type 2 patients at risk for hypoglycemia.[111]

Hospital admission and readmission rates for hypoglycemia exceed those for hyperglycemia among older adults and African American Medicare beneficiaries. According to a study in *JAMA*, hypoglycemia rates were twice as high for older patients (≥75 years) compared with younger patients (65-74 years), and admission rates for both hyperglycemia and hypoglycemia were four times higher for black patients compared with white patients.[112] In the ACCORD (the Action to Control Cardiovascular Risk in Diabetes) study published in the NEJM, hypoglycemia requiring assistance and weight gain of more than 10 kilograms was more frequent in the study group using intensive therapy to target normal glycated hemoglobin levels compared with standard therapy. There was also an increased mortality in the intensive therapy study group, with no significant reduction in major cardiovascular events.[113]

• *Anticoagulants Adverse Events*

Anticoagulants, also known as blood thinners, are medications used to eliminate or reduce the risk of blood clots. They include the traditional ones (warfarin, other coumarins, and heparins) and the newer, potentially safer, novel oral anticoagulants (dabigatran, rivaroxaban, apixaban, and edoxaban).

Anticoagulant medications are among the most common medications that cause ADEs in hospitalized and ambulatory patients. The study "Anticoagulation-Associated Adverse Drug Events" discovered that most anticoagulant-associated ADEs among hospitalized patients resulted from medication errors and were therefore potentially preventable. Also in this study, patients who suffered an anticoagulant-associated ADE and high hospitalization had an elevated 30-day mortality rate and high hospitalization costs.[114]

CDC and Emory University researchers found that the number one medication most responsible for medication-related emergency hospitalizations is warfarin (see Figure 5.8). Almost all of the hospitalizations from warfarin were the result of unintentional overdoses or interactions with other drugs. Too much warfarin also resulted in gastrointestinal bleeds and brain hemorrhages.[115]

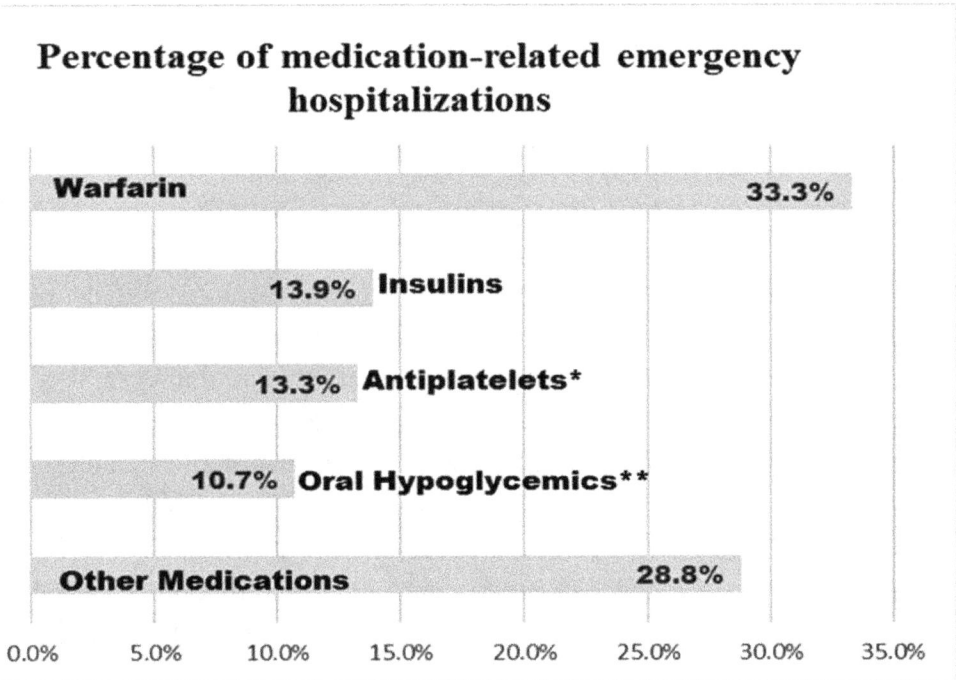

Percentage of medication-related emergency hospitalizations

Medication	Percentage
Warfarin	33.3%
Insulins	13.9%
Antiplatelets*	13.3%
Oral Hypoglycemics**	10.7%
Other Medications	28.8%

*   Aspirin, Clopidogrel, others   ** Glipizide, glyburide, metformin, others

*Figure 5.8: The most common medications contributing
to medication-related emergency hospitalizations*

- *Antibiotic/Antimicrobial Resistance*

The rise in antimicrobial-resistant infections is a growing threat and is becoming a global health crisis. This is primarily a result of overprescribing and prioritizing the use of newer, more broad-spectrum drugs over cheaper antibiotics. Another cause of antibiotic resistance is the use of antibiotics in food-producing animals to cure and stave off disease, or to promote weight gain in livestock without having to increase their food intake.[116]

According to the CDC, infections from these "superbugs" (antimicrobial-resistant infections) now resistant to one or multiple antibiotics are responsible for about 700,000 deaths worldwide every year—with more than 23,000 deaths and 2 million illnesses occurring within the United States.[117] About 30% of antibiotics prescribed in this country were deemed unnecessary for the conditions they were prescribed for, according to a study in *JAMA*.[118] Another study found that between 2006 and 2012, there was little change in the rate of antibiotic use and a significant increase in the use of broad-spectrum antibiotics, which are drugs of last resort for the worst infections.[119]

2. *Inappropriate Medication Use in the Elderly*

Inappropriate medication use is a major issue in the elderly population in the United States and around the world. Over 50% of elderly patients have more than one disease condition and are usually on multiple medications (polypharmacy), which can increase their chances of having medication-related problems and adverse outcomes. Inappropriate prescribing is also now more prevalent in elderly population, and according to R. Maher, nearly 50% of older adults take one or more medications that are not medically necessary.[120] This increases their risks for ADEs, drug interactions, functional status and cognitive impairment issues, falls, medical costs, and healthcare utilization.

In a study on adverse drug events in the outpatient setting, patients taking five or more medications had a 6.2% increase in prescription drug expenditures, and those taking 10 or more medications had a 7.3% increase. Also, outpatients taking five or more medications had an 88% increased risk of experiencing an ADE, compared to those who were taking fewer medications.[121]

In nursing home residents, rates of ADEs have been noted to be twice as high in patients taking nine or more medications, compared to those taking fewer.[122] In a study on the clinical consequences of polypharmacy in the elderly, evaluating unplanned hospitalizations in older veterans found that patients taking more than five medications were nearly four times as likely to be hospitalized from adverse drug events.[123] In a study in the *Annals of Pharmacotherapy* on the prevalence and risk of potential cytochrome p450-mediated drug-drug interactions in older hospitalized patients with polypharmacy, the probability of a drug-drug interaction increased with the number of medications. Specifically, a patient taking five to nine medications had a 50% probability; the risk increased to 100% when a patient was found to be taking 20 or more medications, which could be a cause of preventable ADEs and medication-related hospitalizations.[124]

Functional decline has been seen in elderly patients on multiple medications. In a study on medication use and functional decline among community-dwelling older women, increased prescription medication use was associated with diminished ability to perform instrumental activities of daily living and also decreased physical functioning.[125] In another study on association of polypharmacy with nutritional status, functional ability, and cognitive capacity, patients taking 10 or more medications had diminished functional capacity and trouble performing daily tasks.[126]

As part of the Women's Health Initiative Observational study, polypharmacy was associated with incident disability in older women.[127] Cognitive impairment, seen with both delirium and dementia, has been associated with polypharmacy. The study "Delirium Risk Factors in Elderly Hospitalized Patients" reported that the number of medications were a risk factor for delirium.[128] The study "Clinical Consequences of Polypharmacy in Elderly" discovered 22% of patients taking five or fewer medications were found to have impaired cognition as opposed to 33% of patients taking six to nine medications and 54% in patients taking 10 or more medications.[129]

3. Inappropriate Medication Use in the Pediatric Population

Safe medication use is often challenging in pediatric and adolescent populations (children up to the age of 18), because most prescription and over-the-counter medications that are prescribed for children have not been tested in that population. Therefore, their use is usually off-label, not evidence-based, and sometimes inappropriate.[130] According to TJC, safe medication use is complicated in these populations because most medications used in the care of children are formulated and packaged primarily for adults. Therefore, medications must often be prepared in different volumes or concentrations within the healthcare setting before being administered to children.[131]

According to WHO, unsafe medication use in children worldwide is further complicated by teenage abuse of prescription medications. It is also complicated by new therapies with pediatric indications but without evidence of long-term benefit and risk. Additionally, in resource-poor countries, there may be no treatments available, especially during times of war and civil strife. Counterfeit medicines are rampant, sometimes with deadly effects especially when unintentionally used for the treatments of endemic infectious diseases such as HIV/AIDS, malaria, and tuberculosis and for parasitic diseases.[132]

These safe medication use challenges have resulted in wrong dosage, short-term toxicity or treatment failure, administration of altered dosage forms of medications because of the unavailability of appropriate pediatric formulations, and unfortunate administration errors (intravenous drips running fast, errors in dosage calculation, and dilution). When the formulations of strengths suitable for administration to neonates, infants, and young children are not available, accidental poisoning and injuries by parents or caregivers who are unaware of the appropriate doses can occur, especially if there are cultural or health literacy challenges. Long-term safety problems—for example, long-term use of inhaled corticosteroids in early infancy—may increase the risk of growth retardation and/or osteoporosis, co-morbidity, or malnutrition exacerbating the medication toxicity, and may increase the risk for contamination from trying to reconstitute nonsterile oral powder for pediatric use.[133]

Strategic Overview for Implementation of MAB Rx

A better understanding of the current healthcare environment, challenges, and opportunities allows for the development of an MAB

Rx strategic plan that will support organizations in effectively meeting the goals of the new value-based healthcare system—optimizing healthcare value by achieving better care, smarter spending, and creating healthier communities. This can be accomplished by the following:

- Successfully implementing and integrating MAB into the care delivery system and spreading it across the continuum of care
- Developing, building, and/or augmenting the right infrastructures to support MAB's success, spread, and sustainability over time.

When implemented successfully, the MAB Rx will be a major contributor to the optimization of healthcare value across the continuum of care to achieve the Triple Aim, and it will contribute to the goals of NQS, the CMS Quality Strategy, and other quality strategies worldwide. So, what is the best way to implement the MAB Rx?

Consider the work of Dr. Sam, the director of pharmacy operations in a large healthcare system. His key focus is threefold: to align the pharmacy's priorities with the organization's vision, mission, and core strategies; contribute to transforming the care delivery system; and support the successful transition of the organization from a primarily fee-for-service world to an alternative payment model, ready to thrive in the new value-based healthcare environment. He plans to accomplish this over time by doing the following:

- Creating high-performing, effective leadership, provider, and staff teams that are engaged and aligned with the new realities and focused on the new goals, priorities, and strategies needed to transform the healthcare delivery system and thrive in the new healthcare environment
- Partnering with key stakeholders to implement identified critical strategies that will contribute to the organization's goals
- Building the right infrastructures and having the right tools in place to ensure success, scalability, and sustainability

In 2015, Dr. Sam had a strategic retreat with his leadership team, key stakeholders from different departments, and key physicians, clinicians, and pharmacy staff teams to learn about the new healthcare landscape and the organization's strengths, weaknesses, opportunities, and threats (SWOT) in this new healthcare environment; and to renew their commitment to the organization's mission, vision, and purpose. Also, during this off-site, the teams reviewed and discussed many different pharmacy strategies and initiatives that would support the priorities of the organization in this new era of healthcare.

Subsequently, over a few brainstorming sessions, the key stakeholders and teams identified the implementation of the MAB Rx as the major strategy to accomplish the following:

- Positively contribute to the mission, core priorities, and strategic direction of the organization
- Align and positively impact the Medicare Parts C and D, Pay-for-Value, HEDIS, MACRA, TJC, and other quality goals for the organization
- Contribute to optimizing the new payment bonuses, and minimize the penalties under the new alternative payment model goals
- Meet the goals of the Triple Aim, NQS, and the CMS quality strategy
- Help improve operational efficiencies that are important to the organization
- Demonstrate a significant return on investment and a relatively high implementation feasibility
- Contribute to transforming the care delivery model
- Positively impact regulatory requirements

Next, Dr. Sam and his team developed a proposal to get organization-wide support. Over the next three months, the team worked with leaders, additional key stakeholders, staff, and patients to identify the following strategic anchors, strategies, and initiatives for the successful implementation of the MAB Rx:

- *Care Delivery Transformation*: Integrate and optimize MAB in the new models of care to improve the health outcomes of MCC patients
- *Engaged People*: Activate and engage healthcare consumers while developing high-performing, effective healthcare teams to ensure the success of MAB
- *Performance Outcomes*: Identify regulatory and quality measures that MAB would impact to demonstrate value (improved quality and service/reduced cost) in MCC patients and organizations
- *Solid Infrastructures*: Build/optimize/consolidate infrastructures and business capabilities to successfully implement, support, and sustain MAB
- *Committed Leadership*: MAB sponsorship, partnerships, and alliances to optimize health outcomes in MCC patients nationally and globally

Then, the teams and key stakeholders focused on identifying the specific initiatives that would link to the strategies and strategic anchors that will support the successful implementation of MAB. These initiatives could be modified based on the organization needs and priorities. From these initiatives, an action plan was developed that included what was to be done, who was accountable, and when the initiative was due. Figure 5.9 gives an overview of how the strategic anchors, strategies, and initiatives align to enable organizations to successfully implement and integrate MAB.

The following chapters provide a more in-depth study of some of the initiatives that are critical for MAB success.

The Medication A.R.E.A.S. Bundle (MAB) Strategic Plan:
Contributing to Healthcare Value to Achieve the Triple Aim

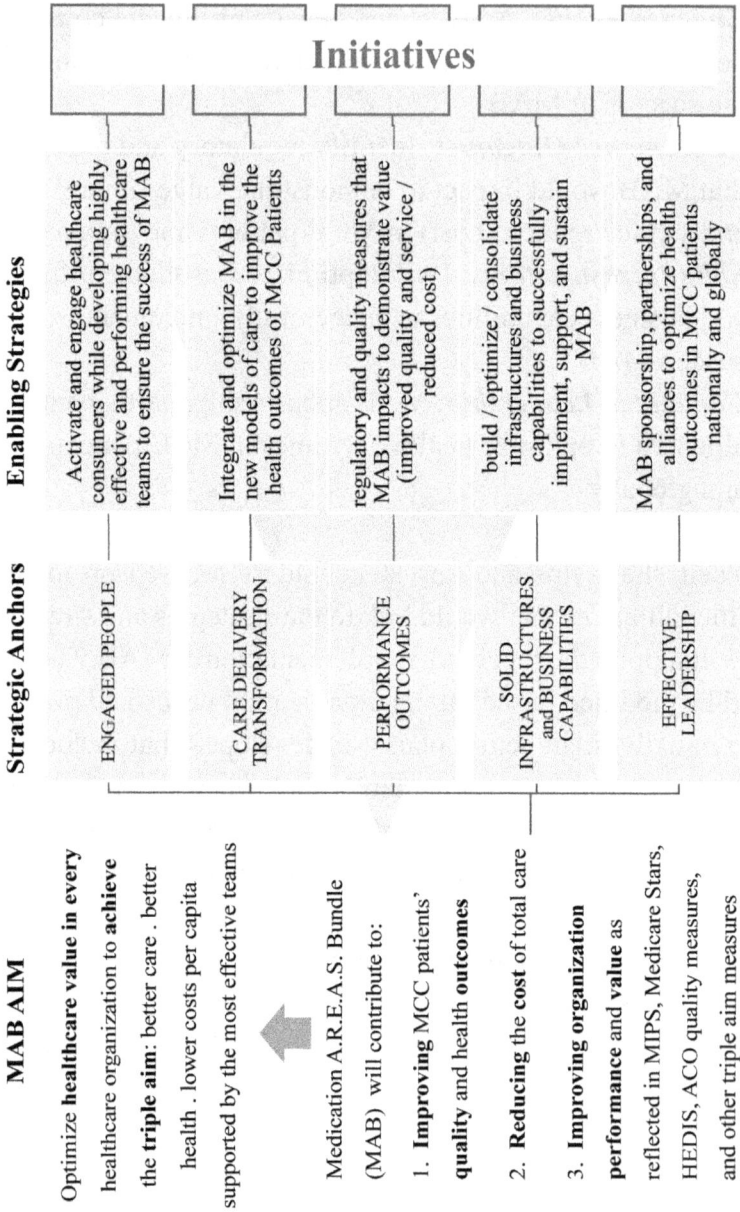

Initiatives

MAB AIM

Optimize **healthcare value in every** healthcare organization to **achieve** the **triple aim**: better care . better health . lower costs per capita supported by the most effective teams

Medication A.R.E.A.S. Bundle (MAB) will contribute to:

1. **Improving** MCC patients' **quality** and health **outcomes**

2. **Reducing** the **cost** of total care

3. **Improving organization performance** and **value** as reflected in MIPS, Medicare Stars, HEDIS, ACO quality measures, and other triple aim measures

Strategic Anchors

ENGAGED PEOPLE

CARE DELIVERY TRANSFORMATION

PERFORMANCE OUTCOMES

SOLID INFRASTRUCTURES and BUSINESS CAPABILITIES

EFFECTIVE LEADERSHIP

Enabling Strategies

Activate and engage healthcare consumers while developing highly effective and performing healthcare teams to ensure the success of MAB

Integrate and optimize MAB in the new models of care to improve the health outcomes of MCC Patients

regulatory and quality measures that MAB impacts to demonstrate value (improved quality and service / reduced cost)

build / optimize / consolidate infrastructures and business capabilities to successfully implement, support, and sustain MAB

MAB sponsorship, partnerships, and alliances to optimize health outcomes in MCC patients nationally and globally

Figure 5.9: The diagram of a draft MAB strategic plan

Chapter 6:
Framework for the MAB Rx
Implementation Across the Continuum

"No medication works inside a bottle. Period.
And drugs don't work in patients who don't take them."
Dr. C. Everett Koop[1]

Topics Covered:

- The BSMART Checklist framework and its elements
- Utilizing the BSMART Checklist framework to reliably implement the MAB Rx

To effectively implement MAB, a proposed framework draws upon and combines the following elements: motivational interviewing techniques to facilitate change; patient-provider relationships; ongoing reinforcement of new habits; patient involvement in the decision-making and goal-setting processes, empowering and encouraging patients at every point of contact; recognition for achieving goals; and having social support, tools, and training. These elements can be condensed into a multifaceted framework that will help providers and staff have a reliable and consistent thought process for successfully addressing and implementing all elements of MAB at every point of care. This multifaceted framework is known as the BSMART Checklist. The components of the BSMART Checklist include the following:

- *Barriers*: Identify barriers and assess readiness to change
- *Solutions*: Provide solutions to the identified barriers

- *Motivation*: Skills to help patients help themselves—short- and long-term
- *A.R.E.A.S. tools*: Provide tools to keep patients on track and make it easier for providers to do the right thing
- *Relationships*: Develop optimal relationships with patients and the healthcare team members
- *Triage*: Refer patients to other resources in the healthcare system and communities for ongoing support and care

The BSMART Checklist can help providers address MAB, from the hospital setting to the provider's office to other healthcare infrastructures (pharmacy, care management, and others) and in the home setting.

BARRIERS

Identifying barriers is the first step in determining what solutions and interventions a patient's team will use to optimize medication use and health outcomes. The following are some common barriers that prevent patients from receiving appropriate medication use:

Adherence Barriers
- *Patient-related factors*: Some common adherence barriers include beliefs or concerns about disease or medications, patients with asymptomatic conditions, cultural and religious beliefs, depression, forgetfulness, confusion, patients who cannot communicate well (for example, the unconscious, babies and young children, or people who speak foreign languages), and negative experiences with medications in the past or knowledge of someone who experienced this.
- *Healthcare team–related factors*: These include a poor relationship between patient and physician; lack of clear instructions from health professionals; disparity between the health beliefs of the healthcare provider and those of the patient; lack of ongoing positive encouragement and reinforcement by the provider

or staff; poor provider communication skills, contributing to lack of patient knowledge or understanding of the treatment regimen; poor support of nurses, pharmacists, or other team members; and staff members multitasking.

- *Socioeconomic-related factors*: There is a lack of social support especially for patients on chronic medications, for the homeless, and for those without access to providers and/or pharmacies.
- *Health system–related factors*: These problems include frequent changes in formulary medications, poor access to care, and a lack of or inadequate materials to educate patients.
- *Medication therapy–related factors*: These include adverse effects from use of medications, complex treatment regimens (number of concurrent medications, frequency of taking medication), a lack of clear instructions on how to take the medications, a lack of immediate positive effects from taking the medication, medications that have been socially stigmatized (for example, medications for depression), medications that require significant lifestyle changes, and perceived or actual significant side effects.[2]

Reconciliation Barriers
- *Systems factors*: effective tools and decision support to make the medication reconciliation process simple
- *Patient-related factors*: having multiple providers writing their prescriptions and filling them in multiple pharmacies
- *Healthcare team–related factors*: Obtaining barrier information from patients is sometimes time-consuming for most providers; getting all the patients' information from the multiple sources can also be challenging; and knowing who is responsible for doing the medication reconciliation is sometimes unclear and differs depending on the practice setting.

Engagement Barriers
- *Patient-related factors*: lack of knowledge and understanding of the disease and/or medication, not taking an active interest in being

informed about their own health and medicines, life stresses, or low health literacy

Affordability Barriers
* Affordability of medications, healthcare benefits structure, very high deductible plans
* No generics available

Safe Medication Use Barriers
* ***The prescribing stage***: errors from miscalculating dosage; miscommunication, including poor handwriting or confusion of drugs with similar names; inappropriate use of zeroes and decimal points; confusion of metric and apothecary systems; use of inappropriate abbreviations; ambiguous or incomplete orders; inadequate written or verbal communication; the prescribing of potentially inappropriate drugs for older adults; not entering the data when using computerized prescribing; pressure to overprescribe or over-treat, for example, opioids; not identifying the patient's factors, allergies, or other medications the patient may be taking; poor documentation; illegible or incomplete scripts; or lack of knowledge about the drug
* ***The transcription stage***: incomplete or illegible prescriber orders; incomplete or illegible nurse handwriting; the use of abbreviations; lack of familiarity with drug names, dose, route, or frequency; or preparing a medication administration record in an environment that is noisy or poorly lit
* ***The preparation* stage**: medication dosing errors; illegible handwriting by the provider; wrong dosages of a medication, either lower or higher than what was ordered by a prescriber; confusing medications that are similar in appearance or packaging, or that have similar spellings or phonetics (for example, the insulin products —Novolin, Novolog, and Novolin 70/30; clonidine and Klonopin; vinblastine and vincristine; hydroxyzine, hydralazine, Hydrodiuril); or, for intravenous medications, —preparing the

doses with the wrong diluent, failing to dilute a medication such as potassium liquid with water prior to administration, or poor aseptic methods when preparing IV medicines (disinfecting vials, cleaning the preparation area, washing hands or wearing sterile gloves, and making sure that windows are closed in the preparation area)[3]

- *The dispensing/supply of medication stage*: patient information (diagnoses, lab values, allergies, and drug contradictions) often unavailable to pharmacy, nursing, and medical staff prior to dispensing the medications; time constraints and hurrying, leading to dispensing the wrong medication or misinterpreting the prescription dose, directions, or units; illegible handwriting by the provider; dispensing the wrong medication due to similar packaging or labeling, similar strengths, dosage forms, frequency of administration, similar clinical use; or physical environment of the pharmacy, such as small or cramped space, a noisy environment from the radio, other issues already raised by patients or pharmacy staff, noise of robotic equipment, poor lighting, or extreme temperatures in the pharmacy

- *The administration stage*: the 5Ws—a drug given to the wrong patient, by the wrong route, at the wrong time, in the wrong dose, or the wrong drug used; omission or failure to administer; or inadequate documentation leading to administration duplication

- *The monitoring stage*: failure to recognize symptoms of addiction or patterns of overuse; lack of monitoring for side effects; drug not stopped if not working or if the course of therapy is completed; drug stopped before the course is completed; drug lab levels not measured or not followed up on; or communication failures when changes are made in therapies from one practice setting to another[4]

Questions to Ask to Identify Barriers

Providers can choose one or two from the following questions below to help better understand a patient's medication-taking behaviors and determine what barriers their patient may have:

Adherence

- During the last week, how many days have you missed taking any of your medications?
- During the last week, what percentage of your medication have you taken?
- Have you stopped or started taking any of your medication on your own?
- Have you ever had difficulty taking your medication as prescribed and, if so, why?
- What gets in the way of taking your medications on some days?
- Have you experienced any problems or had any side effects while taking your medication?

Other screening tools, like the Morisky Medication Adherence Scale, have been used to screen for appropriate medication use. The Morisky Scale is composed of the following four questions:

- Do you ever forget to take your medications?
- Are you careless at times about taking your medications?
- When you feel better, do you sometimes stop taking your medications?
- Sometimes, if you feel worse when you take your medications, do you stop taking them?[5]

Reconciliation

- How many pharmacies do you use to get all your medications?
- When last did you get a complete list of all your medications?

Engagement

Questions to identify patients with inadequate health literacy include the following:

- How often are medical forms difficult to understand and fill out?
- How often do you have difficulty understanding the written information your healthcare provider gives you?

- How often do you have problems learning about your medical condition because of difficulty understanding written information?
- How confident are you filling out your healthcare/medical forms by yourself?
- How confident do you feel you are able to follow the instructions on the label of a medication bottle?
- How often do you have someone else help you read your health materials?[6]

Affordability

It is sometimes embarrassing or challenging for patients to admit that they cannot afford their medications. Some clues healthcare providers can look out for include patients with high deductible plans, lost jobs, and patients not adherent to their medications. Sometimes, patients will ask how much a medication costs. When they do, or if you suspect they are having challenges affording their medications, you can confirm by asking the following:

- Are you having a problem paying for your medications?
- Do you need help affording your medications?

Safe Medication Use

To identify the discrepancy between how patients are taking their medication versus how their provider prescribed it, ask the patient these two questions:

- I see you are taking medication X. Tell me how you are taking this medication.
- How did your doctor tell you to take this medication?

Exploring Readiness to Change

To ensure optimal outcomes, it's critical to assess whether a patient is ready to accept a condition and utilize the prescribed medications as part of the overall healthcare plan. This is especially necessary to assess in patients who will be taking medications for an extended period of time (for example, patients taking antihypertensive medications). It is critical the provider elicit any and all perceived barriers and obstacles to medication adherence. The word "but"—as in, "I know I have to take my medications, but ..."—should alert the provider that the patient has some ambivalence.

A tool that can be used to assess readiness is the readiness assessment ruler (see Figure 6.1). The readiness ruler, with a scale from 0 to 10, is an efficient tool for measuring how a patient feels about taking a medication for a long period of time. Exploring readiness helps patients uncover and build their motivation to change habits and accept new therapy. In addition, it guides the clinician to effectively tailor the intervention to support movement toward change.

The readiness questions: To assess readiness and/or improve a patient's readiness, you can ask the following questions:

Readiness Ruler – The Three Stages:

Not Ready	Unsure	Ready to take action

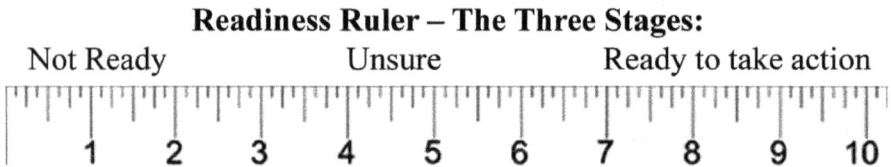

1   2   3   4   5   6   7   8   9   10

Figure 6.1: Readiness assessment ruler: Circle one answer for each medication.

- On a scale of 0 to 10, how ready are you to start taking the medication?
- What is your understanding of the disease or condition you have?
- What are your personal reasons for wanting to get better, reach a specific goal concerning your condition, and/or control your disease or condition? How else can I help you?[7]

These questions can elicit patient perspective and help patients plan goals and solve problems. Using a nonjudgmental and positive tone will help a patient open up. Stay away from the word "why" because it has a judgmental connotation.

Readiness Stages

- *Not ready (readiness ruler: 0 to 3)*

The patient is not even thinking about the need to change. He or she may respond to these questions by saying, "I don't really have a problem" or "The doctor fixed it already." At this point, it may be best to help the patient become more aware of his or her condition and link disease and consequences. It is also important to point out the benefits of early treatment.[8]

- *Unsure (readiness ruler: 4 to 6)*

The patient is considering change but is ambivalent and has not yet taken any action. Responses to these questions may include, "I know I need to take my medication, but I don't have the time to change." For these patients, it's best to reinforce their understanding of the need to change while teaching them skills and providing the necessary tools. This is the "yes, but" stage in the change process. Use of the readiness ruler and the script outlined below will help the patient to move toward action. If patient is a 4 to 6, as most are when considering a personal health behavior change, ask the following:

- What does a 4, 5, or 6 mean to you?
- What are some reasons why you want to start taking this medication?
- What positive benefits do you think might come from taking this medication?
- What negative consequences do you think might come from not taking it?

Summarize the positives and negatives, then ask the patient, What do you need to move to a 7 or 8? Summarize what the patient said it would take to change, then ask, How confident do you feel about making that change now?

- *Ready to take action (readiness ruler: 7 to 10)*

The patient is ready to make the necessary changes to improve his or her health. These patients need help with goal setting, medication plans, and progress diaries, as well as support when pitfalls occur. Reinforcing goals at each visit and providing positive feedback will help improve outcomes. The more encouraging the provider, the better the outcome. Motivation, recognition, and rewards can be as simple as congratulatory praise, an encouraging word, or even a handwritten note. "Cheerleading" from the provider at each encounter will help sustain success.

SOLUTIONS

Once the barriers have been identified and patients assessed for readiness, the next step is tailoring the patient's action plan with interventions related to the identified barriers. For many patients with MCC, more than one barrier is often involved, so the solutions and interventions must be multifaceted and must be addressed at each point along the continuum (hospital → physician's office→ pharmacy →care management →home) with patient/caregiver involvement.

HOSPITAL Medication A.R.E.A.S. Solutions

Adherence

The transition from hospital to home is a vulnerable time for patients, and nonadherence to prescribed medication regimens after discharge can increase the risk of complications. Studies have shown that one in five hospitalizations is complicated by post-discharge adverse events, and 66% of these events are related to medications.[9] Additionally, 33% to 69% of medication-related hospital admissions are due to medication nonadherence, with a resultant cost of approximately $100 billion per year.[10] Therefore, educating patients on the importance of medication adherence to prevent complications and readmissions is vital before discharge, and, in cases of high-risk patients, a follow-up call is essential to address issues and concerns and to reemphasize the importance of taking the medication as prescribed.

Reconciliation

Medication reconciliation is the process of comparing a patient's medication orders to all of the medications that the patient has been taking. This reconciliation is done to prevent medication errors such as omissions, duplications, dosing errors, or drug interactions. It should be done at admission, each time a patient moves from one setting to another where orders change or must be renewed, and upon discharge where new medications are ordered or existing orders are rewritten.

- *Upon admission*: Get the best possible medication history (BPMH). According to The Joint Commission's accreditation of healthcare organizations, getting the BPMH is a five-step process:

  □ Develop a list of current medications.
  □ Develop a list of medications to be prescribed.
  □ Compare the medications on the two lists.
  □ Make clinical decisions based on the comparison.
  □ Communicate the new list to appropriate caregivers and to the patient.[11]

- *Transitions between hospital settings*: Because some medications are not appropriate in every setting, when a patient is moved from one level of care to another, it is important that the nurse reviews the medication administration record and compares the medications the patient was taking prior to admission against the medications ordered in the transfer. If any pre-transfer medications are not ordered again or explicitly declared to be inappropriate, a nurse or pharmacist will contact the patient's physician. The physician will then either order the medication or formally confirm the omission was deliberate.

- *Discharge*: At discharge from the hospital, it is important to reconcile the discharge instructions and prescriptions with the medication administration record and the home medication list, because a patient may continue taking some medications at home that may be a duplicate of the new medications ordered at discharge. If a medication the patient received in the hospital is not in the discharge instructions, and there is no adequate documentation indicating why that medication has been omitted, then a nurse or pharmacist should contact the patient's physician to verify whether the patient should discontinue the use of the medication.

- *Roles:*
  - The *physician's role* in medication reconciliation is to ensure that the patient's medication orders on admission, transfer, and discharge are completed as accurately as possible. Any changes to medications should be documented in the chart and any discrepancies resolved. The AMA published an online medication reconciliation education document for physicians, available at https://bcpsqc.ca/documents/2012/09/AMA-The-physician%E2%80%99s-role-in-Medication-Reconciliation.pdf.
  - The *pharmacist's role* in medication reconciliation is to coordinate the process. The pharmacist, wherever possible, should take primary responsibility for ensuring proper communication of medication information to patients and other healthcare providers on admission, transfer, and discharge. When certain medications the patient was using at home are not supplied by the pharmacy because they are not on the hospital formulary, the pharmacist needs to communicate this with all providers and staff. Formulary alternatives may be prescribed; or, depending on a hospital's policies, the patient's own medications may be used. All this should be documented appropriately and taken into account upon discharge to prevent adverse outcomes from duplication or other errors. The pharmacist should also ensure the medications ordered are appropriate, based on the patient's clinical condition(s) and other factors.

▫ The *nurse's role* in the medication reconciliation process is essential. The nurse must have a good understanding of all the medications a patient is to receive and why. When medications a patient was using at home are not supplied by the pharmacy, because the medications are not on the hospital formulary, communication between the pharmacist and the nurse is critical to discuss alternative options. The College of Nurses of Ontario Medication Practice Standard 2015 includes medication reconciliation and can be found at http://www.cno.org/docs/prac/41007_Medication.pdf.

▫ The *pharmacy technician's role* in medication reconciliation is still fairly new and not widespread. However, there is evidence that in hospital settings, pharmacy technicians are effectively doing medication reconciliation upon admission with successful results. In 2009, a pilot program at the Inova Alexandria Hospital's ED found that after two years of medication reconciliation done by the pharmacy technician, the error rate was less than 5%.[12] The contributing factors for this success included the support and cooperation of hospital staff and leadership, and the pharmacy technician having an excellent knowledge of medications as well as recognizing that his or her role is to help, not to prove anyone wrong.

Engagement

Research shows that when patients are engaged in their healthcare, it can lead to measurable improvements in safety and quality. The Agency for Healthcare Research and Quality has developed the "Guide to Patient and Family Engagement in Hospital Quality and Safety," an evidence-based resource to help hospitals partner with patients and families to improve quality and safety through stronger engagement. It recommends hospitals do the following:[13]

• Work with patients and families as advisors and show how they can also work with them as advisors at the organizational level

- Promote better communication among patients, family members, and healthcare professionals from the point of admission
- Implement safe continuity of care by keeping the patient and family informed through nurse bedside change-of-shift reports
- Engage patients and families in discharge planning throughout the hospital stay and post-discharge

While many organizations invest in hotel-like amenities to improve the patient experience, a new study published in *Management Science* suggests leaders would be wiser spending their resources on improving the caregiver-patient engagement and communication, the number one factor in preventable readmissions. This study showed that hospitals could reduce their 30-day readmission rates by 5% if they helped their caregivers/providers develop interpersonal skills and empathy to improve communication with patients, in addition to complying with evidence-based care.[14] Also, patients need information about their medications, such as why they are taking them and how the medications will help them have a better quality of life. A well-informed patient and/or family can help prevent medication errors by hospital staff and are less likely to make medication errors at home. Adherence to the medication regimen is another goal achieved through patient engagement and education.

When educating a patient about medications, it is important to assess readiness to take the medication. This can be done using the readiness ruler (discussed earlier) or, more effectively, through motivational interviewing. This method works on facilitating and engaging the intrinsic motivation within a patient in order to change behavior through exploring and resolving ambivalence. Motivational interviewing techniques and methodologies can be found online at https://www.accp.com/docs/bookstore/psap/p7b08.sample01.pdf and http://drugtopics.modernmedicine.com/drug-topics/news/boost-med-adherence-rates-motivational-interviewing. You can also search YouTube for motivational interviewing training.

When consulting and educating patients about their medications, consider using the following outline and tips:

- *Provide patients with both the generic and brand names of the medication*: This is important to help patients identify their medications when a generic equivalent is substituted for a brand-name version, and it prevents patients or providers from making sound-alike errors when giving or documenting a medication history.
- *Identify the purpose of the medication*: When patients understand the purpose of the medication being prescribed, it significantly increases their chances of taking it as prescribed. Patients should be informed of the benefits of the medication as well as the consequences for not taking it. For example, when they know that lowering their high blood pressure can prevent another heart attack, they are more likely to take their blood pressure medication.
- *Explain how to take the medication*: To optimize the benefits from taking the prescribed medication and minimize any adverse events or outcomes, patients must know the dosage unit (for example, tablespoon versus teaspoon, and milligrams versus meters), what time of day to take it, how to take it (on an empty or full stomach), side effect management, what to do if they miss their medication(s), and the duration of time they will be taking the medication. Provide adherence tools, such as a pillbox, to help patients keep track of their medications.
- *Point out significant drug interactions or potential adverse reactions*: Inform the patient if there are serious drug interactions (for example, Coumadin), food-drug interactions (such as with grapefruits or other foods), or environmental-drug interactions (for example, excessive sun exposure causing a severe dermal reaction).
- *Explain proper storage conditions*: To maintain efficacy and potency, medications need to be stored properly. Inform patients of medications that need to be refrigerated or that should not be stored in the bathroom cabinets due to humidity.
- *Monitor/follow-up care*: Patients should be made aware of any lab tests or ongoing monitoring that's required because

of the medications they are on (such as warfarin, digoxin, and amiodarone). These tests will help providers adjust doses, change medications, and discontinue the medications when necessary.[15]

Other general information:

- Encourage patients and caregivers to be active participants when medications have been prescribed, so they are engaged and informed.
- Tell patients not to take expired medications or someone else's medications.
- Tell them not to discontinue medications without first speaking to their provider.
- And tell them to always let providers know if they are taking herbal or over-the-counter medications, to ensure safety.

Engaging patients is not just a one-time occurrence; it should be ongoing (in a nonintrusive or annoying way) to build trust and a long-lasting relationship. It is important to remember that engaging patients and families requires more than a series of simple steps or a checklist of activities. Meaningful patient and family engagement is about creating a partnership culture within the healthcare system. With the support of leadership, the collaboration of providers and teams, and the perseverance within the system, organizations can create cultures centered on patients and families, with the goals of improving patient experience, improving quality of care, and reducing cost.[16]

Affordability

There are opportunities to improve medication affordability in hospitals including the following:

- *Waste*: Biologics, hepatitis C, and oncology medications are among the most expensive for both hospitals and patients, yet studies show that many hospitals are throwing away millions of dollars of medications each year, and these costs are indirectly passed on to patients.[17] This waste has primarily been driven by single-dose vials of infusion drugs that are too large for individual patients. In some cases, as much as one-third of a vial is left over after a patient is treated. The issue of drug costs hits close to home for many patients, who can face huge bills for care related to these medications even if they have insurance. Some drugs, such as bortezomib (used to treat multiple myeloma), come only in 3.5-milligram vials in the United States, even though 2.5 milligrams is the standard dose. Some $309 million is lost in annual sales due to discarded doses. Yet, 1-milligram vials of the drug are available in the UK, which could minimize waste and cost (if the cost is not offset by the cost of single-dose vials versus multidose vials).[18]

- *Use of patient's own medications*: Another way to save costs for patients in hospitals is to use patients' own medications. This has been shown to minimize waste and medication costs charged to patients post-discharge.[19] According to a study by Gigi Wong, patients who used their own multidose medications instead of medications dispensed in the hospitals resulted in a savings of 74% for the hospital, even when labor costs for verification by a pharmacist were included.[20]

- *Patient education prior to discharge, focusing on*:
  - Eliminating unnecessary drugs
  - Prescribing generics when available
  - Using combination therapies that are less expensive than the individual components—for example, using Prinzide (a combination tablet of Lisinopril and Hydrochlorothiazide)
  - Tablet splitting for medications that can be safely split (they are usually scored)

Safe Medication Use

In the hospital, administering, transcribing, and prescribing errors are the most common errors that occur. To prevent these and other errors, the American Hospital Association (AHA), in collaboration with several organizations and resources, has developed a list of successful practices for improving medication safety and the medication use processes within our hospitals and health systems. The following systems should be put in place that will support providers, staff, and patients:

- Develop a positive patient identification process.
- Develop special procedures and written protocols for high-alert drugs.
- Educate staff and patients about safe medication practices.
- Ensure the availability of pharmacy expertise to tailor medications based on patients' conditions.
- Ensure the availability of up-to-date drug information.
- Fully implement unit dose systems.
- Implement an EHR with an effective computerized physician order entry system.
- Limit the variety of devices and equipment.
- Perform medication reconciliation upon admission, transitions in care, discharge, and ambulatory care settings.
- Longer-term changes (systems redesign):
  - Develop a voluntary, nonpunitive system to monitor and report adverse drug events.
  - Optimize the use of computers in the medication administration system.
  - Institute 24-hour pharmacy service, if possible.[21]

A focus on simplifying and standardizing medication system processes, prescribing, and communication practices is also critical in preventing medication errors and adverse outcomes. A complete explanation can be found at http://www.aha.org/advocacy-issues/tools-resources/advisory/96-06/991207-quality-adv.shtml.

The Institute for Safe Medication Practices (ISMP) has also developed 11 best practices—realistic practices already adopted by many organizations—upon which hospitals and ambulatory healthcare systems can focus their medication safety efforts over the next few years. The purpose of the Targeted Medication Safety Best Practices for Hospitals is "to identify, inspire, and mobilize widespread, national adoption of consensus-based best practices for specific medication safety issues that continue to cause fatal and harmful errors in patients, despite repeated warnings in [previous] ISMP publications."[22] Read more about these best practices at http://www.ismp.org/Tools/BestPractices/TMSBP-for-Hospitals.pdf.

There is now ample evidence that healthcare systems that use information technology (IT)—such as computerized physician order entry, automated dispensing cabinets, bedside bar-coded medication administration, and electronic medication reconciliation—are key components of strategies to prevent medication errors. IT systems reportedly have the potential to save up to $88 billion over 10 years in costs in the United States, with increasing adoption.[23] In his research, Abha Agrawal concluded there is now ample evidence that healthcare systems that use automated notes and records, order entry, and clinical decision support have been shown to have fewer complications, lower mortality rates, and lower costs.[24]

How can patients help prevent or minimize medication errors in the hospital and other healthcare settings? Patients or caregivers should:

- Bring their medications or a list of medications with them when going to the hospital, to help the hospital staff and providers know what they are currently taking.
- Ask about each medication being given and the reason for the medication.
- Make sure the nursing staff checks the patient's hospital identification bracelet before administering any medication, to prevent the patient from getting someone else's medications.
- Ask prior to any test or procedure if it will require any dyes or medicines, to avoid any allergic reactions.
- Have the nurse or pharmacist explain each medication and address any issues before discharge and after they get home.
- Make sure their medication list is updated whenever there is a change or modification.

What happens if an error does occur?

- Inform the patient and family: Many providers are afraid to notify patients and family members for fear of a negative impact on the patient-provider relationship and of putting themselves at higher risk for malpractice lawsuits. According to a study published in the *Journal of Health & Life Sciences Law*, when patients and their families are notified of serious mistakes, the chances of them reactively suing are reduced. Providers also have an ethical duty to let their patients know of any errors that occur, regardless of the consequences of making the error.[25]
- Notify the rest of the healthcare team and management leadership: Informing them is crucial in order to: better handle any immediate, significant, negative patient outcomes; reduce any further mismanagement; and provide insights that will prevent the error from occurring in the future.
- Document the error: Report it to the hospital peer review committee and/or patient-safety committee (based on hospital policies) for an independent review and recommendations to minimize future errors.

PHYSICIAN / PROVIDER OFFICE: Medication A.R.E.A.S. Solutions

Adherence

The role of the provider in improving medication adherence and increasing a patient's likelihood of picking up their first prescription is critical. Research has shown that when providers take the time to educate patients about their medications, they are more likely have patients who get their medications filled and take them as prescribed.[26] When prescribing new medications, providers should support patients with the following information:

- *Name*: Tell them the brand and generic names of the medication(s) being prescribed, to avoid confusion and duplication.

- *Why*: Help them understand the reason behind taking this medication; this will increase the value of the medication and help the patient link the disease or illness with treatment.
- *Effects*: Inform them of the common side effects and what to do if they occur.
- *Affordability*: Write generics, or refer patients to financial assistance programs or co-pay assistance programs to help them afford their medications. This is especially important in this era of high-deductible benefit plans.
- *Triage*: Refer patients to other services and resources to support their ongoing medication management.

Reconciliation

The process of reconciling medications in outpatient settings (ranging from the physician's office, outpatient surgery, and dialysis facilities to outpatient oncology clinics and emergency departments for patients who are not admitted) involves similar steps outlined by the Joint Commission for getting the BPMH:

- Develop a list of current medications based on the medications the patient is currently taking at their place of residence, which can be done by the medical assistant or nurse prior to the patient seeing the physician or provider.
- Compare it to the list of medications in the patient's chart or EHR.
- Ensure there are no interactions, duplications, or other errors (the EHR can support this).
- Determine if there should be any additions, modifications, or deletions to the medication list based on the outcome of the visit.
- Communicate the new, updated medication list to the patient and caregiver.

Physicians should encourage patients to keep an up-to-date, accurate medication list with them at all times, and, as part of that effort, routinely provide the patient with an accurate, reconciled list. The newly reconciled list should include the date and time of the reconciliation, identify the person making the reconciliation, and, when possible, include that person's contact information. The patient may use this new list as a personal reference, review or update it with physicians who prescribe the medications, and present it to other physicians and providers for inclusion in the patient's medical record(s).

Engagement

In this new value-based healthcare system, providers and teams will be responsible for the outcomes of their patients. This has caused a lot of concern because of the fear that some patients will not follow the provider's recommendations. To significantly increase the chances of patients adhering to the recommendations

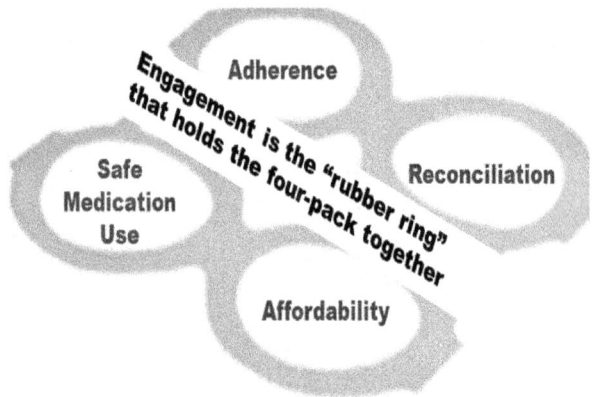

Figure 6.2: Engagement as the "rubber ring" that holds MAB together

given, and to get the outcomes desired, providers and teams are going to have to focus on engagement to build trust and create an environment where patients feel safe enough to be honest about the issues and challenges preventing them from following prescribed recommendations.

With MAB, providers must engage patients at each point of care—to increase the chances of them adhering to their medication regimens, keeping an updated medication list, being able to pay for their medications, and taking their medications safely. One of the best ways to view engagement is to think of the ring that holds a four- or six-pack of soda together (see Figure 6.2). With MAB, engagement is the "ring" that allows the adherence, reconciliation, affordability, and safe medication use components to come together and stay together effectively. Below is a list of additional tips and tools for providers to use when engaging patients:

- *Patient education*: When educating patients on "why" they are taking a prescribed medication, give them online tools that are readily available, so patients have a resource to use if they forget what was discussed.
- *Telehealth and telemedicine strategies*: To engage patients in remote or distant locations, providers can bring patients "closer" by using telehealth and telemedicine tools provided by the organization. According to mHealth Intelligence, new telehealth legislation is pushing adoption of the technology across the country and by organizations.[27]
- *Storytelling*: There is a growing body of research suggesting that sharing personal stories engages patients and improves their overall health. Providers can encourage patients to attend sessions to hear and share experiences about their condition with others. When complex information is woven into stories and experiences related by other people with similar issues, patients can better grasp these complex concepts. To support this concept, Massachusetts General Hospital Paul S. Russell Museum has launched a kiosk called The Sharing Clinic, where people have the opportunity to listen to the stories of other patients and record their own comments. Having a space to listen and share stories has allowed patients to engage with their disease and treatment in a new way.[28]
- *Mobile health tools*: As of October 2014, 90% of American adults own a cellphone, and 64% own a smartphone.[29] In this age of mobile technology, mobile health tools have become a fast way of increasing patient engagement. mHealth Intelligence reported that mobile health tools allow patients to keep in touch with their primary care physician more efficiently than ever before, and the medication apps are helping patients more effectively remember to take their medications as prescribed.[30]

Affordability

In a January 2009 medication survey by *Consumer Reports*, nearly half of the people interviewed said their doctors did not consider cost when prescribing medications.[31] And earlier *Consumer Reports* surveys of doctors found physicians ranked price as their least important consideration when prescribing drugs. (How well the drug worked was their first concern.)[32] However, this is changing as providers are balancing how well the medication works with the patients' ability to afford it, because there is little use prescribing a medication the patient cannot afford. Some strategies providers can use to make medications more affordable for patients include:

- Elimination of unnecessary drugs
- Using combination medications
- Using generics and/or formulary preferred medications
- Alternative medications in the same class that are less expensive with similar outcomes
- Tablet splitting (when appropriate)
- Focusing on non-pharmacological solutions, such as diet, exercise, and sleep
- Minimizing or avoiding free samples, as these would most likely be an expensive, brand-name medication and end up costing patients more in the long run if they stick with it

Safe Medication Use

In the provider's office, prescribing errors are the most common of the six key medication use stages where medication errors can occur. This happens due to errors from miscalculating dosage, miscommunication, poor handwriting, confusion of drugs with similar names, inappropriate use of zeroes and decimal points, pressure to overprescribe or overtreat, not identifying the patient's factors, or lack of knowledge about the drug. To prevent prescribing errors, providers should do the following:

- Use an EHR with decision support and alerts to support their prescribing.
- If using paper prescriptions, limit each script to one to two medications.
- Approach medication names with caution (for example, the similarity between clonidine and Klonopin).
- Eliminate drug abbreviations (like HCTZ for hydrochlorothiazide).
- Use metric measures for dosages.
- Avoid writing "as directed," especially with pain medications.
- Eliminate abbreviations in routes of administration.
- Specify the therapeutic duration.
- Specify the indication (there are few exceptions where this should not occur).
- Prescribe specific quantities, rather than dispensing, for time periods.
- Remain aware of medications with narrow therapeutic indexes (for example, warfarin).
- Remain aware of potentially lethal doses of medications (for example, overdosing on opioids).
- Have a pharmacist on your team to augment your prescribing efforts.[33]

PHARMACY: Medication A.R.E.A.S. Solutions

Adherence

To increase the chances of patients taking their medication, the pharmacy consultation should include the following components at a minimum (this is not all inclusive of the law):

- *5Rs*: Ensure the right patient is getting the right medication, right indication, right direction, and right duration of therapy.
- *Why*: Explaining why a medication has been prescribed is critical to helping patients link the disease/illness with the treatment.
- *How*: A brief description of how the medication works can further help patients link the disease/illness with treatment (for example, explain how a bronchodilator works to open the airway passages).

- *Value*: Patients who understand the value and benefits of the medications they are taking have been found to have less side effects and improved adherence.
- *Side effects*: Address the important side effects and include side effect management tips to improve adherence.
- *Reaffirm the value of the medication*: Close the consult by answering questions the patient may have and providing patient-centric written materials that augment the consultation.

Reconciliation

The pharmacist in the community practice setting should be involved in the medication reconciliation process. In a study by Jeff Freund on the process of medication reconciliation in the community pharmacy setting, he gave insight into the feasibility of a workflow process for pharmacists and pharmacy technicians to conduct medication reconciliation for patients undergoing transitions in care.[34] This study showed the medication reconciliation workflow in the community pharmacies, which included the following steps: patient identification, gathering documents, entering medications into computerized pharmacy management systems, verifying medications with pharmacy patient profiles, resolving discrepancies/changes, organizing prescriber calls/faxes, and providing patient counseling. This workflow took 27 minutes, on average, and, because many medication discrepancies were identified during the transition of care, it was highly valuable for community pharmacists to perform medication reconciliation services.[35] Also, to ensure that the medication reconciliation is effective, pharmacists highly recommend that patients get all their prescriptions from one pharmacy. If that is not possible, patients should inform their primary pharmacist of where they are getting their other medications and what they are, so the primary pharmacist can enter all that data into the pharmacy management system and provide patients with the best possible medication list.

Engagement

Patient education and engagement has emerged as a critical strategy for improving patients' health outcomes. Therefore, pharmacists are doing the following to enhance that engagement and support patient knowledge about their therapies:

- CVS Caremark research has shown that a pharmacist in a face-to-face setting is the most effective healthcare professional at encouraging patients to take medications as prescribed. This is in part because pharmacists understand many of the contributing factors, which range from cost and side effects to the inherent challenges of taking multiple medications, and can help address these challenges most effectively. CVS pharmacy's CARE 1on1 program offers patients dedicated one-on-one time with a pharmacist to engage patients about medication adherence, tools to stick to a medication routine, cost savings, medication safety, and side effect management, when their prescription is transferred or filled for the first time.[36]

- Between October 2009 and April 2010, researchers from Harvard University and Brigham and Women's Hospital assisted the CVS Caremark researchers in analyzing the pharmacy claims data of benefit members at a large Midwestern manufacturing company and focused on interventions with diabetic patients. In their research, they estimated that the employer saved more than $600,000 through healthcare cost avoidance with the intervention group, while expenditures for the counseling totaled $200,000, a return on investment of $3 for every $1 spent on additional counseling. The researchers concluded: "In a health care system eagerly seeking programs that can reduce costs and improve care, such simple, pharmacist-based counseling programs to improve adherence to existing medication regimens and initiate missing therapies should be of great value."[37]

Affordability

Pharmacists can definitely help patients save on their overall prescription costs. In addition to the ideas already mentioned, pharmacists can ensure that members and patients get the best prices possible, avoid waste and adverse outcomes (leading to more expensive healthcare resource usage), and, at the same time, help reduce healthcare's total cost of care by doing the following:

- *Perform a medication review to address polypharmacy or duplication issues*: When patients receive multiple medications from several different prescribers, there is a chance that at least a couple of the medications may be unnecessary, inappropriate, or duplicates. After doing the medication review, the pharmacist will identify and address these issues, such as eliminating unnecessary drugs, leading to better patient outcomes and lower costs.
- *Recommend patients and caregivers use verified and trusted websites like GoodRx.com to compare prices*: Patients can save up to 80%, even if they have insurance or Medicare. GoodRx makes comparing prescription drug prices easy by providing current cash and sale prices, manufacturers coupons, pharmacy discounts, and valuable savings tips for thousands of prescriptions. GoodRx informs patients which pharmacies have popular generic drugs for less than $4 per fill, where certain prescriptions are available for free, and where many of their savings coupons can be used from within the app.
- *Recommend generics as a substitute for brand-name drugs, if available*: Using generics can save patients a significant amount of money because they are usually much cheaper yet just as safe and effective as their brand-name counterparts. If a generic isn't available, substitute a different, cheaper medication (usually in the same class) that works just as well.
- *Encourage patients to fill 90-day prescriptions using home delivery services*: Once patients are stable on a chronic medication, they will most likely save money by filling a 90-day

prescription instead of the standard 30-day prescription using the home delivery system (such as mail order). When using insurance, patients filling a 90-day prescription will only have one or two co-pays, instead of three co-pays for the same amount of medication. They would also only have to make one trip to the pharmacy every three months or, even better, get it delivered to their home.

- *Give patients the option to process their prescription(s) without going through insurance*: Many retail pharmacies offer some common generics at prices as low as $4 for a 30-day supply and $10 for a 90-day supply, if patients are willing to pay out of pocket. Patients should be aware that these costs, not processed through their insurance, will not count toward their deductible.

- *Recommend tablet splitting when safe and appropriate*: For medications that can be split, patients will save money if the provider prescribes a pill that's twice the normal dose, so patients can split it in half. Pharmacists should take the time to explain which medications can be split safely and accurately.[38]

- *Use combination therapies where possible*: For example, using Metaglip (a combination tablet of metformin and glipizide) instead of taking metformin and glipizide separately.

- *Effective management of specialty drugs*: With the explosion of specialty drugs in the outpatient setting, organizations are launching specialty drug services to focus on patient quality while reducing costs where possible. With the complexities and toxicities sometimes associated with specialty medications, these organizations believe that their patients can be managed better by the clinical pharmacists who are working with the rest of the patient's care team using a shared EHR.

Safe Medication Use

Dispensing errors account for 19% of all inpatient errors. According to researcher Rama Nair, the following are some strategies to reduce or minimize dispensing errors:

- Focus on correct entry of the prescription.
- Confirm the prescription is correct and complete.
- Beware of look-alike, sound-alike drugs.
- Be careful with zeros and abbreviations.
- Organize the workplace.
- Focus on reducing stress and balancing heavy workloads.
- Take the time to store drugs properly.
- Thoroughly check all prescriptions.
- Always provide thorough patient counseling.[39]

The goal of every pharmacist is to minimize dispensing errors. Patient counseling is the last point of contact between the patient, pharmacist, and medication in the dispensing process, so it is the most important strategy every pharmacist must adopt in order to minimize dispensing errors. In addition, reporting errors as they occur and when they occur will help in learning from the mistakes and ultimately prevent such errors in the future.[40]

POPULATION HEALTH MANAGEMENT: Medication A.R.E.A.S. Solutions

To address the new focus on health, value, and patient outcomes, healthcare systems and physician groups are implementing population management, care management, and care coordination programs to manage the health of their populations, especially their high-risk patients. The goals of these programs are to keep the identified patient population as healthy as possible; improve patient quality and health outcomes; minimize the need for expensive interventions such as emergency department visits, hospitalizations, imaging tests, and unnecessary procedures; and meet the goals of the Institute for Healthcare Improvement's (IHI) Triple Aim. To do this, many of these programs have care managers who spend time with patients to tailor their interventions by addressing specific medical and socioeconomic challenges and issues. As part of the medical interventions, addressing the Medication A.R.E.A.S. issues is critical, especially in high-risk patients, to ensure optimal outcomes. Because of the extra time care managers in population health management programs usually have compared to other team members in the hospitals, physician offices, and pharmacies, they are able to further address the following.

Adherence

In addition to the solutions discussed in the hospital, physician office, and pharmacy sections, care managers can support patients by giving additional attention to the following:

- *Barriers*: Identify additional adherence barriers by using tools such as motivational interviewing, the Beliefs About Medications Questionnaire (BMQ), or the Morisky Scale, and address any concerns.
- *Readiness to change assessment*: To ensure optimal outcomes, care managers can work with patients to determine their readiness to take their medications as prescribed using the readiness assessment ruler (see Figure 6.1). The ruler's scale from 0 to 10 is an efficient tool for measuring how a patient feels about taking a medication for a long period of time. Exploring readiness helps patients uncover and build their motivation to change habits and accept new therapy. In addition, it guides the clinician to effectively tailor the intervention to support movement toward change.
- *Adherence tools*: Recommend adherence tools—pillboxes, telephone reminders, eReminders, and apps—to keep patients on track and make it easier for them to fill and refill prescriptions.

Reconciliation

Care managers and home health providers should work with their patients' providers and pharmacists to reconcile patients' medication lists. In some organizations, care managers and home health providers connect with pharmacists remotely via iPads or other eTools to do an effective medication reconciliation while with the patient. This has been very beneficial because the healthcare professional in the patient's home can gather all the medications the patient is on and work with an expert remotely to address drug interactions, duplications, and any discrepancies between what is on the patient's profile and what they are actually taking—thus enabling the patient to have the best possible medication reconciled list.

Engagement

In addition to the engagement solutions discussed in the hospital, physician office, and pharmacy sections, care managers can further engage patients by doing the following:

- *Educate patients to focus on the markers of the disease (for example, LDL lab tests and blood pressure) instead of just the symptoms, as predictors for how well they are doing.* This is especially important for chronic diseases that have few to no symptoms.
- *Provide patients with a written medication action plan that summarizes their prescriptions, including name and dose.* Written action plans are great tools to augment adherence because they remove the burden of trying to memorize instructions.
- *Collaborate with other resources to address the socioeconomic challenges of patients.* This includes social support, housing, food, income, education, and employment. These collaborations are crucial to the overall care.
- *Educate patients so they understand the treatment plan and do not become disengaged.* Studies are showing that organizations with success practices around patient education and engagement have the following traits:
  - Teaching efforts are consistently targeted to the appropriate key learner.
  - Educators consistently evaluate patients' understanding of the information provided.

- The organizational culture supports efforts to prioritize patient education.
- Strategies and technologies are adopted to make patient education activities fit easily, if not automatically, into hospital employees' work flow.
- Education materials are designed thoughtfully with the patient in mind.[41]
- Patients' education about why they are taking the prescribed medication(s) is augmented with online tools that are readily available. Then patients can have resources to use if they forget what was discussed.

Affordability

Care managers can help address the affordability issues by working with other team members to ensure the following are in place for patients:

- Eliminating unnecessary, inappropriate, or duplicate medications
- Placing patients on generics as a substitute for brand-name drugs, when available
- Encouraging patients to fill 90-day prescriptions
- Giving patients the option to process their prescription(s) without going through insurance
- Splitting tablets when safe and appropriate
- Putting patients on combination therapies when possible

Safe Medication Use

Care managers can facilitate safe medication use and practices by following up with patients to make sure that the right medication has been prescribed for the right patient—including the right indication, right dose and directions—and that patients understand the purpose of the medication. Care managers are also excellent team members to monitor patients for any side effects or adverse events during each visit or telephone visit with the patient.

HOME/RESIDENCE: Medication A.R.E.A.S. Solutions

Adherence

When patients get to their place of residence and start taking their medications, what causes them to stop taking the medications after a period of time or change the directions given by the provider? The most common challenges and barriers that cause secondary nonadherence include forgetfulness, poor or no relationships with healthcare team members, affordability/cost of ongoing therapy, waning motivation over time, and medication-related challenges such as side effects or other negative experiences. To improve secondary medication adherence:

- *Healthcare team members (physician, pharmacist, nurse, others) focus at every point of contact*: At each point of contact, providers and staff should proactively: address any issues the patient has with their medications; encourage adherence by reemphasizing the benefits and value of the therapy; congratulate the patient when their outcomes are moving in the right direction or meeting the established goals; and empathize and inquire when patient is not on track.
- *Use reminder outreaches*: To support primary adherence, outreach calls should be made to high-risk patients within three to five days of them getting their prescription, to ensure patients are on track and not experiencing any issues that will prevent them from taking the medication as prescribed. Since forgetfulness is the most common reason for secondary nonadherence, sending an automated reminder call or text a few days before the prescription needs to be refilled has been shown to be helpful.
- *Engage patients*: Patients should engage in self-management and keep these three words in mind: understand, organize, and monitor.
  - *Understand*: After a prescription is obtained, it is important they have the ability to learn how to take the drug safely and appropriately.

- *Organize*: In addition to understanding how to take a medication correctly, it is essential for them to organize and plan their medications around their daily schedules to improve adherence and remembrance. This should include both prescribed and non-prescribed medications.
- *Monitor*: Patients should have knowledge of potential side effects and risks that will allow them to connect symptoms to medication use and seek appropriate action before an adverse event. They should alert their physician or pharmacist if they experience any side effects or have any issues with their medications, to ensure safe use and prevent nonadherence behaviors.

Reconciliation

The medication reconciliation process is a shared responsibility of healthcare providers in collaboration with patients and caregivers. Patients are in the best position to know what they are taking and how their medications affect them. One major solution patients can be involved in to reduce harm, increase clarity and effectiveness, and improve safe medication use is for them to continuously and consistently maintain an accurate, up-to-date list as discussed. The medication list should have the following: the name of the medication, strength, directions on how and when to use, why (the reason for taking it), and the name of the provider who prescribed it.

To ensure that all providers and team members have the most accurate medication list, patients and caregivers should do the following:

- Take their medicine containers to each appointment to show their providers.
- Be honest about the medicines they are taking and how they are taking them.
- Maintain a current list of medicines (including OTC and complementary medicines).
- Speak up if they are unsure about their medicines or suspect a medication error.

Engagement

When patients and caregivers are engaged in their healthcare and medication use, there is the potential for improved health outcomes and patient satisfaction. To stay engaged, here are some questions patients should ask their healthcare provider:

- What are the brand and generic names of the medication?
- What is the purpose of the medication? What is the strength and dosage?
- What are the possible adverse effects? What should I do if they occur?
- Is there any other medication I should avoid while using this product?
- I am allergic to (name of the medication). Should I take this medication?
- How long should I take this medication? What outcome should I expect?
- When is the best time to take the medication?
- How should I store the medication?
- What do I do if I miss a dose?
- Should I avoid any foods while taking this medication?
- I'm also taking _____ (which I got at another pharmacy). Can I take both safely?
- Is this medication meant to replace any other drug I am already taking?
- May I have written information about this drug?

Affordability

Consumers, patients, and caregivers can do the following to best manage their medication costs effectively and safely:

- *Work with their pharmacist, who will help them by doing the following*:
  - Perform a medication review to eliminate any unnecessary, inappropriate, or duplicate medications

- ▫ Recommend generics as a substitute for brand-name drugs, if available
- ▫ Encourage patients to fill 90-day prescriptions
- ▫ Give patients the option to process their prescription(s) without going through insurance
- ▫ Recommend tablet splitting when safe and appropriate
- ▫ Use combination therapies where possible

- *Compare prices*: Shop around and check websites such as onerx. com, www.goodrx.com, and others that can help compare drugs and prices. Patients should be wary of international drug sites on the Internet as they are unregulated and may sell counterfeit or contaminated drugs. Patients should stick to pharmacies that carry the Verified Internet Pharmacy Practice Sites (VIPPS) seal, awarded by the National Association of Boards of Pharmacy.

- *Be wary of TV drug ads*: They usually pitch the newest drugs, which are not only more expensive but also often work no better than the older ones. In addition, drug ads often omit safety or side effect information. See the *Consumer Reports* "AdWatch" series for examples of how some TV drug ads omit or minimize safety and side effect information.[42]

- *Get the right insurance*: The right drug plan can save consumers significant amounts of money.

- *Get help*: Pharmaceutical companies offer a certain amount of free or low-cost medications through their patient assistance programs. Use the online directory RxAssist to see if there's one that can help you.

- *Pay attention to where the medication is administered*: For some medicines, it can make a big difference in the cost if the medication is administered at a doctor's office, a hospital outpatient center, an infusion center, or by a nurse who comes to the patient's home. According to a study by Aetna Healthcare, the costs for the exact same medication and dose are, on average, twice as high when given in a hospital outpatient setting as they would be in a doctor's office or in the home. Most patients don't need the level of care available in a hospital or outpatient center; instead, less intensive settings (such as an outpatient home infusion setting, provider office, or home visit) are sufficient. Patients who are paying a percentage of the cost now have to pay more money out of pocket unnecessarily. It also means higher costs for the patient's employer or health plan, which can lead to higher premiums for everyone.[43]

Safe Medication Use

The following safe medication use recommendations from the Institute for Safe Medication Practices, the FDA, the Agency for Healthcare Research and Quality, and the American Society of Health-System Pharmacists will help patients significantly reduce their chances of having adverse events and outcomes.[44]

Medication Use:

- Before taking the first dose, read the label. Make sure that the medication you have received is the one that your doctor ordered. If there is any difference in the appearance or shape of your medication between refills, do not take it until you've discussed it with a pharmacist. Remember, many medications have names that sound or look alike.
  Read the directions on the label and any written information you've been given. If any of it seems to contradict what you already know about the medication, call your doctor, pharmacist, or nurse.
- Do not chew, crush, or break capsules or tablets unless instructed to do so.
- With liquid medication, use only the measuring device that came with it. Many household teaspoons and tablespoons are not accurate.
- Do not take medications in the dark. Although you may think you know exactly what the bottle on your nightstand contains, turn on a light to be sure.
- Never take another person's prescription medication or share yours with anyone, even if the other person appears to have the same medical condition as you.

- Take the medication exactly as prescribed, and do not discontinue without first checking with your physician or pharmacist.

Side Effects:

- If you develop itching or swelling, or if you have trouble breathing after taking a new medication, seek medical help immediately.
- Tell your provider, pharmacist, or caregiver if you do not feel well after taking a medication, and ask for help immediately if you think you are having a side effect or reaction.

Storage:

- Keep medications in their original, labeled containers. This can help you to identify each pill and follow the proper directions.
- Do not store medications in the bathroom medicine cabinet or in direct sunlight, because humidity, heat, and light can affect a medication's potency and safety.
- Do not store medicines in the refrigerator unless instructed to do so, and keep liquid medicines from freezing.
- Store medications where children cannot see or reach them (for example, in a locked box or cabinet), and teach children that medications can be dangerous if misused.
- Keep medications for people separate from pet medications and household chemicals.
- Do not keep tubes of ointments or creams next to a tube of toothpaste. They may feel similar when you grab one quickly.

Others:

- At every appointment and upon admission, bring all of your medications/pill bottles or a complete up-to-date list of your medications for your provider to review. This should include any herbal over-the-counter medications, vitamins, supplements, and natural remedies, in addition to your prescription medications.
- Get all your medications from one pharmacy when possible.
- Keep phone numbers for your doctors and pharmacist, along with the numbers of your local emergency medical and poison

control centers, in a convenient location. Know the locations of pharmacies that are open 24 hours a day in case of an emergency.

- Check the expiration date on all medications.
- Throw away outdated products.
- Invest in a reference book on medications. Several are available in low-cost paperback editions, and your healthcare provider can make a recommendation.

There are many solutions to improve medication adherence, but solutions will only work when a patient's barriers are identified. For example, addressing financial issues in a patient whose barrier is primarily a religious belief system is meaningless, potentially harmful, and a waste of time. So it is critical that solutions be aligned with the identified barriers to improve adherence and patient outcomes. Also, the Medication A.R.E.A.S. Solutions have some similarities and uniquenesses across the continuum of care—ranging from the hospital setting, the physician/provider office, the pharmacy, and the care management/population management services to the home or residence of the patient. So whenever possible and meaningful, leverage solutions that cut across most or all practice settings.

MOTIVATION

For people to be motivated to change and maintain the change, they must have a strong sense of purpose and meaning that will motivate their decision to change. Some examples of deep motivators include the following:

- A grandmother hopes to live long enough to see the her grandkids graduate and get married.
- A graduate student starts eating healthier when she realizes her new job in front of the camera will require her to look and feel her best.
- A young volunteer gives up milk shakes in order to save a certain amount of money for his mission trip.

- A married father takes his hypertension medications to prevent erectile dysfunction, a consequence of uncontrolled hypertension.

Healthcare providers must help their patients recognize their personal reasons and desires for wanting to get better. A deep personal motivator (like the examples above) can be used to encourage patients to take medications consistently, change their diets, and exercise. The motivator can also be linked to specific health goals—for example, to help a diabetic man get his HbA1c to under 7 so he can stay healthier and work for a longer period of time. Whatever health goal is set, the patient is more likely to follow through on the necessary health behaviors that will make the goal a reality if it's linked to strong personal motivators.

Linking the importance of getting better to the identified motivators should be done in a warm, nonjudgmental style of interaction. This can be accomplished through motivational interviewing (MI). MI is a technique used to understand patient challenges, help patients come to terms with the challenges and changes occurring in their lives, help them link the new behaviors with a strong personal motivator, and use "change talk" techniques to get patients on the right track to improving their health outcomes.

These are the key aspects of MI:

- The "*why*" behind the principles of motivational interviewing: an overview–EFEP:[45]
  - Engage–Engagement is essential.
  - Focus–Focus on something the patient is willing to work on.
  - Evoke–Evoke the desire for action.
  - Plan–Create an action plan and focus on commitment.
- The "*how*" behind the principles of motivational interviewing when resistance is encountered: REDS[46]
  - Rolling with resistance—helping patients focus on solutions
  - Expressing empathy—reassurance, compassion, and understanding

- Developing discrepancy—recognition of discrepancies to motivate
- Supporting self-efficacy—reinforcing the potential for positive change
- The *"what to do"* to ensure a successful MI interaction–RULE[47]
  - Resist the "righting reflex."
  - Understand your patient's motivations (then link the motivation to the new behavior).
  - Listen to and understand the patient.
  - Empower and support the patient to increase his or her belief in the ability to change the current challenging behaviors and habits, and adopt new self-managing skills.
    Below is an application of MI—helping patients come to terms with the changes they need to make in their lives after an event—called OARS.[48]
- Open-ended questions: Allows for richer, deeper conversations. For example, "Tell me more about the circumstances that led to your heart attack."
- Affirmation: Recognizing and reinforcing. For example, "You showed a lot of commitment to want to start a medication regimen."
- Reflection: Seek, clarify, and deepen understanding. For example, "It sounds like you want some help to keep you on track as you start your new medication regimens, exercise program, and diet."
- Summary: Use summaries to understand, reinforce, and capture key points, and to reinforce the patient's commitment to the adoption of a healthier lifestyle. Teach him or her how to stay on track when challenges or roadblocks arise.

Since the main goal of motivational interviewing is to increase intrinsic motivation for change ("I will change because I want to"), helping the patient become aware of the discrepancies between current behaviors and highly cherished personal motivators, values, and goals is critical.[49] There are many courses and articles that can be found on the Internet that teach providers and team members the motivational interviewing techniques needed to help patients improve their intrinsic motivation to change.

The Marathon Runner Versus the Sprinter

Think of running a 26.2-mile marathon but without the following: spectators to cheer you on, water or drinks along the way to keep you hydrated, and other participants running alongside you. With none of these supportive infrastructures, do you believe you would successfully complete the 26.2 miles? While some people can, many cannot. Many marathon runners have attributed a part of their success to the motivation of other runners, the support along the way, and spectators cheering them on. Now, imagine yourself as a sprinter, running a 100-meter dash that lasts a few seconds. Would you really need as much support as someone running a grueling marathon over the course of several hours?

A patient who is given a seven-day course of antibiotics is similar to a sprinter. He or she does not always need motivators to take medication over a short period of time. However, a patient who is on medication for a chronic condition is more like a marathon runner. Because outcomes aren't always felt or visible, and the medication must be taken for a long period of time, this type of patient will need more motivation and support to keep going.

Some tools and resources that can help motivate and keep patients on track with their medication regimens include:

- Mailed reminders, newsletters, and letters from providers encouraging patients to stay on track and reminding them about the purpose of taking their medications
- Live, follow-up phone calls offering encouragement, help, and support regarding side effect management or other concerns
- Lifestyle coaches and care managers to address any Medication A.R.E.A.S. issues
- Email or text reminders
- Health education classes

- Support groups (live or virtual)
- Educational tools and self-care resources
- Web-based tools

Also, to keep this motivation alive, there has to be ongoing feedback. In a Stanford University study, Albert Bandura found patient motivation and confidence increased when they had challenging goals and received ongoing feedback on their progress.[50] Having confidence in one's ability to succeed often leads to success. Feedback should be congratulatory when the patients are on track, or empathetic when the patients have problems that prevent them from achieving their goals. Therefore, at each visit, the provider should review the health goals, link goals to something important to the patient, provide tools and resources when appropriate, and provide feedback along the way. This will give patients the support needed to continue striving toward their goals and to succeed.

Goal Setting

People who write out their goals and have a stepwise action plan to achieve these goals are as much as 10 times more likely to achieve their goals than those who only think about them.[51] To help patients use their medications appropriately, providers should set clear health goals with patients, in a collaborative manner, and encourage them to write these down. Each time the patient has contact with a provider or members of the healthcare team, the patient's goals should be reviewed with feedback provided.

Providers, with the support of the healthcare team, should help patients set goals in stages, so they can celebrate every small step that is achieved toward their larger goal. For someone who is 50 pounds overweight, setting a goal of losing 10 pounds may be much more attainable than asking the patient to start with a goal of losing all 50 pounds. For patients who are physically inactive, an initial goal could be to walk a short distance every day for a week, building up to a mile or more. For a diabetic who forgets to test blood sugar, the initial goal may simply be daily glucose testing; once this is achieved and sustained for some time, the patient can move on to other diet and lifestyle changes to support a healthy blood sugar range.

Educating, Empowering, and Encouraging Feedback

Educating patients about their disease conditions and medication treatment plans is essential if patients are to successfully use their medications appropriately to achieve the optimal therapeutic outcomes. Educating patients includes providing concise and focused verbal information about their conditions and medication treatment plans. Written information to reinforce what's been discussed should also be provided whenever possible. In addition, behavioral tools, such as follow-up phone calls and reminder postcards must be used to help patients take their medications as prescribed. Last but not least, encouragement and support from providers and family members will help patients exert greater effort. Providers can create a positive interaction that motivates patients to excel by encouraging goal sharing, setting clear objectives, discussing goals at each visit, and providing positive feedback. The value of a provider recognizing and acknowledging when patients reach both small goals and large milestones cannot be understated. Research shows the combination of education, empowerment of patients by providing tools and feedback, and ongoing encouragement given to patients will significantly improve adherence to therapy plans and improve outcomes more than any one component alone.[52]

Medication Action Plan (MAP)

MAPs are tools designed to help patients manage their chronic conditions by helping them set and implement goals. Once the patient and provider develop a MAP, the provider should track the patient's progress, acknowledge any improvement, and provide incentives (if applicable) to help motivate the patient. When a patient does not meet a certain goal, the provider should work with the patient to identify the issues or barriers and to help the patient get back on track.

A.R.E.A.S. Tools

There are many tools and resources to help keep patients on track once they start taking their medications. These include apps, reminder tools, memory tools, safety resources, written information, and many others.

Example of Tools

Memory tools

Adherence devices such as pillboxes, calendars, and diaries can help patients remember when to take their medications—and if they have taken their medications—and reduce a complex regimen. Also, linking doses to a patient's daily habits can simplify complex regimens because the habits serve as triggers, reminding patients to take their medications. This linking has been associated with improved outcomes.

The most commonly used reminder devices are the pillboxes that organize pills by days and times to be taken. These boxes simplify complex drug regimens and help people remember to take their medications. They can also be used as a double-check system to see if the medication has been taken. Calendars and diaries can also accomplish similar objectives. More complex electronic devices have alarms or beepers that can be programmed for the time the patient needs to take his or her medications. These electronic devices beep at the assigned time, reminding the patient to take his or her medications. Adherence devices can help improve appropriate medication use, when used with other tools.

Written information

Written information about a medication can reinforce the verbal information given by the provider and help patients remember once they have left the provider's office or pharmacy. Studies have shown that patients fail to remember up to 50% of the information given by their healthcare provider.

Follow-up management

Complex medication regimens contribute to a revolving door of rehospitalizations for patients with heart failure and other comorbidities. Therefore, it's important to call patients who have complex medication regimens within a 3-to-5-day period of receiving their medication to review their treatment plan. This can significantly reduce the errors that could result in a readmission. Follow-up management can be also very helpful for patients on chronic medications. There are software programs that can help providers identify patients who are not picking up their medications on time. These programs can automatically alert a provider if a patient is overdue in picking up a medication, based on the day's supply entered in the system. Phone calls (automated or live) can be used or postcards/letters can be generated that will serve as gentle reminders to patients.

Follow-up management is particularly effective when a patient has a good relationship with his or her provider. Research has shown that mailing reminders to patients taking chronic medications can increase compliance over time by about 28%. While it is expensive to mail reminders to all patients on chronic medications, targeting patients who demonstrate certain nonadherence tendencies (for example, patients with diabetes who do not pick up medications three or more times) may be a good start. In addition, newsletters and informative letters can provide patients with the knowledge boost they need to stay on track. Many of the pharmacy patient data computer systems can identify patients who demonstrate patterns of nonadherence. Patients who miss appointments often or are not at goal (for example: LDL > 100 or HbAic >9) could be targeted. Patient permission will be needed to send them emails, including reminders.

Visual aids

Visual aids are important tools to help patients remember information about their medications. For visual learners, a picture is worth a thousand words. Pictures can help patients understand how a medication works and remember what they've learned. Medication charts can also help improve a patient's understanding about how to use medications through visual imagery. They are very beneficial for patients who have low literacy or are non-English speaking. A sample medication card can be viewed at www.picturerxcard.com.

Medication instruction labels

The universal illustrations on medication instruction labels make it easier for patients to understand and remember instructions. These labels explain how to use the medication, the method of administration, and any potential side effects.

The teach-back method

The teach-back method is an effective way to check patient understanding. In this method, the provider explains the medication directions and asks the patient to explain them back. For example, a provider might say, "We've discussed some strategies for taking your medication regularly. To help me know whether I've explained things thoroughly, please tell me how you plan to take your medications." Based on the patient's response, the provider can determine if additional explanations or interventions are necessary.

Care managers and lifestyle coaches

Care managers and lifestyle coaches can be very effective in helping patients change their behavior and adapt to the changes that need to be made to improve their health. They do this by listening, supporting, and advising patients about medical choices, treatment plans, preventive care, and overcoming barriers.

Health education classes

Health education classes have been shown to keep patients healthy by giving them the knowledge and tools to stay healthy, prevent disease, and treat medical conditions. Providers can also recommend adjunct tools such as written materials, DVDs, websites, and information about classes and other programs are also provided to help patients reach their goals and improve outcomes.

Support groups / Social media / Patient portals

Support groups, social media, and patient portals can be very beneficial to patients, especially those with chronic conditions. By sharing their experiences, support group members who have successfully managed their conditions can help provide hope to newcomers and calm their fears. Support groups in-person, on social media, and patient portals can also help patients by:

- Answering questions about their condition
- Providing an opportunity to discuss feelings
- Enabling them to develop coping skills
- Allowing them to work through complex emotions and feelings
- Offering support from others who are in the same situation or condition
- Helping them deal with negative thoughts and feelings
- Providing a support infrastructure

In addition, having a "partner in health" (such as a family member) is also very beneficial to improving patients' confidence and helping them achieve their goals. This partner can provide long-term encouragement and support, especially when patients feel they cannot do it alone.

Educational tools and self-care resources

Lao Tzu, the founder of Taoism, said, "Give a man a fish, and you feed him for a day; teach a man to fish, and you feed him for a lifetime." His wise words can be applied to a patient with a chronic condition. Prescription medications can only go so far. It's also important to teach patients how to properly use their medications and best manage their conditions. This will provide them with the tools and confidence to achieve their health goals. There is robust evidence from a recent systematic review that self-care manuals, when regularly used, are associated with increases in self-efficacy (or confidence in performing recommended actions), self-care skills, and overall patient satisfaction. The benefits of self-care interventions are increased when reinforced by a clinician in a group or individual visit, in both English- and Spanish-speaking populations.

Affordability Tools
Tools for patients to find the best cost for prescriptions:

- http://www.goodrx.com Compare prescription drug prices and find coupons at more than 60,000 US pharmacies
- http://www.consumerreports.org/drugs/6-tips-for-finding-the-best-prescription-drug-prices/ Read the article "Save Money on Meds: 6 Tips for Finding the Best Prescription Drug Prices"

Safe Medication Use Tools, for providers, team members, and patients from ISMP
The Institute for Safe Medication Practices (ISMP) offers a wide range of resources and information to help healthcare practitioners in a variety of healthcare settings prevent errors and ensure that medications are used safely. For a complete and comprehensive list, go tohttp://www.ismp.org/tools/.

- Brochure for consumers on medication misuse
- Community pharmacy medication safety tools and resources
- Do-not-crush list
- Error-prone abbreviations toolkit
- Guidelines for preventing medication errors in pediatrics
- Healthcare 411 by AHRQ
- High alert medications consumer leaflet
- Improving medication safety with anticoagulant therapy
- Patient-controlled analgesia: making it safer for patients
- Throw away your old medicines safely
- *ISMP Medication Safety Alert* and *Safe Medicine* newsletters

Technology Tools: Medication Management Apps and A.R.E.A.S. Genius Bar (GB), linking patients' devices to better engagement and outcomes
The purpose of medication management apps is to help patients take their medication(s) as directed, empower them by providing daily motivation tips, and keeping them on track by reminding them to take their medications at specific times. Some key features to look for in apps include security to protect patient information, reminder alerts that can be programed, the space and flexibility to put in various forms of medications (i.e., inhaler, liquids, pills), and availability for the smartphone or tablet being used.

Additional features that may be helpful (usually for a fee) include the ability to track missed doses, an alert about side effects if too much medication is taken (especially for medications with strict dose limits), sharing information with healthcare providers and family caregivers, reminders for more complicated medication schedules, a searchable medication database, and accessibility online (http://www. scriptyourfuture.org/home/the-consumers-guide-to-finding-good-medication-management-apps/). While these apps can help patients take their medication as directed and keep them on track, with the number of apps and features growing, it can be tough to select an app that will help patients address their own medication A.R.E.A.S. challenges.

One new concept that is being investigated by some community pharmacies is the idea of an A.R.E.A.S. Genius Bar (A Bar), a concept derived from the Ochsner Health systems GB (who got the concept from Apple). The A Bar is a new concept for pharmacies to leverage technology to engage patients and improve health outcomes by having an A Bar in the pharmacy staffed by a technician or clerk. Based on the consultation with the pharmacist, the patient will be given a "script" with their own medication A.R.E.A.S. challenges which will be given to the technician at the A Bar, who will then inform patient about the mobile apps appropriate for them. The A Bar will also have wearable devices that are bluetooth-enabled such as a blood glucose monitor, a wireless weight scale, or a wireless blood pressure monitor.

The technician will then involve the patient in setting up the apps and training them on what to do. As Benjamin Franklin said, "Tell me and I forget, teach me and I may remember, involve me and I learn." The value of these medication apps, coupled with wearable devices and optimized with training from the technician, will lead to greater patient engagement, better outcomes, and better health in the long run (http://www.hhnmag.com/articles/7502-health-systems-genius-bar-links-patients-devices-for-better-engagement-outcomes).

Web-Based Tools

Research shows that web-based tools can augment provider teaching. There is evidence that use of online self-care information may increase skills and self-efficacy. In a random, 2000 survey of Kaiser Permanente members-only website users, 50% said the site helped them become better informed about an illness, 49% reported it saved them a call to the advice nurse, and 35% said it helped prepare them for an office visit. Also, more than half the nation is now online, and Internet use is increasing for people regardless of income, education, age, race, ethnicity, or gender. Recent studies found 40% to 52% of Internet users go online for information about healthcare, rating it equal to or better than information obtained during a doctor's visit. However, patients' self-care practices vary and are not always optimal because they don't know which websites are accurate.

While it's best to advise patients to see their primary care provider for their conditions, when patients ask for online information, it's important to recommend trustworthy websites. Some websites that you can recommend include:

- Mayo Clinic: www.mayoclinic.com
- National Institutes of Health Medline Plus: http://medlineplus.gov
- National Council on Patient Information and Education: http://talkaboutrx.org
- Web MD: www.webmd.com

RELATIONSHIPS

In a study published in *JAMA Internal Medicine* in 2012, patients who felt their doctors listened to them and involved them in decisions gained their trust quicker, which contributed to patients following their doctor's orders more often and taking their drugs as prescribed. "By supporting doctors in developing meaningful relationships with their patients, we could help patients take better care of themselves," said the lead author Dr. Neda Ratanawongsa, an assistant professor at the University of California San Francisco Department of Medicine.[53]

A positive patient-provider relationship is one of the strongest predictors of whether patients will take their medications as prescribed. Studies show that patients who have good relationships with their healthcare providers and do not feel judged by them will be more honest about their medication use.[54] These patients will also be more likely to tell their provider about issues and barriers that prevent them from using their medications appropriately. When a patient tells a provider about any medication barrier, the provider can do the following:

- Explore readiness to change through motivational interviewing techniques.
- Engage patients in setting goals related to their medication use and overall health. Involve family members or caregivers whenever possible.
- Explain the purpose of the medication, how it works, its benefits, and what results or side effects to expect. This will help patients anticipate what to expect from their medications, which can be very empowering.
- Let your patients know you believe in them and their abilities to take their medications as prescribed.
- Encourage questions from patients.

TRIAGE

Once the provider has identified barriers and applied various solutions to improve a patient's appropriate medication use, he or she may need to coordinate the patient's medication therapy management plan with broader healthcare-management services. This will help ensure that the patient receives continuous support. Patients will be linked to specific services based on their needs. These services can provide additional support through more in-depth screening for nonadherence, identify issues and barriers, explore readiness to change, encourage goal setting, and provide more in-depth education. Many healthcare organizations have some or all of the services listed below to enhance the patient-provider relationship:

- *Care/case management*: This is a collaborative process that assesses, plans, implements, coordinates, monitors, and evaluates the options and services required to meet patients' needs. Care/ case management promotes quality and cost-effective interventions and outcomes, enhances access to care for patients with chronic conditions, and improves the continuity and effectiveness of services.
- *Behavioral and social medicine*: Referrals to the behavioral or social medicine departments will be reviewed on a case-by-case basis using criteria that supports social service or behavioral health intervention.
- *Health education classes*: Health education classes provide patients with additional opportunities to learn about the importance of medication adherence for a healthier lifestyle.
- *Community programs*: There are many support programs in the community to assist patients with their chronic conditions. Usually, the community services or public affairs departments can supply providers with information for their patients. The various departments may also provide this information to members through publications or alliances with other organizations or programs.

The BSMART Checklist is an example of a framework that can help providers systematically and consistently implement MAB across practice settings successfully. It does this by remembering to identify **barriers**, tailor **solutions** to the barriers, **motivate** patients at every point of contact, provide **A.R.E.A.S. tools** to help patients stay on track, build positive **relationships** with patients, and **triage**/leverage the larger healthcare system and communities to optimize MCC patients' health outcomes, reduce total healthcare costs, and improve organizational performance.

Chapter 7:
Transforming Care Delivery Using the MAB Rx for MCC Patients and Populations

"You never change things by fighting the existing reality. To change something, build a new model [or framework] that makes the existing model obsolete."
R. Buckminster Fuller[1]

Topics Covered:

- Implementing the MAB Rx in moderate and high-risk populations with MCC
- Core MAB actions to address low-risk MCC populations
- Using a lean operational infrastructure and a continuous improvement process to focus on operational efficiency and effectiveness
- Implementing a new pharmacist-provider care delivery model and outpatient pharmacy clinical services to optimize MAB

1. Implementing the MAB Rx in a High-Risk Member (Mr. MT) Using the BSMART Checklist

The following is a case study: MT is a retired 62-year-old computer engineer with a history of diabetes, coronary artery disease, and uncontrolled hypertension. He smokes one pack of cigarettes daily and is about 45 pounds overweight. One evening on his way from a function, he drove himself to the emergency room with complaints of chest pains. Upon admission, he was diagnosed with a mild heart attack and was admitted to the cardiac unit. Two days later, he was transferred to the med-surg unit, and two days after that was discharged with an appointment to follow up with his primary care physician (PCP) in four days. At his PCP visit, his labs were as follows: glycated hemoglobin (HbA1c, a diabetes marker) = 10.2; low-density lipoprotein (LDL) = 162; and blood pressure (BP) = 146/92. MT's medication list included the following:

Old Medication List (not all inclusive)	New Medication List after medication reconciliation	Comments
Lisinopril 20 mg daily		Combined to reduce number of medications
Hydrochlorothiazide 25 mg daily	Prinzide 20-12.5 mg daily	When MT complained of dizziness and nausea, the pharmacist realized he was taking duplicative medications: lisinopril, Prinzide, and hydrochlorothiazide. The lisinopril and hydrochlorothiazide had been discontinued at the hospital, but MT started taking them again because he had been taking them before his hospitalization.
Atenolol 50 mg daily	Atenolol 50 mg daily	MT had stopped taking his atenolol because it made him feel too tired. He will now take it at night time to reduce daytime drowsiness.
Metformin 1,000 mg twice daily	Metformin 1,000 mg twice daily Added glipizide10 mg daily	Morning dose: MT had experienced a stomachache and diarrhea with his morning dose, so he reduced the dose to half; he occasionally forgot to take his evening dose with dinner.
Aspirin 81 mg daily	Aspirin 81 mg daily	
	Warfarin 5mg daily	To be monitored by anticoagulation clinic
Vicodin 1-2 tablets every 4 hours as needed for pain	Vicodin 1-2 tablets every 4 hours as needed for pain	Vicodin and Tylenol are for his ongoing knee pain and chronic arthritis pain, but it was an excessive amount of Tylenol and he was no longer experiencing good pain control. So the pharmacist referred MT to the Pain Management Program.
Over-the-counter Tylenol 500 mg up to 3 times a day as needed for pain		
Spironolactone 50 mg daily	Spironolactone 50 mg daily	
Lipitor 10 mg daily	Atrovastatin 10 mg daily	Changed to generic
Three other medications and vitamins		In general, MT expressed that he was on too many medications (about 13) and had difficulty remembering them and affording all of them.

Figure 7.1: MT's medication list – old and new.

MT is not unique in his medication-taking behaviors or with the challenges he is experiencing. He has medication adherence challenges; his medication list has not been reconciled with what he is actually taking; he has financial challenges; he is not aware of the importance of the lifesaving medications he had stopped taking; and he had several other challenges. So how did his physician, pharmacist, and healthcare team use the BSMART Checklist to address his Medication A.R.E.A.S.

challenges and improve his overall health outcomes, while at the same time improving their organizations' quality goals? This is how his medical team did it at every point of contact across the continuum of care.

BARRIERS

What are MT's barriers that prevent him from getting the optimal health outcomes from his medications (see Figure 7.1)?

The Medication AREAS <u>Barrier Identification Questionnaire</u> the pharmacist used with MT:

Adherence
- ☐ Have you stopped or started taking any of your medication on your own?
- ☐ What gets in the way of taking your medications on some days?
- ☐ Have you experienced any problems or had any side effects while taking your medication?

Reconciliation
- ☐ How many pharmacies do you use to get all your medications?
- ☐ When last did you get a complete list of all your medications?

Engagement & Education
- ☐ How often do you have difficulty understanding the written information your pharmacists give you about your medication?
- ☐ How confident do you feel you are able to follow the instructions on the label of a medication bottle?

Affordability
- ☐ Do you need help affording your medications?

Safe Medication Use
- ☐ MT, I see you are taking atenolol. Tell me how you are taking this medication. How did your doctor tell you to take this medication?

Figure 7.2: The Medication A.R.E.A.S. barrier identification questionnaire

- Lack of understanding of the benefit versus risk of critical medications
- His belief system and concerns
- Affordability of his medications
- Did not have his most up-to-date prescription list
- Got his medications from more than one pharmacy
- Forgetfulness
- Was taking duplicate medications
- Was on very high doses of Tylenol
- Had experienced negative side effects
- Had some unhealthy habits (for example, smoking)

MT's pharmacist used the medication AREAS barrier identification questionnaire (see Figure 7.2) to identify his barriers and used the readiness assessment ruler to determine his readiness to make changes. MT's readiness assessment number was 7, so he was ready to make the necessary changes to improve his health.

SOLUTIONS

Once we have identified barriers and assessed patients for readiness, the next step is tailoring the patient's action plan with interventions related to the identified barriers. Because more than one barrier is often involved, the solutions and interventions must be multifaceted and must be addressed at each point (from the hospital → his physician's office → pharmacy → care management → home) with the patient/caregiver involvement.

Hospital

Adherence: Prior to discharge, the pharmacist educated MT and his caregiver about his medications, including directions, side effects and how to manage the side effects should they occur, the duration of therapy, and the importance of adhering to his medication regimens to prevent adverse outcomes, including being readmitted for the same or similar issue. It is critical that all patients be educated about the importance of medication adherence to prevent complications and readmissions, and this needs to start while the patients are still in the hospital, to help them and their caregivers become familiar with the medications and the importance of taking them as prescribed.

Reconciliation: When MT was admitted to the hospital, the pharmacy technician got a list of all the medications he was taking prior to admission. This list was then compared and reconciled with the list of admission medications ordered by the hospitalist. When one of MT's preadmission medications was not ordered, the pharmacist contacted the physician to see if the medication had been accidentally omitted or if the omission was deliberate (if deliberate, then the reason should be documented).

When MT was transferred from one unit to another, the prescriber wrote new medication orders. Before the actual transfer, a nurse reviewed the medication administration record. She compared the medications he was taking prior to admission and those that had been ordered in the initial unit against the medications in the transfer orders. Upon discharge, the physician and nurse reconciled MT's medications, with a final review by the pharmacist, before the pharmacist consulted with MT and gave him a copy of his most up-to-date medication list.

Engagement: To more effectively engage MT after his discharge, the team nurse followed up with him and his caregiver to connect, address any issues, empower and encourage him to follow his health and medication regimens as prescribed, and link him to resources to support him as he got better. Also, the nurse educated MT to focus on the markers of the disease (LDL and BP), in addition to the symptoms of the disease, to predict how well he was doing (some of his diseases have no symptoms) and set some goals with him.

Affordability: One of MT's complaints was he felt he was on too many medications. Upon reconciling his medications, the team was able to help him reduce his costs, improve his adherence, and reduce safety issues by:

- Eliminating the unnecessary drugs: This both saved money and reduced his risk for adverse outcomes from multiple medications.
- Using combination therapies where possible—for example, using Prinzide (a combination of lisinopril and hydrochlorothiazide), which was cheaper than taking lisinopril and hydrochlorothiazide separately.
- Using generics: This saves patients a significant amount of money because they are usually much cheaper, and just as safe and effective, as their brand-name counterparts. If a generic isn't available, substitute a cheaper medication (usually in the same class) that works just as well.

Safe medication use: When the pharmacist did the full medication reconciliation process with MT and his caregiver, she found that he was on high doses of Vicodin for his ongoing knee pain and was not adherent to his critical medications. These issues increased his chances of having an adverse event. Further exploration revealed that he had different providers prescribing his medications and had his prescriptions filled at different pharmacies. Therefore, a reconciliation of all his medications had not been done, and he was not monitored by anyone in between his primary care physician's visits.

Upon discharge—in addition to eliminating his unnecessary medications, using combination therapies where possible, and educating him and his caregiver about the importance of why he needed to take his medications as prescribed—the pharmacist put in a referral to the pain clinic to have MT's pain assessed and see if alternative, non-opioid medications could be used to treat his chronic knee pain.

Physician/Provider Office

The role of the provider in improving medication adherence is critical. Research has shown that when providers take the time to educate patients about their medications, they are more likely to get their prescriptions filled and take the medication as prescribed.[2] When MT met with his doctor five days after his discharge from the hospital, his physician reviewed his medical history, reasons for admissions, and his medications. The doctor did the following for the new medications prescribed:

- *Name*: Informed MT of the brand and generic names of the medications, to avoid confusion and duplication.
- *Why*: Helped MT understand the reason behind taking the medication prescribed, to link his illness with treatment and improvement of his quality of life.
- *Effects*: Informed MT of the common side effects to expect and what to do if they occurred.
- *Affordability*: Prescribed generics where possible.
- *Triage*: Referred MT to a health education class (and other healthcare services) and to a clinical pharmacist for further follow-up and education.

Pharmacy

To increase the chances of MT taking his medication after leaving the pharmacy, the pharmacist consultation included the following (this is not all inclusive of the law):

- *5Rs*: This means ensuring the right patient is getting the right medication, right indication, right direction, and right duration of therapy.
- *Why*: Explaining why a prescribed medication should be taken is critical to help patients link the disease/illness with treatment.
- *How*: A brief description of how the medication works can further help patients link the disease/illness with treatment (for example, how a bronchodilator works to open the airway passages).
- *Value*: Patients who understand the value and benefits of the medications they are taking have fewer side effects and improved adherence.
- *Side effects*: Improving adherence includes addressing the important side effects and offering tips on side effect management.

- *Consult*: To augment the consultation, the pharmacist should reaffirm the value of the medication, answer questions the patient may have, and provide patient-centric written materials.

Care/Population Management/Other Resources
MT was referred to the care management team for further monitoring and adjustment of his therapies. Additional emphasis was placed on the following:

- *Value* (same as previous page)
- *Markers*: Educated MT to focus on the markers of the disease (for example, LDL lab tests and blood pressure), instead of just the symptoms, as predictors for how well he was doing. This is especially important for chronic diseases that have few to no symptoms.
- *Adherence tools*: Recommend adherence tools to keep MT on track—a pillbox and telephone reminders.
- *Action plan*: The care manager gave MT an updated written action plan that summarized his visit and outlined his prescriptions, his conditions, his goals and targets, key contacts if he had questions or issues, and future upcoming appointments.

Home/Residence
The healthcare team worked with MT in the home to improve secondary medication adherence in the following ways:

- At each point of contact, providers (physician, pharmacist, nurse, others) proactively addressed any issues MT had with his medications, encouraged adherence by reemphasizing the benefits and value of the therapy, and congratulated him when his outcomes were moving in the right direction or meeting the established goals.
- Since forgetfulness is the most common reason for secondary nonadherence, the care manager sent an automated reminder call or text a few days before MT's prescription was due, to remind him to reorder it.

- The care manager reminded MT how critical his role was in helping his provider keep an up-to-date and accurate medicines list, being honest about the medicines he was taking, and speaking up if he suspected an error had occurred.

MOTIVATION

To motivate people to change, we must first help them recognize their personal reasons for wanting to do so. We can do this by linking their problem to things they care about or some identity they aspire to, while maintaining a warm, nonjudgmental style of interaction.

For MT, the care manager used motivational interviewing (MI), one of the many tools to help MT improve his intrinsic need to change. The care manager used MI to accurately understand MT's challenges and help him come to terms with the changes he needed to make by focusing on OARS:[3]

- Open-ended questions: Allows for richer, deeper conversations—"Tell me more about the circumstances that led to the heart attack."
- Affirmation: Recognizes and reinforces a patient's efforts—"You showed a lot of commitment to want to start your medication regimen."
- Reflection: Seeks, clarifies, and deepens understanding—"It sounds like you want some help to keep you on track as you start your new medication regimens, exercise program, and diet."
- Summary: Use summaries to understand, reinforce, and capture key points. This reinforces MT's commitment to the adoption of a healthier lifestyle and helps him stay on track when challenges or roadblocks arise.

The care manager also used the MI REDS technique when she encountered resistance from MT:

- *Rolling* with any resistance encountered, to avoid arguing and instead help MT focus on solutions
- *Expressing* empathy over MT's reluctance to change in a few areas
- Recognizing *discrepancies* to motivate
- Supporting *self-efficacy* by reinforcing the potential for positive change

Since the main goal of motivational interviewing is to increase intrinsic motivation for change ("I will change because I want to"), helping MT become aware of the discrepancies between his current behaviors and his highly cherished personal values and goals was critical.

Finally, the care manager worked with MT to increase his belief in his ability to change his current medication-taking behavior, diet, and smoking habit. She did this by acknowledging his readiness to change, empowering and encouraging him to adopt new self-managing skills, reinforcing his commitment to adopting a healthier lifestyle, and showing him how to stay on track when challenges or roadblocks arise.

A.R.E.A.S. TOOLS

Tools are incredibly important in helping patients stay on track with their medication regimens. For MT, the following tools helped him stay on track:

- *A pillbox* organized his pills by days and times to be taken. It simplified his polydrug regimen and helped him remember to take his medications. The pillbox also served as a double-check system to see if he had taken his medication.
- *Written information* about a medication reinforced the verbal information he received from his provider.
- *Follow-up management* is vital. Complex medication regimens contribute to a revolving door of rehospitalizations for patients with heart failure and other comorbidities. Therefore, MT's care manager followed up with him within 72 hours of his discharge to address any issues he was having with his condition or medications.

- *A congratulatory letter* from his physician emphasized how well he was doing, as reflected in his lab results, and reminded him why it was important to keep taking his medications.
- *Reminder calls* were made about picking up medication refills.
- *A community support group* created a venue for him to share his experiences, learn from others who had successfully managed their conditions, be in a safe environment to discuss his feelings (and maybe fears), develop coping skills, and get support from those who shared a same situation or condition.
- *Trusted web links* were suggested to help him self-care his conditions.

RELATIONSHIPS

A positive patient-provider relationship is one of the strongest predictors of whether a patient will take his or her medications as prescribed. Studies show patients who have good relationships with their healthcare providers and do not feel judged by them will be more honest about their medication use. These patients will also be more likely to tell their provider about issues and barriers that prevent them from using their medications appropriately. MT always felt his healthcare team encouraged, empowered, and educated him on what he needed to do to successfully improve his health and quality of life.

TRIAGE

MT was referred to the following resources in the broader healthcare system:

- Care/case management: to promote quality and cost-effective interventions and outcomes, enhance access to care for patients like MT with chronic conditions, and improve the continuity and effectiveness of services

- Pain management: to address MT's uncontrolled pain management challenges, examine his medications, and provide him with a regimen that lessened his pain and improved his quality of life
- Health education classes: to provide MT with an additional opportunity to learn about his conditions and pharmacological and nonpharmacological therapies for a healthier lifestyle, and to emphasize the importance of medication management

MT Nine Months Later

- *Barriers and solutions to his barriers:*
  - Takes his metformin with breakfast and dinner
  - Takes his beta-blocker at night to reduce dizziness
  - Changed to combo medication (prinzide) for blood pressure
  - Takes glipizide once daily
  - Uses a pillbox
  - Has his medication reconciled every time there is a change in his therapies or a new medication is added
  - Is on target with the following objective measures:
    - Labs: HbA1c = 7.7, LDL = 101, BP = 124/80
    - Lost 15 pounds and is walking one mile daily
    - In the best shape in over 10 years
- *Motivation*
  - Successfully used his action plan with goals to improve his health in the following ways:
    - Reduced smoking, now down to one cigarette a day with plans to quit completely
    - Is developing healthy eating habits and lifestyle
    - Got feedback and encouragement from his provider and healthcare team
    - Sets new diabetes goals every three to six months with his provider

- *A.R.E.A.S. tools*
  - Uses pillboxes to stay on track
  - Sometimes receives an interactive voice response (IVR) call to remind him to pick up his medications
- *Relationship*
  - Is encouraged by his provider and healthcare team at every visit, which helps keep him on track
  - Very satisfied with care from his doctor and staff
- *Triage*
  - Attended a health education class where he learned how to control his chronic conditions and gained a better understanding of the disease process
  - Worked with a nutritionist to create a diet plan

MT's Economic, Clinical, Humanistic Outcomes (ECHO)

Economic outcomes:
- Overall prescription costs significantly lowered due to switching to generics, consolidating some medications, and finding the best prices for all of his medications in one pharmacy
- Wasn't readmitted to the hospital, so the hospital avoided the associated penalties
- Eventual economic advantages to come from reducing the progression of his disease conditions and adopting a healthier lifestyle

Clinical outcomes:
- Improvement in the diabetes, hypertension, and cholesterol quality measures
- Positive contribution to the Medicare Stars, HEDIS, and other quality measures related to his conditions
- Positive impact on the readmission rate

Humanistic outcomes (care experience):
- Contributed to positive patient satisfaction scores reflected on the CAHPS survey
- Contributed to positive patient satisfaction scores reflected on the pharmacy survey

2. Implementing MAB in High-Risk Populations: Diabetes in African Americans

According to the American Hospital Association's 2017 Environmental Scan, studies have shown that if Americans with chronic conditions could achieve "six normal" ranges (for low-density lipoprotein cholesterol, blood pressure, blood sugar, waist-to-height ratio, stress management, and tobacco toxins) with or without medication, there would be a subsequent reduction in chronic disease by 80% to 90% over 10- to 30-year periods. If only 65% of individuals achieved the six normals, the nation would save over $600 billion in healthcare spending per year.[5]

Diabetes is one of the most prominent of all the chronic conditions that if treated effectively would make a significant difference in health outcomes and total healthcare costs. The prevalence of type 2 diabetes continues to increase at an alarming rate around the world, and more people are being affected by prediabetes. Although the origination and development of type 2 diabetes, and its long-term complications, are known, its treatment has remained challenging, with only half of the patients achieving the recommended hemoglobin A1c target of 8 or less.

In the United States, between 1974 and 2014, the number of type 2 diabetics increased from 3.2 million to 29 million and now represents nearly 10% of healthcare expenditures.[6] Much of the economic burden of diabetes is related to its increased hospitalizations and complications, including amputation, blindness, kidney failure, heart attack, stroke, uncontrolled hypertension, sexual dysfunction, and vascular dementia. Experts predict that if major steps are not taken to manage this disease, by 2050, 120 million to 180 million Americans will have diabetes—a sixfold to tenfold increase in the US population.[7] These statistics, coupled with the poor quality of life, the adverse outcomes, and the economic burden associated with the complications of uncontrolled diabetes, requires that the prevention and effective management of diabetes become a national priority.[8]

One of the ethnic groups that is disproportionately affected by diabetes is the African American population. According to the American Diabetes Association:

- In 2006, African American men were 2.2 times more likely to start treatment for end-stage renal disease related to diabetes than non-Hispanic white men.
- In 2006, African Americans with diabetes were 1.5 times more likely to be hospitalized and 2.3 times more likely to die from diabetes than non-Hispanic whites.
- African Americans are almost 50% more likely to develop diabetic retinopathy than non-Hispanic whites.
- 4.9 million African American adults, or 18.7% of all African Americans 20 years of age or older, have diagnosed or undiagnosed diabetes, compared to 7.1% of non-Hispanic white Americans.[9]
- The risk of diabetes is 77% higher among African Americans than among non-Hispanic white Americans.[10]

Case Study

In the SAFER Healthplan, 18% (2,220 people) of the total population with type 2 diabetes were adult African Americans. Of this group of African Americans, 333 (15%) were enrolled in the care management programs based on the following criteria:

- HbA1c greater than 9: All had this in the last 12 months.
- Access to health services: Many were unable to take off work for healthcare appointments, and others did not have transportation to get to their appointments.
- Age: They ranged in age from 35 to 67 (the mean age was about 49 years).
- Hospitalization: They were hospitalized at least once in the last six months.
- Comorbidities: They also had at least one of these conditions— hypertension or dyslipidemia.

- Diet: Less than 30% had ready access to purchasing fresh fruits and vegetables.
- Disease knowledge: Less than 30% understood the adverse outcomes of having diabetes.
- Exercise: Less than 5% consistently exercised more than 60 minutes per week.
- Labs: About 85% had their diabetes screening tests done in the last 12 months.
- Medication use: 45% were taking their diabetes medications (including oral agents and insulin) as prescribed six months after starting the medication, and 60% had experienced a side effect.
- Personal and family medical history: More than 70% had a family history of cardiovascular disease.
- Psychological well-being: About 10% had been diagnosed with clinical depression.
- Tobacco use: 15% smoked one-half to one pack of cigarettes daily.
- Weight: 60% were overweight, and of those, 37% were obese.

The effective management of diabetes is multifaceted, comprised of education, nutritional management, exercise, and medications. Using the BSMART Checklist, let us implement MAB (alongside the other components of diabetes management) in our high-risk populations to help reverse or minimize some of these complications, slow down the progression of the disease, improve the care and health of the population, and contribute to reducing the total cost of care burden associated with diabetes.

BARRIERS

To better understand the MAB barriers in the African American group, three focus groups were set up with patients from the care management group. These were the most common barriers identified:

- Lack of understanding of diabetes and the need for medications (beliefs that diabetes was due to high sugar ingestion, so there was no need to take medications—just reduce the sugar intake)
- They were not sure if the best medications had been prescribed for their conditions
- Had experienced negative side effects from other medications
- Co-pays for medications were too high
- Challenges of getting an up-to-date prescription list, primarily due to the use of multiple pharmacies
- Challenges between brand and generic names of medications
- Did not trust nutritional plans, which were not reflective of what they were used to eating
- Labs were not open at the hours convenient for them (early mornings or late in the evenings or weekends), which prevented them from getting their lab tests done

These barriers were then incorporated into the barrier questions asked by the care managers of all the African American diabetes patients enrolled in the care management program. Their readiness assessment scores ranged from 3 to 8, which were dealt with individually with the care manager.

SOLUTIONS

Once the barriers were identified and the readiness assessment completed, the care manager (CM) tailored each patient's action plan with interventions related to the identified barriers and focused on the following:

- Education: The CM educated patients about diabetes and the importance of the medications in treating diabetes. The CM also focused on the value and benefit of their medications as well as the markers of the disease (for example, HgbA1c lab tests and blood glucose self-monitoring tests), instead of just the symptoms of the disease, as predictors for how well they were doing.

- Diet: The CM worked with dietitians to modify the diet tools used to teach patients about their diabetic diets. These new tools incorporated general foods eaten by African Americans, in addition to the suggested foods featured in the booklets.
- Office hours: The CM team worked with the lab to open earlier and close later by staggering shifts.
- Adherence tools: The CM recommended adherence tools to keep patients on track, such as pillboxes, medication apps, and telephone reminders.
- Action plan: The CM gave patients updated written action plans that summarized their visits and conditions, outlined their prescriptions, reflected their goals and targets, listed key contacts if the patients had questions or issues, and detailed future appointments.

MOTIVATION

The providers and CMs of the African American patients used the following tactics to motivate their patients to be more engaged and more adherent to their therapies and action plans.

- Motivational interviewing, to find out what motivated them, then reflecting that reason back and highlighting the perceived benefits to improve their intrinsic need to change
- Educating them about the disease process, and making a positive link between being adherent to the treatment, nutritional and exercise plans, and glucose monitoring and experiencing positive outcomes and overall health
- Financial incentives for taking their medications
- Using social networking to create online communities that help reinforce patients' motivation
- Leveraging the use of storytelling that focused on overcoming medication use challenges, to help reinforce patients' motivation to adhere

- Using pictures and stories to stress the acute and chronic complications that occur when patients do not follow their action plan or take their medications as prescribed (such as cardiovascular disease, eye damage or blindness, foot damage or possible amputation, hearing impairment, infections, kidney damage or dialysis, nerve damage, and sexual dysfunction)

A.R.E.A.S. TOOLS

Tools are incredibly important to help patients remember when and how to take their medications, to remember if they have taken their medications, to remind them of the importance of taking their medications, to prevent patients from having adverse outcomes when taking their medications, to empower patients to self-manage their conditions, and to help reduce a complex regimen. The following tools helped the African American group stay on track:

- Pillboxes
- Storytelling CD to listen to at home
- Written information about the medications
- Follow-up management
- The medication app for the patients with a smartphone or tablet
- Reminder calls
- Safe medication use tools

RELATIONSHIPS

The patients felt their healthcare team and CMs encouraged, empowered, and educated them at every point of contact and gave them the tools and resources needed to successfully improve their health and quality of life.

TRIAGE

The patients were enrolled in the care management program and health education classes. The patients were also encouraged to join the community support group and enroll at the local gym at a significant discount.

The African American Diabetic Group—Nine Months Later

Sixty percent of the patients had HbA1c less than 7 by doing the following:

- *Barriers and solutions*
    - After their barriers were addressed, 85% were taking their medications as prescribed.
    - More than 70% had access to fresh fruits and vegetables as they learned about farmers' markets and other avenues for getting their fresh produce.
    - They increased their knowledge of their disease. Over 95% of them understood the adverse outcomes of having diabetes and the positive outcomes if they optimized their complete regimens.
    - One to two days a week, an evening clinic was established, and the lab opened earlier and closed later to accommodate the needs of all patients who had access challenges during the day.
    - More than 45% consistently exercised more than 60 minutes per week, and more than 90% consistently exercised for a total of 30 minutes a week.
    - More than 95% had a diabetes screening in the last nine months.
    - Only 2% continued to have a diagnosis of clinical depression.
    - Less than 3% of the population had readmission, and none had a readmission due to the diabetes condition.

- *Motivation*
  - Successfully used their action plans with goals to improve their health:
    - Tobacco use: Less than 5% smoked one-half to one pack of cigarettes daily.
    - Weight: Over 80% of the patients lost 10 pounds or more.
    - Tips: The patients utilized tips to develop healthy eating habits and lifestyle.
    - Goals: The CMs and providers helped the patients set new diabetes goals every three to six months.
    - Congratulatory letters: The patients received congratulatory letters from their providers and CMs every time they reached a goal.
- *A.R.E.A.S. tools*
  - Everyone had a pillbox to stay on track.
  - Sometimes patients received an IVR call to remind them to pick up their medications.
  - About 30% of the patients started using the medication management app to monitor their adherence, keep their medication lists current, and get health tips. The app included a link for them to find their medications at the lowest price. For medications with a low therapeutic window, like warfarin, the app allowed alerted patients to double-check their dose before taking their medications.
  - Over 90% were consistently checking their blood sugar daily with the free glucose meters they were provided to monitor their symptoms.
- *Relationship*
  - They were encouraged by their providers, CMs, and healthcare team at every visit, which helped keep them on track.
  - They were very satisfied with care they received from their doctors and healthcare teams.
- *Triage*
  - Over 70% attended a health education class where they learned

to control their chronic conditions and better understand the disease process.

▫ Nutritionists provided diet plans that included foods the patients were used to in addition to the foods in the traditional diabetes diet plans.

The African American Diabetic Group ECHO

Economic outcomes:
- Lower cost prescriptions
- Lower readmissions, so no associated penalties for the hospital
- Disease progression reduced, healthier lifestyles, and healthier communities resulting in eventual economic advantages for the organization

Clinical outcomes:
- Improvement in the diabetes, hypertension, and cholesterol quality measures
- Positive impact on Medicare Stars, HEDIS, and other quality measures related to diabetes
- Positive impact on the readmission rate

Humanistic outcomes (care experience):
- Improved patient satisfaction scores reflected in CAHPS survey
- Improved patient satisfaction scores reflected in pharmacy survey

3. Core MAB Actions to Address Low-Risk MCC Populations

The number of people with multiple chronic conditions (MCC) has risen significantly, resulting in one out of four Americans having an MCC. Chronic conditions are responsible for seven out of every 10 deaths, killing more than 1.7 million Americans every year.[11] For 88% of the population with MCC, medications are a first choice for medical intervention.[12]

How can healthcare providers and teams increase the chances of MCC patients taking their medications as prescribed and increase appropriate use of medications to ensure better care and health outcomes? With the number of MCC patients overall, it would be virtually impossible to spend an extensive amount of time on every patient using the BSMART Checklist to implement MAB at every point of contact. The BSMART Checklist is reserved for moderate- to high-risk patients; however, there are core MAB actions every provider can use for lower-risk patients to address the most common MAB barriers. These include not understanding or accepting their conditions, unreconciled medication lists, lack of engagement around treatment plans, unaffordability of medications, and perceived or actual side effects.

So, at each point of contact with lower-risk MCC patients, providers and qualified team members should do the following to optimize MAB when prescribing or consulting on a medication:

- Always emphasize and reinforce the value and benefit of therapy: Evidence shows that patients who understand their disease condition and the purpose of their medications are more likely to be adherent.
- Educate: Focus on the markers of the disease, instead of symptoms, as predictors for how well patients are doing (many diseases have no symptoms) and set goals.
- Address financial issues: Some 40% to 60% of patients have higher out-of-pocket costs due to having high-deductible health insurance coverage.
- Engage: At each point of contact, it is important to encourage, empower, and educate patients and caregivers.
- Tools: Provide tools such as pillboxes and apps for self-monitoring.
- Relationship: Maintain a healthy, positive relationship with patients.
- Triage: Direct patients and caregivers to online resources or other healthcare services such as health education and nutrition classes where they can learn more about the disease process, treatment options, nutritional plans, blood sugar monitoring, exercise plans, and other strategies to promote better health.

Including these core elements in your consultation with patients will address key MAB barriers in low-risk MCC patients in a very short period of time (two minutes on average) and will help reduce their chances of becoming your moderate- to high-risk patients who require more intensive interventions.

Providing Resources to Support Operational Efficiency and Effectiveness
When a new program or strategy is introduced, many teams automatically ask for more resources for implementation. While some programs and strategies may require new resources, most organizations do not have the luxury of providing them. Over the last several years, many organizations have been focusing on what to stop doing instead of just doing more. Some organizations make this an annual review and reward teams that are able to take a look at the organizational and operational infrastructures to assess for efficiency and effectiveness. Questions being asked include: What three things can we stop doing that will not impact patient care? What can we stop doing or repurpose to more effectively meet the Triple Aim on behalf of our members? As Steve Jobs said, "Deciding what not to do is as important as deciding what to do."[13]

Each year, many organizations automatically add a percentage of dollars to the previous year's budget, which perpetuates the idea that to do more, we need more. Imagine, however, your institution's budget for the following year was cut by 3%, and you wanted to implement one or two new strategies that would bring tremendous value to the organization but would require resources. What would you do?

This was the dilemma faced by Dr. Sam, the pharmacy director mentioned in Chapter 5 who wanted to implement the MAB prescription strategy and have the new MAB care delivery model, but had a 3% reduction in his budget. Fortunately, a few years prior, his organization had adopted a program that focused on lean techniques to improve efficiencies and identify projects and initiatives that had very little value-add and needed to be eliminated. Over the past two years, the pharmacy team had implemented the lean review to identify the non-value-added processes and projects that they could eliminate. They were now going to repurpose most of the savings and resources toward implementing the new MAB Rx strategy and care delivery model.

The Lean Review

The lean review is an adaptation of the Toyota Production System (TPS). TPS was developed by top Toyota executives in the late 1940s to improve the company's manufacturing processes and is now used by companies across various industries to reduce inefficiencies, eliminate waste, improve the cost structure, and enhance the overall value of their end product to customers. The TPS elements have been transferred to healthcare to accomplish these same goals.

Dr. Sam worked with his team members and the staff in each pharmacy to focus on these five steps at their 28 pharmacy systems: assess the current state, determine the future workflows, identify the future organizational structure, pinpoint priorities, and develop a plan to move forward.[14]

The following six-step plan helped them identify priority activities to: eliminate non-value-added activities, optimize key activities, leverage technology areas, implement continuous improvement activities, standardize key processes, and train and develop staff to keep improving the processes. These new activities would be continuously reviewed by each pharmacy team with an official evaluation (proposed every 18-24 months) by the Rx Lean Team, to assess how they had reduced inefficiencies, eliminated waste, improved the cost structure, and enhanced the overall value of care.

1. Eliminate non-value-added activities:
   - By using work stream and process mapping to evaluate all the steps in the prescription-filling to the prescription-dispensing processes, they were able to improve efficiency of filling prescriptions.
   - Eliminating the non-value-added steps resulted in reduced wait times and decreased the prescription processing time.

2. Optimize key activities:
   - Working with the supply chain organization and leveraging technology, the team implemented a "just-in-time" inventory strategy, which aimed to reduce inventory and associated carrying costs. They were able to reduce their inventory costs by 15% due to fewer medications left sitting on the shelves, increasing turns, and significantly eliminating outdates.
   - They improved the return-to-stock process, which saved staff resources and inventory.
3. Leverage technology (see Chapter 9 for more details):
   - The teams adopted this modified saying from a senior leader in the organization: Old Organization + New Technology or New Processes = Costly Old Organization (OO + NT or NP = COO).

     So focus on: Old Organization + New Culture (including New Technology or New Processes) = New Value Organization (OO + NC [NT or NP] = NVO).

Old Organization + New Technology or New Processes = Costly Old Organization (OO + NT or NP = COO)	$\Longrightarrow$	**Old Organization + New Culture (leveraging New Technology or New Processes) = New Value Organization (OO + NC [NT or NP] = NVO).**

   - Automated dispensing systems were put in the large pharmacies to increase efficiencies.
   - An "operations effectiveness room" was created to support workload balancing, remove administrative and nonessential activities out of the pharmacies (for example, drug reviews), and monitor stores for optimal effectiveness.
   - They more effectively leveraged their PBM to receive better prices, became part of the preferred network of pharmacies, and combined their central specialty and mail services with the PBM to improve operating and purchasing efficiencies for both organizations.

4. Implement continuous improvement activities:

    As part of the overall operations, teams were given time to take an identified process that could be stopped and operationalize it. The teams also were encouraged to quarterly ask the following three questions about the core activities of their pharmacies:

    - *How good are we relative to the best?* Often teams have no idea. They look at their own processes and performances, but they don't know there is a gap between what they are seeing on their data and what the best are doing. Acknowledging that gap can be profoundly motivating for teams.

    - *Do we know where our variation exists?* Why ask this? Because hidden in the average number the team typically pays attention to lies both good and bad performance—exceptionally good and exceptionally bad sometimes. When the team started to look at variation, it gave them real insight. To remove that variation, they would need the poor performers to learn from the better ones.

    - *Are we looking at our rate of improvement over time?* We think we may be improving, but in looking at the data over time, we might not be. We may be flat, or we could actually be improving dramatically.

    These questions helped the teams focus their attention on the right measures, set the right priorities, and stay focused.

5. Standardize key processes:

    Standardization is still a controversial topic in healthcare as many providers and teams believe it removes their ability to personalize care and adversely impacts innovation. Research, however, shows that standardizing practices and processes in healthcare can—when done correctly—be very effective in reducing costs for health systems, promoting quality patient care at an affordable cost, and positively impacting patient outcomes.[15] The challenge is to know what to standardize, when to standardize, and, simultaneously, how to remain flexible to change processes in the advent of new information.

When proposing standardization in any organization, it is best to start by identifying processes that will yield operational efficiency, are evidence-based, and currently cause confusion and errors, due to the significance in variation. For example, clinical pathways, surgical checklists, the medication dispensing process, back room operations, and other processes are good examples of things to be standardized. When the right processes are standardized, spread, and embedded into the operational workflow—and additional waste is taken out of the system—there is reduction in errors and unwarranted variations. This leads to improved operational effectiveness and potential resources, which can be used to fund and take on new opportunities. The pharmacy team experienced this when they standardized the prescription-filling and dispensing process, the inventory system, drug use management processes, and other processes identified by the teams.

6. Train and develop staff to keep improving the processes:
   ▫ The pharmacy trained its staff on lean principles and involved them in analyzing the pharmacy and patient workflows.
   ▫ Staff identified over 20 processes that could be stopped, along with 15 initiatives that improved efficiencies and inventory management without adversely impacting care. Stopping these processes and initiatives actually improved their service.

The savings allowed the team to reinvest and repurpose the resources needed for new services and innovations and to build a competitive advantage.

Implementing and Optimizing MAB in Care Delivery

With the resources gained from the operational efficiencies implemented and the positive Triple Aim outcomes of the MAB pilots with patients and populations, Dr. Sam and key physician leaders in the organization proposed that clinical pharmacists work alongside providers to implement MAB in moderate- to high-risk patients. They also proposed to have clinical pharmacists in the outpatient pharmacies implement the core MAB actions in low-risk MCC populations, regardless of the chronic disease condition. They also proposed implementing the Enhanced MTM (medication therapy management) pilot program they were selected for by CMS. The clinical pharmacists would be supplemented with nurses, medical assistants or pharmacy technicians, so they would work at their highest scope of practice at least 80% of the time.

1. MAB Clinical Pharmacists (MCP)—Advanced Care Delivery Model

Dr. Sam, in collaboration with key stakeholders, put forward a proposal for a new collaborative care delivery model: for every 10 physicians/providers budgeted for in the organization, there would be one MCP budgeted in the primary care setting, and one MCP to five providers in the specialty settings (for example oncology, endocrinology, infectious disease) where medications were a significant mode of treatment.

This MCP, under the governance laws and under approved protocols in collaboration with providers, would manage a select MCC population and provide the following services:

- *Adherence*: Work with the selected MCC population to encourage patients to take their medications at least 80% of the time (higher for certain drugs) as measured using PDC or MPR.
- *Reconciliation*: Ensure the MCC patients have the best possible reconciliation medication list at all times—upon admission, transfer between units, at discharge, and in the ambulatory setting when medication therapies or doses change.
- *Engagement*: Engage and educate patients about their medications, provide tools, encourage healthy behaviors, teach skills to help patients self-manage their conditions, and motivate them through

encouragement, empowerment, and empathy at each point of contact.

- *Affordability*: Address affordability and drug costs at every point of contact through the use of generics, consolidation, alternative therapies, and elimination of therapies when possible. Refer patients to the medical financial assistance programs within the organization or other sources when needed, and contribute to the minimization of prescription waste in all practice settings through vial maximization, appropriate medication utilization, and inventory control.

- *Safe medication use*: Promote safe medication use practices and medication safety by ensuring appropriate prescribing practices. Focus on abuse potential and carefully monitor medications with narrow therapeutic windows. Ensure effective transcribing processes, including double checks for narrow therapeutic window medications like warfarin, chemotherapy, and opioids. Promote effective dispensing practices including automation, storage, and consultation on new medications. Ensure optimal conditions when medication is being administered by other providers and staff through the transcription process to the dispensing and administration processes.

The MCP's activities would be augmented by:
- Working with providers to improve their clinical knowledge and skills
- Utilizing the integrated pharmacy information management system (iPIMS) where the adherence rates are populated next to the medications and can be used to document the MCP's activities
- Aligning or integrating the iPIMS system with the electronic medical record using interconnectivity systems, so the MCP can get a holistic picture of the patient and can provide physicians and other clinicians with patient MAB information and recommendations
- Using analytics to identify the appropriate set of patients to

refer to the MCPs in addition to the referrals received from the providers—"slice and dice" data for appropriate segmentation and interventions—and to predict population risk for effective and timely interventions

- Supplementing gaps in care through coordinating care with other practitioners and resources in the organization and/or community
- Leveraging other pharmacy infrastructure and business capabilities (see Chapter 9)

2. Outpatient Clinical Pharmacists—Collaborative Care Delivery Model

Dr. Sam proposed all outpatient clinical pharmacists use the core MAB actions when the pharmacy system identifies a patient as potentially having medication adherence issues with key chronic medications, starting with MCC patients with cardiovascular diseases (diabetes, hypertension, and dyslipidemia). For more complex patients who met the MCP criteria, the outpatient clinical pharmacists (OCP) would refer the patient to the MCP service for further follow up.

3. Enhanced MTM Services

Dr. Sam's organization was one of the selected groups to participate in the new CMS demonstration model to test changes in the Medicare Part D program. The changes made in the new Enhanced MTM services were "designed to better align the standalone prescription drug plan sponsor and government financial interests, while also creating incentives for more robust investment and innovation in targeting medication therapy interventions."[16] The goal of the Enhanced MTM model is to deliver greater value and better health outcomes for Medicare Part D beneficiaries and Medicare.[17] The team believed that MAB would unlock the potential of this Enhanced MTM program to make good on its goal.

Benefits of the MCP and OCP Care Delivery Models

Dr. Sam proposed these new clinical pharmacists in collaboration with other providers would be an initial investment for the organization (using the resources gained from the operational efficiencies put in place), but the organization would see the following in 12-18 months:

- *Improvement in adherence rates* → directly and indirectly leading to better treatment outcomes, better patient outcomes, and better organizational performance in HEDIS, MIPS, Medicare Stars, and other treatment-related quality measures
- *Reduction in medication-related readmissions* → reducing the HRRP penalties, reducing hospital costs, and improving hospital Medicare Stars ratings
- *Improvement in patient care coordination and engagement* → leading to better service scores and improved and sustained patient outcomes
- *Bending the curve of total costs of care and per-member-per-month (PMPM) costs* → from effective drug use management and prescribing recommendations
- *Improved patient safety outcomes and measures* → fewer medication-related adverse events and admissions, and improved organizational performance in patient and medication safety

Chapter 8:
Performance Outcomes—
MAB Impact on Quality Measures,
to Improve Outcomes
and Demonstrate Value

*"Achieving high value for patients must become the overarching
goal of health care delivery, with value defined as the health outcomes
achieved per dollar spent. This goal is what matters for patients
and unites the interests of all actors in the system. If value improves,
patients, payers, providers, and suppliers can all benefit while the
economic sustainability of the health care system increases."*
Michael Porter[1]

Topics Covered:

• The Triple Aim measures that MAB impacts–quality, service, &
affordability
• How MAB demonstrates value by positively impacting the NQS
• How to leverage performance reports to address data transparency

To improve performance, create accountability, and demonstrate value,
organizations must have shared goals, agreed-upon measures to evaluate
the goals, and critical strategies to impact the identified goals. In this
new value-based healthcare system, our shared goal must be creating
value for every patient by implementing the Triple Aim: improving
patients' experience of care, enhancing the health outcomes of patients
and populations, and reducing the per capita cost of healthcare.[2]

Organizations that achieve high value for patients take this pursuit very seriously and have rigorous disciplined measurement processes, accountability, and the right measures to assess their progress and continuously drive improvements. Currently, structural and process measures are used most often, with few outcome measures used. However, there is a major focus in healthcare to develop more outcome and patient-centered measures to assess the value of care being provided and the outcomes of care being delivered.

Many organizations are also developing or adopting critical strategies to improve patient health outcomes and reduce total healthcare costs. This results in improved organizational performance as reflected by key quality and regulatory measures. As described in Chapter 7, one key strategy to achieving organizational success is MAB. MAB has been shown to improve patient outcomes and achieveing organizational success is the MAB Rx. MAB has been shown to positively impact many key measures in Medicare Stars, HEDIS, QPP, ACO quality measures, PQRS, HRRP, patient safety, Consumer Assessment of Healthcare Providers and Systems (CAHPS), and many other Triple Aim measures.

Medicare Stars—Quality Measures

One of CMS's most important strategic goals is improving the quality of care and health status for Medicare beneficiaries. CMS publishes the Part C and D Star Rating Measures each year to drive improvements in Medicare quality, incentivize quality improvement in Medicare Advantage (MA) and prescription drug plans (PDPs or Part D plans), assist beneficiaries in finding the best plan for them, and determine MA Quality Bonus Payments.[3] Medicare plans are rated on a scale of one to five stars, with one star for poor performance, three for average, and five for excellent. MA with prescription drug coverage (MA-PD) contracts are rated on up to 44 unique quality and performance measures; MA-only contracts (without prescription drug coverage) are rated on up to 32 measures (Part C); and stand-alone PDP contracts are rated on up to 15 measures (Part D).[4]

For plans covering health services, the overall rating for the quality of many medical/healthcare services falls into five categories under Part C. For plans covering drug services, the overall rating for the quality of prescription-related services falls into four categories/domains. The performance measures are derived from plan and beneficiary information collected from HEDIS, CAHPS, HOS (hours of service), and administrative data.[5]

- Part C Categories/Domains:
  - Domain 1—Staying Healthy Screenings, Tests and Vaccines
  - Domain 2—Managing Chronic (Long-Term) Conditions
  - Domain 3—Member Experience with Health Plans
  - Domain 4—Member Complaints and Changes in the Health Plan's Performance
  - Domain 5—Health Plan Customer Service

- Part D Categories/Domains:
  - Domain 1—Drug Plan Customer Service
  - Domain 2—Member Complaints and Changes in the Drug Plan's Performance
  - Domain 3—Member Experience with the Drug Plan
  - Domain 4—Drug Safety and Accuracy of Drug Pricing

MAB directly or indirectly impacts 25% to 30% of the measures under the Part C and Part D domains. For example, under Part C Domain 2, MAB impacts the following measures:

- C09—Care for Older Adults, Medication Review
- C12—Osteoporosis Management in Women Who Have Had a Fracture
- C15—Diabetes Care, Blood Sugar Control
- C16—Controlling Blood Pressure
- C17—Rheumatoid Arthritis Management
- C19—Plan All-Cause Readmissions

Under Medicare Stars, Part D Domain 4, MAB impacts the following measures:

- D11—High-Risk Medication
- D12—Medication Adherence for Diabetes Medications
- D13—Medication Adherence for Hypertension (RAS Antagonists)
- D14—Medication Adherence for Cholesterol (Statins)
- D15—MTM Program Completion Rate for CMR (comprehensive medication reviews)[6]

HEDIS—Quality Measures (2016)

The Healthcare Effectiveness Data and Information Set (HEDIS) is a tool used by more than 90% of America's health plans to measure performance on important dimensions of care and service. HEDIS consists of 81 measures that are divided into five domains of care (subject to change):

- Access/Availability of Care
- Experience of Care
- Utilization and Risk-Adjusted Utilization
- Relative Resource Use
- Effectiveness of Care

MAB can impact a significant number of measures under the effectiveness of care domain, such as (not all-inclusive):

- Adherence to antipsychotic medications for individuals with schizophrenia
- Annual monitoring for patients on persistent medications
- Antidepressant medication management
- Appropriate treatment for children with upper respiratory infections
- Asthma medication ratio
- Avoidance of antibiotic treatment in adults with acute bronchitis

- Cardiovascular monitoring for people with cardiovascular disease and schizophrenia
- Comprehensive adult diabetes care
- High blood pressure control
- Diabetes monitoring for people with diabetes and schizophrenia
- Disease modifying anti-rheumatic drug therapy for rheumatoid arthritis
- Follow-up after hospitalization for mental illness
- Follow-up care for children prescribed ADHD medication
- Medication management for people with asthma
- Medication reconciliation post-discharge
- Metabolic monitoring for children and adolescents on antipsychotics
- Osteoporosis management in women who have had a fracture
- Persistence of beta-blocker treatment after a heart attack
- Potentially harmful drug-disease interactions in the elderly
- Statin therapy for patients with cardiovascular conditions
- Statin therapy for patients with diabetes
- Use of high-risk medications in the elderly
- Use of multiple, concurrent antipsychotics in children and adolescents

MACRA/QPP

MAB will directly or indirectly impact a significant number of the QPP's 271 quality measures (168 high-priority measures) under the following NQS domains: Communication and Care Coordination (CCC), Community/Population Health (CPH), Effective Clinical Care (ECC), Efficiency and Cost Reduction (ECR), Patient Safety (PS), and Person and Caregiver-Centered Experience and Outcomes (PCEO).[7]

Below is a list of many of the QPP measures that MAB can impact to improve patient health outcomes (not all-inclusive):

MEASURE NAME	NQS DOMAIN	MEASURE TYPE
All-Cause Hospital Readmission	CCC	Outcome
Medication Reconciliation Post-Discharge	CCC	Process
Melanoma: Coordination of Care	CCC	Process
Pain Assessment and Follow-Up	CCC	Process
Parkinson's Disease: Rehabilitative Therapy Options	CCC	Process
Childhood Immunization Status	CPH	Process
Immunizations for Adolescents	CPH	Process
Preventive Care and Screening: Influenza Immunization	CPH	Process
Preventive Care and Screening: Screening for Clinical Depression and Follow-Up Plan	CPH	Process
Preventive Care and Screening: Screening for High Blood Pressure and Follow-Up Documented	CPH	Process
Preventive Care and Screening: Tobacco Use: Screening and Cessation Intervention	CPH	Process
Preventive Care and Screening: Unhealthy Alcohol Use: Screening and Brief Counseling	CPH	Process
Tobacco Use and Help with Quitting Among Adolescents	CPH	Process
Weight Assessment and Counseling for Nutrition and Physical Activity for Children and Adolescents	CPH	Process
Adult Kidney Disease: Blood Pressure Management	ECC	Intermediate Outcome
Controlling High Blood Pressure	ECC	Intermediate Outcome
Diabetes: Hemoglobin A1c (HbA1c) Poor Control (>9%)	ECC	Intermediate Outcome
Door to Puncture Time for Endovascular Stroke Treatment	ECC	Intermediate Outcome
Hypertension: Improvement in Blood Pressure	ECC	Intermediate Outcome
Ischemic Vascular Disease: All or None Outcome Measure (Optimal Control)	ECC	Intermediate Outcome
Clinical Outcome Post Endovascular Stroke Treatment	ECC	Outcome
Depression Remission at Six Months	ECC	Outcome
Depression Remission at Twelve Months	ECC	Outcome
HIV Viral Load Suppression	ECC	Outcome
Optimal Asthma Control	ECC	Outcome
Surgical Site Infection	ECC	Outcome
Acute Otitis Externa: Topical Therapy	ECC	Process
ADHD: Follow-Up Care for Children Prescribed Attention-Deficit/Hyperactivity Disorder (ADHD) Medication	ECC	Process
Anti-Depressant Medication Management	ECC	Process

Medication A.R.E.A.S. Bundle

MEASURE NAME	NQS DOMAIN	MEASURE TYPE
Atrial Fibrillation and Atrial Flutter: Chronic Anticoagulation Therapy	ECC	Process
Chronic Obstructive Pulmonary Disease: Long-Acting Inhaled Bronchodilator Therapy	ECC	Process
Coronary Artery Disease: Angiotensin-Converting Enzyme (ACE) Inhibitor or Angiotensin Receptor Blocker (ARB) Therapy—Diabetes or Left Ventricular Systolic Dysfunction (LVEF < 40%)	ECC	Process
Coronary Artery Disease: Antiplatelet Therapy	ECC	Process
Coronary Artery Disease: Beta-Blocker Therapy-Prior Myocardial Infarction or Left Ventricular Systolic Dysfunction (LVEF <40%)	ECC	Process
Depression Utilization of the PHQ-9 Tool	ECC	Process
Documentation of Signed Opioid Treatment Agreement	ECC	Process
Evaluation or Interview for Risk of Opioid Misuse	ECC	Process
Heart Failure: Angiotensin-Converting Enzyme (ACE) Inhibitor or Angiotensin Receptor Blocker (ARB) Therapy for Left Ventricular Systolic Dysfunction	ECC	Process
Heart Failure: Beta-Blocker Therapy for Left Ventricular Systolic Dysfunction	ECC	Process
Hematology: Multiple Myeloma: Treatment with Bisphosphonates	ECC	Process
Initiation and Engagement of Alcohol and Other Drug Dependence Treatment	ECC	Process
Ischemic Vascular Disease: Use of Aspirin or Another Antiplatelet	ECC	Process
Opioid Therapy Follow-Up Evaluation	ECC	Process
Osteoporosis Management in Women Who Have Had a Fracture	ECC	Process
Perioperative Anti-platelet Therapy for Patients Undergoing Carotid Endarterectomy	ECC	Process
Persistence of Beta-Blocker Treatment after a Heart Attack	ECC	Process
Proportion Receiving Chemotherapy in the Last 14 Days of Life	ECC	Process
Rheumatoid Arthritis: Functional Status Assessment	ECC	Process
Rheumatoid Arthritis: Glucocorticoid Management	ECC	Process
Statin Therapy at Discharge after Lower Extremity Bypass	ECC	Process
Statin Therapy for the Prevention and Treatment of Cardiovascular Disease	ECC	Process

228

MEASURE NAME	NQS DOMAIN	MEASURE TYPE
Stroke and Stroke Rehabilitation: Discharged on Antithrombotic Therapy	ECC	Process
Stroke and Stroke Rehabilitation: Thrombolytic Therapy	ECC	Process
Acute Otitis Externa: Systemic Antimicrobial Therapy— Avoidance of Inappropriate Use	ECR	Process
Adult Sinusitis: Antibiotic Prescribed for Acute Sinusitis (Overuse)	ECR	Process
Adult Sinusitis: Appropriate Choice of Antibiotic: Amoxicillin with or without Clavulanate Prescribed for Patients with Acute Bacterial Sinusitis (Appropriate Use)	ECR	Process
Appropriate Treatment for Children with Upper Respiratory Infection	ECR	Process
Avoidance of Antibiotic Treatment in Adults with Acute Bronchitis	ECR	Process
Medication Management for People with Asthma	ECR	Process
Adherence to Antipsychotic Medications for Individuals with Schizophrenia	PS	Intermediate Outcome
Documentation of Current Medications in the Medical Record	PS	Process
Elder Maltreatment Screen and Follow-Up Plan	PS	Process
Perioperative Care: Selection of Prophylactic Antibiotic— First or Second Generation Cephalosporin	PS	Process
Perioperative Care: Venous Thromboembolism Prophylaxis (When Indicated in All Patients)	PS	Process
Use of High-Risk Medications in the Elderly	PS	Process
Pain Brought Under Control Within 48 Hours	PCEO	Outcome
Psoriasis: Clinical Response to Oral Systemic or Biologic Medications	PCEO	Outcome
CAHPS for PQRS Clinician/Group Survey	PCEO	Patient Engagement/ Experience
Hepatitis C: Discussion and Shared Decision Making Surrounding Treatment Options	PCEO	Process
Osteoarthritis: Function and Pain Assessment	PCEO	Process

ACO Quality Measure Benchmarks (2015 Reporting Year)

Before an ACO can share in any savings created, it must demonstrate that it meets the quality performance standard for that year. CMS does this by measuring the quality of care in ACOs using 33 nationally recognized quality measures under the four key domains, including: patient/caregiver experience (eight measures); care coordination/ patient safety (10 measures); preventive care (eight measures); and at-risk population, which covers diabetes (two measures evaluated as one composite measure), hypertension (one measure), ischemic vascular disease (one measure), heart failure (one measure), coronary artery disease (one measure), and depression (one measure).[8]

When the MAB Rx is implemented and integrated into the care delivery system of an ACO, it will support the ACO in meeting many of its quality measures. Some of the key measures that MAB can support in the four domains include:

Measures in the At-Risk Population Domain

- At-Risk Population Diabetes Composite: percent of beneficiaries with diabetes whose HbA1c is in poor control (greater than 9%)
- At-Risk Population Hypertension: percent of beneficiaries with hypertension whose BP is less than 140/90
- At-Risk Population IVD (ischemic vascular disease): percent of beneficiaries with IVD who use aspirin or other antithrombotic
- At-Risk Population heart failure: beta-blocker therapy for LVSD (Left Ventricular Systolic Dysfunction)
- At-Risk Population coronary artery disease (CAD): ACE inhibitor or ARB therapy for patients with CAD and diabetes and/or LVSD
- At-Risk Population Depression: depression remission at 12 months

Measures in the Care Coordination/Patient Safety Domain

- Risk Standardized, All Condition Readmissions
- ASC Admissions COPD or Asthma in Older Adults
- ASC Admission Heart Failure

- Skilled Nursing Facility 30-Day All-Cause Readmission Measure
- All-Cause Unplanned Admissions for Patients with Diabetes
- All-Cause Unplanned Admissions for Patients with Heart Failure
- All-Cause Unplanned Admissions for Patients with MCC
- Documentation of Current Medications in the Medical Record

Measures in the Patient/Caregiver Experience Domain
- Health Promotion and Education
- Stewardship of Patient Resources

Measures in Preventive Care Domain
- Influenza Immunization
- Pneumococcal Vaccination
- Tobacco Use Assessment and Cessation Intervention
- Depression Screening
- Proportion of Adults Who Had Blood Pressure Screened in Past Two Years

PQRS Domains
The Physician Quality Reporting System (PQRS) is a voluntary program that encourages individual eligible professionals (EPs) and group practices to provide information about their quality of care to Medicare. Individual EPs and PQRS group practices choose at least nine individual measures (out of over 280) for at least 50% of the eligible Medicare Part B FFS patients. The chosen measures should cover at least three of the six NQS domains, or one measures group as an option. Individual EPs or PQRS group practices are also required to report one cross-cutting measure if they have at least one Medicare patient with a face-to-face encounter.[9] The 280+ PQRS measures fall under the following six domains:

- Communication and Care Coordination
- Community, Population, and Public Health
- Effective Clinical Care

- Efficiency and Cost Reduction Use of Healthcare Resources
- Patient Safety—Making Care Safer by Reducing Harm Caused in the Delivery of Care
- Person and Caregiver-Centered Experience Outcomes

When the MAB Rx is implemented and integrated into the care delivery system, it will support providers in meeting many of their quality measures. The PQRS entity will be folded into MIPS at the end of 2018.

Hospital Readmissions Reduction Program (HRRP)

The HRRP was established to improve healthcare for people on Medicare by linking what CMS pays hospitals to the quality of the care they provide, and not just quantity of the services they provide in a given performance period. The HRRP now provides financial incentives to hospitals to reduce costly, unplanned, and unnecessary hospital readmissions (within 30 days of the initial admission), especially in these following conditions: acute myocardial infarction, heart failure, pneumonia, acute exacerbation of chronic obstructive pulmonary disease (COPD), elective total hip or total knee replacement, and coronary artery bypass graft surgery.[10] MAB can be leveraged upon admissions, during the pre-discharge and discharge processes and the follow-up process, and in the coordination of care across the continuum to reduce medication-related readmissions and the associated subsequent penalties.

Patient Safety

Medical errors and unsafe care harm and kill tens of thousands of Americans each year. The facts are alarming. Approximately 2 million healthcare-associated infections occur annually, accounting for an estimated 90,000 deaths and more than $4.5 billion in hospital healthcare costs.[11] Unplanned, often preventable, hospital admissions and readmissions cost Medicare and the private sector billions of dollars each year and take a significant toll on patients and families, who suffer from prolonged illness or pain, emotional distress, and loss of productivity.

As a result, the NQS has emphasized making care safer and made it a national priority by focusing on these three goals:

- Reduce preventable hospital admissions and readmissions
- Reduce the incidence of adverse healthcare-associated conditions
- Reduce harm from inappropriate or unnecessary care[12]

MAB can support the practices that will improve the following measures and help meet the NQS goals (some of which have been endorsed by the National Quality Forum):

- Plan of Care to Prevent Future Falls
- Documentation of Current Medications in the Medical Record
- Multifactor Fall Risk Assessment Conducted for All Patients Who Can Ambulate
- INR Monitoring for Individuals on Warfarin after Hospital Discharge
- Medication Reconciliation Post-Discharge

CAHPS Service Measures

CAHPS surveys are designed to reliably assess the experiences of a large sample of patients. They use standardized questions and data collection protocols to ensure information can be compared across healthcare settings. There are a number of CMS CAHPS surveys: Hospital CAHPS; Home Health CAHPS; Fee-for-Service CAHPS; Medicare Advantage and Prescription Drug Plan CAHPS; In-Center Hemodialysis CAHPS; Nationwide Adult Medicaid CAHPS; Hospice, Outpatient and Ambulatory Surgery CAHPS; CAHPS for PQRS; and CAHPS Survey for ACOs participating in Medicare initiatives.[13]

Clinical services emphasizing MAB can positively contribute and impact survey questions in some of the domains. For example, see the

ACO CAHPS survey. It has a total of nine domains with 71 questions focused on the following:

- Getting timely care, appointments, and information
- How well providers communicate
- Patient's rating of provider
- Access to specialists
- Health promotion and education
- Shared decision making
- Health status and functional status
- Courteous and helpful office staff
- Stewardship of patient resources

The CAHPS for ACO-12 survey has 12 domains with 80 questions focused on the same nine areas as above and the following:

- Care Coordination
- Between Visit Communication
- Taking Medications as Directed[14]

For this survey, clinical MAB services will contribute to the following domains: getting timely care, appointments, and information; health promotion and education; shared decision making; stewardship of patient resources; care coordination; between visit communication; and helping take medications as directed.

Affordability—Focusing on Resources and Efficiencies
There are a lack of resource and affordability measures to balance the value equation (Value = clinical outcomes and quality x patient care experience/cost and resources spent). So measures addressing costs and appropriate use of services, including measures of overuse and affordability, have been made a priority under one of the MACRA quality domains. Also, many organizations have affordability and utilization measures, and there are some existing PQRS efficiency and

cost reduction measures that MAB can support and improve. These include the following:

- Appropriate Treatment for Children with Upper Respiratory Infection
- Appropriate Testing for Children with Pharyngitis
- Acute Otitis Externa Systemic Antimicrobial Therapy—Avoidance of Inappropriate Use
- Antibiotic Treatment for Adults with Acute Bronchitis—Avoidance of Inappropriate Use
- Adult Sinusitis—Antibiotic Prescribed for Acute Sinusitis (Overuse)
- Adult Sinusitis Appropriate Choice of Antibiotic—Amoxicillin with or without Clavulanate Prescribed for Patients with Acute Bacterial Sinusitis (Appropriate Use)
- Address Appropriate Use of Medications

Other Programs That MAB Can Impact

MAB can directly and indirectly contribute to quality measures in the following programs:

Other Hospital Reporting Programs
- Hospital Inpatient Quality Reporting (IQR) Program
- Hospital Value-Based Purchasing (VBP) Program
- Hospital-Acquired Condition (HAC) Reduction Program
- Hospital Outpatient Quality Reporting (OQR) Program

Other Health Plan Reporting Programs
- eValue8

MAB Impacting the National Quality Strategy (NQS)

Chapter 4 focused on how the ACA was seeking to increase access to high-quality, affordable healthcare for all Americans, in part through the development of the NQS. This strategy is contributing to a measurable improvement in outcomes of care and in the overall health of the American people by pursuing these three broad aims: better care, affordable care, and healthier people and communities (see Chapter 4).[15]

These three aims have been advanced by the following six priorities based on research, input from a broad range of stakeholders, existing effective quality measures, and practices from around the country:

- Making care safer by reducing harm caused in the delivery of care
- Ensuring each person and family are engaged as partners in care
- Promoting effective communication and coordination of care
- Promoting the most effective prevention and treatment practices for the leading causes of mortality, starting with cardiovascular disease
- Working with communities to promote wide use of best practices to enable healthy living
- Making quality care more affordable for individuals, families, employers, and governments by developing and spreading new healthcare delivery models[16]
  Programs and services using all or some components of MAB have positively impacted some of the above priorities and contributed to the three aims of the NQS.

1. *Making Care Safer Can Be Enhanced by Safe Medication Use*

Adverse medication events cause more than 770,000 injuries and deaths each year, and the cost of treating patients who are harmed by these events is estimated to be as high as $5 billion annually.[17] The NQS long-term goals are to accomplish the following:

- Reduce preventable hospital admissions and readmissions.
- Reduce the incidence of adverse healthcare-associated conditions.
- Reduce harm from inappropriate or unnecessary care.

Healthcare providers are working relentlessly to accomplish these goals, aiming for zero harm whenever possible and striving to create a system that reliably provides high-quality healthcare for everyone. Below are examples of programs and services that are using components of or the whole MAB and are making care safer for all.

- *Antibiotic Stewardship Programs*: Research has shown that up to 30% of antibiotics in the United States are inappropriately prescribed, and the overuse of antibiotics is linked to the increasing number of resistant superbugs.[18] A research team from the Warren Alpert Medical School of Brown University and the Dana-Farber Cancer Institute analyzed 26 studies pertaining to antibiotic use in hospitals, ranging from six months to three years. They found that hospitals with antibiotic stewardship programs had a decrease in the number of antibiotics being prescribed to patients and a decrease in bacterial infection rates and length of stay. The study also showed that in some of the programs, the clinical infection rates decreased by more than 4%, and the length of stay decreased by nearly 9%.[19]

- *Prescription Drug Monitoring Programs (PDMPs)*: PDMPs are state-run electronic databases used to track the prescribing and dispensing of controlled prescription drugs to patients. They are designed to monitor this information for suspected abuse or diversion (for example, channeling drugs into illegal use), and can give a prescriber or pharmacist critical information regarding a patient's controlled substance prescription history. This information can help prescribers and pharmacists identify patients at high risk who would benefit from early interventions. PDMPs continue to be among the most promising state-level interventions to improve opioid prescribing, inform clinical practices, and protect patients at risk. Additional research is needed to evaluate PDMP practices and policies to identify best practices.[20]

- *Pharmacogenomics Programs*: Many of the drugs available today to treat cancer, heart disease, and other conditions are powerful agents that work as intended in most patients. Yet, for some patients, a particular drug at the standard dose might not work well enough or may even trigger a serious adverse reaction because of the patient's genetics. Pharmacogenomics—which involves studying how a person's specific DNA sequence influences their response to medications—is very patient-centered because its goal is to ensure patients get the right drug at the right dose at the right time to obtain the best outcomes. By using a person's unique genetic makeup as a factor when prescribing a drug, a physician can maximize treatment effectiveness while avoiding potentially life-threatening side effects.[21]

2. *Ensuring Person- and Family-Centered Care*

Healthcare delivery in the United States is not often designed around meeting the needs of the patient. However, this is changing as providers are encouraging patients and families to play a more active role in their care. Engaging patients in their own care and taking into account individual and family circumstances, as well as differing cultures, languages, disabilities, health literacy levels, and social backgrounds, will ensure more patient engagement and a better partnership between the provider and patient. Most likely, this will also ensure the following long-term goals:

- Improve patient, family, and caregiver experience of care related to quality, safety, and access across settings
- Develop culturally sensitive and understandable care plans in partnership with patients, families, and caregivers and using a shared decision-making process
- Enable patients, their families, and caregivers to navigate, coordinate, and manage their care appropriately and effectively

Below are examples of programs and services that are using components of or the whole MAB to contribute to person-centered care:

- *CVS Health's Pharmacy Advisor Program*: Through Pharmacy Advisor, pharmacists use technology to identify which patients are at risk of not taking their medications as directed. These patients receive a phone call or, in many cases, an in-person reminder from the pharmacist, who provides them with useful information on how they can better control their conditions by being more aware and mindful of how and when they take their medications. This program has had a major impact in the lives of patients trying to manage the disease.[22]

- *Kaiser Permanente Outpatient Pharmacy Clinical Services (OPCS)*: OPCS was established to improve the screening rates and medication adherence rates and contribute to the health outcomes of patients with diabetes mellitus or coronary artery disease with hemoglobin A1c (HbA1c) or low-density lipoprotein cholesterol (LDL-C) outside clinical goals. Pharmacists engaged identified patients and caregivers with a face-to-face BSMART consult to pinpoint barriers to medication adherence, work on solutions to identified barriers, motivate patients, recommend adherence tools, reinforce the pharmacist-patient relationship, and triage, if needed, refer them to other services, such as health education. By encouraging nonadherent patients to restart their diabetes or lipid medications during face-to-face consults, the OPCS pharmacist was able to influence and improve medication adherence rates, screening rates, and clinical outcomes, particularly among patients with diabetes.[23]

3. *Promoting Effective Communication and Coordination of Care*
Effective communication and care coordination will contribute to achieving these goals:

- Improve the quality of care transitions and communication across care settings
- Improve the quality of life for patients with chronic illness and disabilities by following a care plan that anticipates and addresses pain and symptom management, psychosocial needs, and functional status

- Establish shared accountability and integration of communities and healthcare systems to reduce healthcare disparities

Below are examples of programs and services that are using components of or the whole MAB to contribute to the improvement of effective communication and care coordination.

- *Medication reconciliation at interfaces of care*: Medication errors and poor communication between providers in the inpatient setting and other post-acute care settings (nursing homes, assisted living, and health homes) are some key drivers for readmissions within 30 days. Readmissions are also a major source of patient and family stress and may contribute substantially to loss of functional ability, particularly in older adults. The medication reconciliation process is an effective communication and care coordination tool to optimize patients' health outcomes and reduce readmissions, by preventing medication therapy duplications, interactions, omissions, and other medication errors at interfaces of care.

  To facilitate the coordination of care for patients on multiple medications, pharmacists are working with all of the patient's healthcare providers and pharmacies to streamline the number of medications patients take, have patients go to only one pharmacy for all their medication needs (when possible), and ensure patients always have the most up-to-date list of all their medications. This will improve patient health outcomes, reduce costs, and improve the patient care experience.

- *The Medication Therapy Management Programs*: The University of Florida Medication Therapy Management Communication and Care Center, a student-staffed call center, was established in March 2010 for fourth-year student pharmacists. These students:

  - Performed comprehensive medication reviews (CMR) via telephone
  - Completed patient chart quarterly reviews

- Provided patients with personalized medication lists
- Notified prescribers of potential issues or problems following the review
- Mailed medication-related action plans to patients following the CMR
- Spoke to patients regarding adherence issues[24]

These and other related services are helping improve communication and coordination of care by resolving medication-related and health-related problems, optimizing medication use for improved patient outcomes, and promoting patient self-management of medication and disease states. The university's call center has served more than 400,000 people nationwide and delivered medication therapy management services to more than 50,000 patients since its inception.[25]

4. *Promoting Prevention and Treatment of the Leading Causes of Mortality*

More than 133 million Americans have at least one chronic illness, and many have several. As individuals and health systems feel the strain of this growing trend, preventing and treating a number of leading causes of mortality and illness in adults and children—including cardiovascular disease, cancer, diabetes, HIV/AIDS, premature births, and behavioral health conditions—is crucial. Among these, cardiovascular disease is the deadliest, accounting for one of every three deaths in this country. Over $503 billion is spent annually on cardiovascular disease. Approximately 75 million Americans have high blood pressure, 18 million have a history of heart attack or angina, 6 million have a history of heart failure, and 6 million have a history of stroke.

How can healthcare providers and teams promote the effective, evidence-based prevention and treatment for cardiovascular disease and other diseases? This can be done by promoting cardiovascular health through:

- Community interventions that result in improvement of social, economic, and environmental factors
- Interventions that result in adoption of the most important healthy lifestyle behaviors across the lifespan
- Receipt of effective clinical preventive services across the lifespan in clinical and community settings

Below are examples of programs and services that are using components of or the whole MAB to promote the most effective treatment of leading causes of mortality in patients with cardiovascular disease:

- A 2005–08 CVS Caremark integrated pharmacy study examined the impact of medication adherence (and MAB) in chronic vascular disease on health services spending for patients age 65 and older. It found that the annual total per person healthcare savings were $7,893 for congestive heart failure, $5,824 for hypertension, $5,170 for diabetes, and $1,847 for dyslipidemia. The average benefit-cost ratios from adherence for this group were 8.6:1 for congestive heart failure, 13.5:1 for hypertension, 8.6:1 for diabetes, and 3.8:1 for dyslipidemia.[26]
- An effective intervention for patients with cardiovascular disease is aspirin, blood pressure control, cholesterol reduction, and smoking cessation (the ABCS bundle). However, over 50% of patients on these lifesaving medications are not taking them as prescribed, leading to increased mortality, hospitalizations, progression of disease, and healthcare costs. Implementing MAB, along with healthy lifestyle changes, in cardiovascular disease patients improved their health outcomes.[27]

5. *Promoting Wide Use of Best Practices to Enable Healthy Living*
Health is a state of physical, mental, and social well-being, not merely the absence of disease or infirmity. In addition to biology and genetics, our health is affected by a range of factors, such as individual behavior,

access to health services, and the environment in which we live. The broad goal of promoting better health is one that is shared across the nation to accomplish the following:

- Improvement of social, economic, and environmental factors from community interventions
- Adoption of the most important healthy lifestyle behaviors across the lifespan
- Getting effective preventive services across the lifespan in clinical and community settings

Below are examples of programs and services using components of or the whole MAB to ensure person-centered care:

- *The Walgreens Mental Health Initiative*: In 2016, Walgreens launched a new mental health platform and campaign to help meet the growing need for resources and access to care. The Walgreens mental health platform aims to improve health outcomes through patient engagement and early screening and intervention; to heighten consumer awareness and reduce stigmas associated with mental illness; and to connect more people with clinical resources in their communities. The initiative launches in conjunction with Mental Health Month, observed each May in the US.[28]
- *Immunization services*: Community pharmacy-based immunization programs have become a standard of practice across the United States and are a convenient and accessible option for receiving immunizations. This is an opportunity to provide patient-centered care, improve patient outcomes, and contribute to the overall health of people in the communities.

6. *Making Quality Care More Affordable*

Nearly every year for the past 30 years, healthcare spending has risen at a faster rate than the economy. And over the last few years, the cost of medications has risen even faster than healthcare spending. These rising costs have put a burden on America's families as patients, taxpayers, business owners, and employees watch a growing share of their paychecks go to pay for healthcare. Many organizations are putting affordability strategies in place that will accomplish the following:

- Ensure affordable and accessible high-quality healthcare for individuals, families, employers, and governments
- Support and enable communities to ensure accessible, high-quality care while reducing waste and fraud

Building Effective MAB Scorecards and Reports

Peter Drucker, the great leadership theorist, once observed: "What's measured improves."[29] That has never been truer than when we want to improve patients' health outcomes and organizations' operational efficiencies and effectiveness. Healthcare providers share a common goal: providing high-quality care to their patients. Measuring performance allows for an analysis of where and what changes need to be made to improve performance and the quality of care provided, and allows providers and teams to see what is working well.[30] However, this has led to the development of dozens of performance scorecards and reports in many organizations with hundreds (and, in some cases, thousands) of measures to satisfy multiple stakeholders, internally and externally.

While many of these reports and scorecards may be needed, it is critical for organizations to streamline and prioritize what they are going to measure and to look for opportunities to identify cross-cutting measures that can be used in multiple settings and instances. One of the key places to get the scorecard and report development right is in the care delivery operations. This is where team members need information to address the four IHI continuous improvement questions: How good are we? How do we compare to the best? Where are the variations? Are we improving over time?

To build an effective scorecard or performance report that answers those four questions, one must have:

- *An engaged team*: This team wants to internalize the mission of the organization, understand the purpose of the project or initiative, and has the characteristics of a high performing team (see Chapter 10).
- *The right performance-measurement generating system*: What you measure is what you get. Leaders understand that their organization's measurement system strongly affects the behavior of managers and employees. Therefore, a performance-measurement system should be designed to reflect the basic operating assumptions of the organization. This is especially important for multifunctional teams that may need to slice and dice the data to look at different aspects of the business and meet the changing needs of the organization. The system also needs to be able to generate reports and scorecards that are meaningful to the organization to drive performance.
- *The right key measures*: The measures selected for the scorecards and performance reports should have the biggest return on better quality of life for patients and be aligned with the goals and strategies the organization has set forth to have a competitive advantage to excel. Measures should primarily be a mixture of process (lead) measures and outcome (lag) measures, to help teams understand their processes and to make sure that their processes are helping them get the outcomes they desire.

The fewer measures the better (up to a point); however, this concept has eluded many teams that have so many measures they feel like they are drowning in data and are unable to make an impact. To come up with an effective set of core measures to successfully meet the established goals, organizations should have a strategic, multifunctional group of key stakeholders who can identify all the measures necessary for success. Then these stakeholders should work together to identify the measures that will have the biggest impact on the key organization strategies and focus first on goals that will close the widest gaps.

Build the scorecards: To help teams, managers, and executives effectively use data to improve performance, they should have at least these three types of scorecards or reports: the team scorecard (focused on the Triple Aim), the coach's operational scorecard (focused on processes and management), and the executive level scorecard (focused on the health of the organization).

- The *team scorecard* should be simple, visible, have the right leading and lagging measures that reflect quality of care, service and access, cost, and informs the team immediately whether they are winning or losing.[31]
- The *coach's scorecard* is for the manager and is much more detailed. It is more focused on the operational details with structural, process, and balanced measures to ensure the behaviors, structures, and processes put in place are indeed the right ones to get the team to deliver on the outcomes necessary for success.
- The *executive or senior leaders' scorecard* should have the measures that give them a fast but comprehensive view of the health of the business.

Review the scorecards frequently: A cadence of accountability to improve performance is critical for driving performance. For critical or new projects, teams should meet at least weekly to review the performance scorecard or reports and course-correct as needed. During the meeting, the team should use the four IHI questions as a guide to discuss their measures: How good are we (baseline)? How do we compare to the best (benchmarks and goals)? Where are the variations (both warranted and unwarranted)? Are we improving over time (are our interventions making a difference)? Additional questions that should be asked to evaluate progress include: What's going well? What's not going well? Where are the opportunities for improvement that will create a new positive trend? The goal is to create excitement about achieving better results and improving performance at the same time.

Data Transparency

One of the most effective and powerful methods to improve performance is to provide teams with performance data at the team level and the individual level. Then provide them with comparison data of comparable teams or peers that have been risk-adjusted (when necessary). Evidence has shown that unblinded provider and team data, presented in a respectful way, has led to a decline in errors, reduced unwarranted variation, and improved performance, leading to better patient outcomes.

While there are organizations and providers that are not fully on board with data transparency (for fear of negative repercussions), from an ethical, safety, and economic point of view, data transparency is crucial to promote better patient outcomes. From an ethical point of view, patients have a vital stake in the outcomes of healthcare and therefore need to know how organizations and providers are doing.[32]

From the point of view of improving patient safety, performance transparency is crucial. "It is the cornerstone of the cultural transformation that our health care organizations need to undergo to become safe," says Lucian Leape, MD. "Transparency is essential within an institution if caregivers are to feel safe in reporting and talking about their mistakes. The free flow of information is essential for identifying and correcting the underlying systems failures. Transparency is also the key to successful—and ethical—responses to patients when things go wrong. It is the cover-ups that lead to lawsuits. And transparency is essential for accountability, to show the public that the hospital or system responds ethically to its failures. Internal transparency begets external transparency—and vice-versa."[33]

From an economic point of view, consumer access to full information is a critical element of the value-driven purchase of healthcare. Consumers can make meaningful choices only if they have complete information.[34] In the past, few patients and even fewer doctors paid attention to data when deciding where to get their care. This is now changing in light of the ACA—patients are paying much more for their own healthcare and are paying more attention to the value provided by the healthcare system.

In 2016, CMS began posting quality performance data on individual physicians on its Physician Compare website for the first time. The data included 2014 clinical quality performance measures for about 40,000 individual physicians who submitted information through Medicare's Physician Quality Reporting System. Also, CMS updated quality data on ACOs, group practices, and hospitals.

CMS has now published patient experience and clinical quality data for about 20 Pioneer ACOs and more than 330 MSSP ACOs on Physician Compare. In addition, CMS has added new quality measures to its Hospital Compare website for hospital surgical practices and for certain healthcare-associated infections, and has removed several quality measures for which most hospitals had performed well. According to Dr. Leape, "Transparency is an idea whose time has come, and both hospitals and the public will be better off because of it."[35]

MAB Performance Report Used by Dr. Sam

How did Dr. Sam and the team select the measures for the scorecard? The medical and pharmacy leaders had five buckets of measures aligned to the organizational goals and strategies to measure the outcomes and ROI of the Clinical MAB services. These were Quality, Patient Care Experience (Service), Affordability, Productivity, and People.

Under each bucket, measures, taken from key national and organizational priorities and programs (the associated detailed domains and some key measures are listed earlier in this chapter), were reviewed:

Quality:
- HEDIS
- Hospital Reporting Programs
- Medicare Stars Program
- PQRS
- Patient Safety

Patient Care Experience (Service):
- Patient Experience of Care (CAHPS/CAHPS Survey)
- Pharmacy Standardized Service Survey

Affordability:
- A few measures from the PQRS efficiency and cost reduction domain
- Drug use management measures
- Per-member-per-month (PMPM) costs

Productivity:
- Number of patients seen daily (in person or virtually)
- Changes in patient outcomes monthly

People:
- Team and peer surveys, twice a year
- Quarterly patient satisfaction surveys

Measures were also taken from the following: Pay for Value—MIPS Quality Measures (focusing on three of the four MIPS performance categories—quality, resource use, and clinical practice improvement activities) and the ACOs MSSP domains: patient/caregiver experience, care coordination/patient safety, at-risk population, and preventive care.

Once the team identified all the measures necessary for success, they worked together to identify the measures that would have the biggest impact on the key organization strategies and goals and close the widest gaps to demonstrate the value of MAB. Working with providers, IT, and other key stakeholders, the team helped develop the following reports:

- *Medication A.R.E.A.S. Vital Signs Performance Reports*: There were three performance reports developed: the executive vital signs report, the team level report, and the provider level report. Due to multiple reports already in existence, the core measures associated with the Medication A.R.E.A.S. were incorporated into the overall organization vital signs dashboard. The team and provider reports remained because of the value they brought to the teams and providers.

At the team meetings, the MAB pharmacist would share the report with his or her team. Then the team would discuss the progress being made using the four IHI questions as a guide to assess the overall level of quality and to understand how they were driving performance. These questions helped the teams focus their attention on the right measures, set the right priorities, and hold themselves accountable as a team for the outcomes of their populations.

- *Manager Performance Report*: This report helped the manager for the MAB services and each pharmacist see their effectiveness and efficiency, in addition to their outcomes. It had the same measures as the above, with the following added:

  - Productivity, patients seen per hour/per pharmacist
  - Risk adjustment information for the population serviced (from the physician database)
  - Peer and provider survey results (every six months)
  - Outcomes/cost per patient/pharmacist

Throughout the year, the teams modified the reports to ensure they were aligned strategically with the goals and focus of the program and organization, and a new culture of accountability was developed that ultimately benefited the patient.

Chapter 9:
Solid Business Capabilities and Infrastructures—Build/Optimize/ Consolidate Structures to Successfully Implement, Support, and Sustain MAB

"When you don't invest in infrastructure,
you are going to pay sooner or later."
Mike Parker[1]

Topics Covered:

* The purpose of solid infrastructures and business capabilities to support the MAB Rx
* The infrastructures and capabilities needed to successfully implement, support, and sustain MAB
* Integration opportunities of the infrastructures and capabilities

Think about the home you live in and its usual purpose: a place that keeps you secure, enables you to grow and develop, and is an investment for the future. What if you found out that the framework of your house was built with cheap, faulty materials, capable of collapsing on a windy day? What would you do?

Now compare the workplace to this analogy. Imagine your team has just developed an incredible strategy that could help make the organization more secure, achieve a competitive sustainable advantage, and expand its geographic reach and influence. As your team is about to roll out the plan, they realize the infrastructures and business capabilities necessary to support the successful implementation, scalability, and sustainability of this amazing strategy is faulty or weak at best. How successful are you going to be in executing this new strategy? This is what Mike Parker meant when he said, "When you don't invest in infrastructure, you are going to pay sooner or later."

Today in healthcare, many organizations are building strategies and initiatives to improve care delivery and the patient-provider relationship. However, the success, scalability, and sustainability of the outcomes are largely dependent on having the right processes, products, infrastructures, and capabilities in place and made available to support providers and team members—components that many teams sometimes minimize, overgeneralize, or pay little attention to. As organizations strive to be high-performing and provide high-quality, affordable, and well-coordinated healthcare to their patients, they recognize the need for these components to support their innovations and strategies both for the short and long term.

When aligned effectively, an organization's business capabilities (a combination of processes, tools, and structures) will deliver specified outcomes, creating unparalleled value for that organization. The critical capabilities and infrastructures needed to successfully implement, support, optimize, and sustain MAB across the continuum of care include: effective pharmacy benefit management (PBM) and drug use management infrastructures, an evolving drug supply chain management system, "big data" and analytics, efficient health information technology systems, and a solid compliance infrastructure, to name a few.

Pharmacy Benefit Management and Drug Use Management Infrastructures

Healthcare spending in the United States is growing faster than the economy, but prescription medication costs are growing faster still. PBMs have become one of the most effective infrastructures that have contributed to bending the cost trends of prescription drugs, while at the same time contributing to improving patient health outcomes. PBMs are able to do this by providing programs and services designed to help maximize drug effectiveness; improving drug expenditures by appropriately influencing the behaviors of prescribing physicians, providers, and patients; and, in many cases, providing clinical, specialty, or disease management services.[2]

Few large organizations have their own comprehensive PBMs, and some are internalizing many components of the PBM capabilities as they consolidate. But most organizations, health plans, employer groups, unions, and the government still contract with PBMs to handle one or more of the following (known as ABC capabilities):

- *Administrative services*: This involves processing and analyzing claims, billing, enrollments, and data reporting.
- *Benefits management services*: These services develop and manage formularies and prior authorization programs, contract with network pharmacies, manage a maximum allowable costs list, negotiate rebate arrangements, operate mail-order pharmacies and mail-order claims, and perform drug utilization reviews.
- *Clinical services*: Larger PBMs are now offering clinical, medical, and analytic services, such as therapy or disease management programs that incorporate MAB, programs to ensure patient adherence, specialty pharmacy and distribution services, data analytics, and predictive modeling.

The pharmacy benefit management programs—whether integrated into the healthcare system (like Kaiser or the VA), part of retail pharmacies (like CVS or Walgreens), part of specialty pharmacies (like Express Scripts), or part of an insurance company (like UnitedHealth Group)—are now adopting components of MAB as critical strategies to improve patient outcomes.

Most of these organizations have built the following processes, structures, and capabilities to optimize and sustain components of MAB.

Adherence

PBMs now have medication adherence tools and programs to support the improvement of clinical quality and patient health outcomes, to reduce total healthcare costs, and to improve Medicare Stars ratings (and other quality programs) through improved mediation adherence. These programs focus on ensuring patients adhere to prescribed drug therapies for chronic diseases, such as diabetes, asthma, dyslipidemia, and hypertension. Examples of programs that PBMs use are:

- The 90-day fill and refill programs via mail-order service coupled with a lower co-pay, refill reminders, auto-refills, and patient education
- Clinical services with pharmacists and team members addressing patients' barriers, offering customized solutions, motivating them to stay on track, providing them with tools and reminders, and referring them to other resources internally or in the community (BSMART checklist)
- The Optum Adherence Solution, a three-step, proactive program approach[3]
- Predictive analytic services provided by RxAnte and AllazoHealth[4,5]

Reconciliation

Medication reconciliation is a component of the reviews PBMs do in their medication therapy management (MTM) programs. Reconciliation is done to prevent drug interactions and duplications, which can directly or indirectly lead to hospitalizations and readmissions. Also, since medication management and medication reconciliation are included in the Stage 2 and Stage 3 Meaningful Use criteria, reconciliation is seen as a value-added service to health plans and systems.

Engagement

Digital tools, patient portals, and other programs are now transforming the education, empowerment, and engagement of patients and consumers.

Some PBMs are leveraging these programs and tools to keep consumers connected regarding their health—helping them order and manage their prescriptions online, assisting them to better understand plan coverage and prescription drug costs, tracking their medication-related expenses, and monitoring their medication use. Examples of engagement tools include:

- The Briova Community: a program where patients are emailed videos tailored to their conditions and treatment regimens.[6]
- Med Remind: This CVS pharmacy mobile app helps customers stay on track with their medication schedules by enabling them to customize reminders to take their prescriptions at the right time. It also sends notifications to caregivers when a dose is missed. It includes text reminders and the ability to receive reminders on the Apple Watch.[7]
- UBC and DrFirst: UBC, an Express Scripts company, and DrFirst are collaborating to leverage the DrFirst's Patient Advisor platform. It will raise awareness of important programs for providers, improve medication adherence, and transform patient engagement in ways that lead to better decisions and healthier outcomes.[8]

Affordability

PBMs and organizations are able to reduce pharmacy drug expenditures and contribute to reducing the total costs of care through effective drug use management programs. Key components of these programs include:

- *Formularies*: PBMs have established formularies, or preferred drug lists, so purchasing resources can be concentrated on making appropriate drugs (especially generics) available to most plan members, while allowing for medically necessary alternatives for a few select patients.[9] To control prescription drug spending, some of the largest PBMs are now excluding certain medicines from their formularies covered by health insurance.

For example, in 2017 Express Scripts will exclude 85 medicines from its national formulary, with a potential savings of about $1.8 billion.[10]

- *Leveraging generics and, eventually, biosimilar alternatives*: Generic drugs will continue to gain market share as organizations, payers, and health plans seek to reduce costs. Generic drugs already comprise about 70% of the US market by volume, and over 80% in some PBMs. Also, with the advent of potentially less costly biosimilar alternatives, PBMs, delivery systems, and payers are going to leverage these products in place of the high-cost specialty medications. Eventually, they will use them to manage costs where possible and appropriate.[11] Promoting the use of generics and preferred brand medications by using formularies, tiered cost sharing, prior authorization, step therapy protocols, generic incentives, provider outreach, and patient education are also strategies that PBMs and organizations are using to bend the cost curve.[12]

- *Contracts*: PBMs are negotiating effective contracts to get the best prices for organizations and volume discounts. They are also implementing maximum allowable cost pricing with retail and mail-order pharmacies to provide health plan members with convenient access to selected medications.[13]

- *Performance comparisons*: PBMs are implementing, tracking, evaluating, and reporting utilization of targeted medications and medication classes by provider to organizations, which has helped reduce unwarranted variation in prescribing of nonformulary medications. Balanced measures are also used to evaluate impact of initiative work to assure safe, rational, cost-effective prescribing. Clinician or department-level decision support and feedback tools have been developed to effectively engage providers and get support for the formulary process.

- *Medication adherence programs*: Successful treatment of disease with prescription medicines requires the patient consistently use the medicines as prescribed. Adherence to therapy regimen is especially important for management of chronic diseases, such as diabetes, heart disease, arthritis, and cancer. PBMs and organizations have included adherence strategies such as Medicare Part D medication therapy management programs, medication management services for targeted populations, imbedded adherence data into EHRs, and other adherence-type strategies in their drug use management programs in order to create win-win solutions. Patients, employers, insurers, integrated delivery systems, and the public all benefit.

- *Differential co-pays*: To promote the use of formulary or preferred medications, which can be very beneficial to the total costs, many organizations have preferential co-pays for these medications. For example, they charge a $5 co-pay for a 30-day supply of a preferred medication, and a $20 or more co-pay for a 30-day supply of a nonpreferred or nonformulary medication.

- *Education teams*: PBMs now have education teams (sometimes referred to as drug education coordinators) to provide comprehensive drug information in response to clinician and staff inquiries, develop effective drug use management strategies, and promote effective drug therapy use practices among providers. They also work with prescribers to ensure patients are using drugs appropriately. In some cases, they provide high-quality service and information in response to member inquiries regarding general or personalized drug information.

- *Research teams*: PBMs and organizations are having their research teams identify the medications that have the best value and best outcomes at the lowest cost. Based on these findings, they are negotiating value-based contracts or are making the drug manufacturers justify the cost of their products before considering them for the formulary.

- *Other drug price control strategies:*
  - Utilize big data to show value by using claims data to assess patient outcomes versus unit cost or cost to deliver care
  - Leverage genomics to eliminate unnecessary prescribing and

prevent overutilization of high-cost drugs—called precision medicine

▫ Negotiate rebates from drug manufacturers that compete with therapeutically similar brands and generics

▫ Take a stand against the incredible drug price increases that are adding unnecessary costs to health plans and consumers. Some organizations are going to do quarterly or biannual audits to identify products that have unexplainable significant cost hikes, evaluate them, and potentially remove them from the formulary.

▫ Include discount negotiations from retail pharmacies in a plan's pharmacy network. The more selective the network, the greater the discount will be, because each pharmacy stands to gain business.

▫ Leverage mail-service and specialty pharmacy channels that give plan sponsors deeper discounts than retail pharmacies do. These channels also help encourage the use of preferred medications for increased savings.[14]

▫ Reduce waste by performing drug utilization reviews to prevent drug therapy duplications and polypharmacy

▫ Manage high-cost specialty medications through the PBMs' capabilities to safely store, handle, and deliver complex medications that can cost thousands per dose

▫ Provide patient education, monitoring, and support for patients with complex conditions, such as hepatitis C, multiple sclerosis, or cancer

Safe Medication Use

PBMs use their analytics and data systems to monitor prescription safety across all the network pharmacies and to alert pharmacists to potential drug interactions or duplications, even when a patient uses multiple pharmacies within the system.

Drug Supply Chain Management

In the new value-based healthcare landscape, organizations are looking for strategic opportunities to lower costs while improving the quality of patient outcomes and care. In healthcare organizations, pharmaceuticals are in the top three expenditures after labor costs, so organizations are now looking at the drug supply chain to identify opportunities to reduce costs, impact the delivery of healthcare, and serve as value centers within the organization, while simultaneously contributing to optimizing quality.

What is the drug supply chain? The basic drug supply chain is the means through which prescription medicines are delivered to patients, originating with the drug manufacturer (see Figure 9.1). The drug supply chain, however, is much more complex than this basic structure and involves multiple organizations and entities that play differing but sometimes overlapping roles in drug distribution.[15]

The Basic Medication Supply Chain

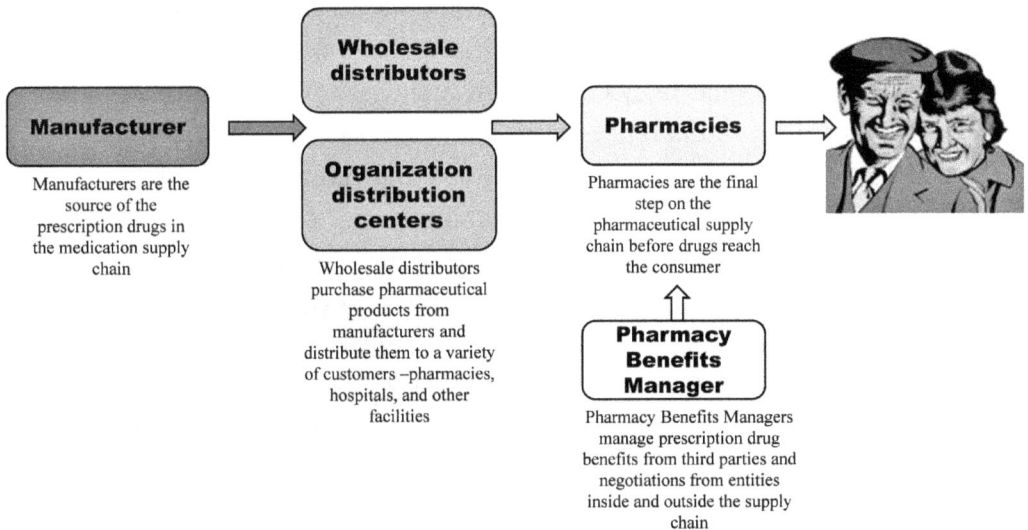

Manufacturer

Manufacturers are the source of the prescription drugs in the medication supply chain

Wholesale distributors

Organization distribution centers

Wholesale distributors purchase pharmaceutical products from manufacturers and distribute them to a variety of customers –pharmacies, hospitals, and other facilities

Pharmacies

Pharmacies are the final step on the pharmaceutical supply chain before drugs reach the consumer

Pharmacy Benefits Manager

Pharmacy Benefits Managers manage prescription drug benefits from third parties and negotiations from entities inside and outside the supply chain

Figure 9.1 Basic Med Supply Chain

The chain also involves contract negotiations, quality and utilization management process screening by PBMs, and various commercial relationships.[16] While there has always been a focus on the supply chain in relation to on-time delivery, there is now increased focus on strategic inventory management, supply chain optimization, and data utilization to control costs and drive value in the midst of shifting regulatory compliance, emerging markets, item-level serialization, and product diversification.[17] An effective drug supply chain infrastructure is critical to support the success, scalability, and sustainability of the following MAB components to create organizational value.

Adherence

The drug supply chain can directly support adherence and indirectly improve organizational quality performance by strategically addressing drug shortages, customizing packaging, and utilizing device developers to impact patient perceptions and attitudes toward their treatment.

- *Drug shortages*: The factors that contribute to drug shortages are complex, including shifts in clinical practices, in wholesaler and pharmacy inventory practices, raw material shortages, changes in hospital and pharmacy contractual relationships with suppliers and wholesalers, adherence to distribution protocols mandated by the FDA, individual company decisions to discontinue specific medicines, natural disasters, and manufacturing challenges.[18] When shortages happen or are anticipated, the supply chain partners and healthcare providers work collaboratively with the FDA to proactively select and use alternative purchasing sources, and work with other manufacturers that make similar products to ramp up production and fill any gaps in the supply, to reduce the chances of patients not receiving their medications. Organizations also work with providers to identify and approve alternative effective therapies to minimize patient care disruptions and prevent adverse outcomes from patients not receiving their medications. These systems and proactive processes, when leveraged, can contribute to improving adherence (or at least, minimize nonadherence) even during challenging times.

- *Packaging*: There are new, smarter packaging options that provide visual dosing reminders for patients and caregivers, decrease dispensing and counseling time, and reduce dispensing errors. For example, Omnicell is a leader in both single-dose and multimed adherence packaging, and offers a range of packaging options, supplies, and equipment to improve medication management and support adherence initiatives.[19] Options like this, however, are currently being used sparingly for starter packs, clinical trials, and some very high-cost medications. While studies have shown the effectiveness of smarter packaging in improving medication adherence, the cost to implement them on a broad scale is still in question.

- *Device developers*: Device developers are increasingly working with drug manufacturers to improve patients' experiences in small, but practical and significant ways. They are focusing on two basic questions: How can we reduce the demands we make of patients? How can we support patients to help them adhere?[21] With these questions in mind, device developers are collaborating with drug and formulation development teams to influence adherence directly and indirectly by supporting the following:
  - The formulation, such as dosing frequency
  - The delivery route from IV to SC, depot implants, wearable devices, and patches
  - The demands on the user associated with dose delivery
  - The support provided to the patients to help them adhere to dosing regimes
  - The patient perceptions, attitudes, and feelings about their treatment[22]

Engagement

Supply chain partners must collaborate and engage to form interdependent partnerships as they work together to transform and optimize the supply chain. Also, supply chain organizations are now reaching out to patients to engage them in product design.

- *Patient engagement*: The rise of consumer interface technologies will help consumers and patients manage their health more effectively. As technology advances, it will allow for increased patient-provider engagement and provide information (with permission) to manufacturers, wholesalers, pharmacies, and others along the supply chain that can be used to design more robust products and services and develop more accurate production and distribution plans.[23]

- *Collaborations with other supply chain entities*: In addition to engaging and collaborating with consumers, the drug supply chain industry will have greater collaboration with other parties involved in the provision of healthcare, helping the industry become safer and more efficient. Currently, there are three distinct supply chains:
  - One for designing, manufacturing, and distributing drugs
  - Another for designing, manufacturing, and distributing medical devices
  - The third for providing healthcare services (including laboratory work and pathology)

Integrating these supply chains so all the upstream and downstream partners can see the full picture enables them to plan ahead more accurately and manage demand more cost-effectively.[24]

Affordability

Cutting costs in the healthcare and drug supply chains has the potential to make pharmaceuticals and medical devices more affordable to more people and to increase healthcare value. Some key areas to focus on include: reducing shortages, cutting manufacturing lead time, reducing obsolescence, using mail-order services, having drug use management programs in place, using big data, and optimizing inventory.[25] Some of these are addressed below:

- *Reducing shortages*: Drug shortages have nearly tripled since 2005, causing providers to pay up to 11% more for drugs that are experiencing shortages and costing hospitals worldwide more than half a billion dollars.[26] By having the supply chain adopt some of the best practices in the industry, patients and consumers will have increased access to drugs and medical supplies, which will support adherence, safety, and better costs.

- *Using mail order services*: Using the mail to deliver medications to patients at their residence enables patients to access medications at a lower cost. Therefore, most pharmacies and benefit managers promote and incentivize the use of mail order for home delivery. For example, a patient's co-pay may be $10 for a 30-day supply if it is picked up at the pharmacy; however, the patient could be offered a 90-day supply delivered to the home by mail for a $20 co-pay, which reduces the frequency of refills. This option is especially beneficial for patients with chronic conditions who might be taking multiple medications.

According to William Fleming, president of Humana Pharmacy Solutions, "Mail-delivery pharmacy is a win-win solution for people who lead busy lives and want to follow their doctor's treatment plan, especially for people who need simplicity in how they purchase their prescriptions. Studies have shown that more than half of consumers buy items online. Mail-delivery pharmacy is a method of purchasing prescriptions that aligns with how they live their lives. By simplifying their lives, we are able to improve affordability and access to medications which should yield better health outcomes."[27]

- *Using big data*: Data is at the core of supply chain innovation, because it enables businesses to measure, monitor, and improve individual supply chain processes while keeping tabs on the performance of the supply chain as a whole. For example, better data leads to better visibility, which is how supply chain leaders can identify and eliminate cost drivers while better understanding how the business can deliver greater customer and patient value. Unfortunately, many businesses are still struggling to make big data practical through integrated data management.

- *Optimizing inventory*: Organizations can have a lower cost structure and save millions of dollars when the following supply chain infrastructures are in place.
  - Organizations that have one common item master and charge master for all drugs have a better understanding of total purchases across the organization and an increased leverage of getting rebates owed from the drug companies.
  - When this item master is combined with a scanning system, organizations have a more accurate inventory, replenishment, and recall management process; understand their inventory and actual costs; and aggregate their spending, which will help them obtain better deals from contractors and manufacturers.
  - Using science to set par levels, reduce inventory levels, improve selection and cycle count, and reorder drug inventory helps reduce waste and inefficiencies, leading to a better cost structure.
  - An effective forecast system should be implemented in the supply chain infrastructure by having inputs from shipment history, purchasing history, dispensing history, return-to-stock, and external factors like seasonality and changes to benefit plans.

Safe Medication Use and Safety

The US drug supply chain is one of the safest in the world. However, the drug supply chain has become increasingly complex as it extends beyond US borders. Threats to the supply chain such as counterfeiting, diversion, cargo theft, and importation of unapproved or otherwise substandard drugs could result in unsafe, ineffective drugs in US distribution. The FDA safeguards the integrity of the drug supply chain through initiatives that help to protect consumers from exposure to substandard drugs and to ensure that safe and effective drugs reach US consumers.[28]

Other ways the drug supply chain is effectively managing the safety of medications include:

- *Global data standards for security*

  Supply chain issues such as shortages and recalls create opportunities for counterfeiters and gray-market vendors, which threaten patient safety and cut into the revenues of legitimate companies. Better supply chain processes are central to increasing patient safety. By adopting a common global data standard and upgrading supply chain processes, organizations could slash counterfeiting in half, returning $15 billion to $30 billion in revenue to legitimate companies for reinvestment in further improvements to patient care.[29]

  In 2013, the Drug Quality and Security Act was signed into law. Title II of the act, the Drug Supply Chain Security Act, outlined critical steps to build a national interoperable system for identifying and tracing drug products through the supply chain. It set national licensing standards for wholesale distributors and third-party logistics providers.[30] This new system further ensures the safety of the drug supply chain by:
  - Enabling the verification of the legitimacy of the drug product identifier down to the package level
  - Enhancing detection and notification of illegitimate products in the drug supply chain
  - Facilitating more efficient recalls of drug products[31]

- *Mail Order and Temperature*

  In very high temperature areas, there has been concern that these conditions may be hazardous to medications in the mail and their potential efficacy. To protect the medications, therefore, manufacturers, suppliers, and pharmacies have taken precautions such as using ice packs and insulated containers to mail medications when temperatures are extreme. Conditions in the home are by no means as extreme, but repeated exposure to moisture and oxygen during normal use can degrade a medication's physical characteristics. Therefore, pharmacists are informing patients about how to appropriately store medications in the home to prevent these issues.

- *Serialization of Drug Packages*
  This has been a hot topic in the last decade to prevent counterfeiting and diversion of medications in commercial supply chains. Proponents of the technology, both inside and outside the industry, highlight the additional business value of inventory control, recall management, and supply chain visibility that accrue to serialized, tracked products. The healthcare industry, however, is looking at a broader picture—one focused on patient safety and improved health outcomes. Medication adherence plays a key role, and perhaps serialization will help.[32]

- *Secure Supply Chain Pilot Program*
  In 2014, the FDA introduced a pilot program to focus its import surveillance resources on preventing high-risk medications from entering the United States. Given the increasingly complex drug supply chain, a collaborative approach by drug companies within their own organizations and with partners across the supply chain became essential to help eliminate counterfeit and high-risk drugs from entering.

  In collaboration with internal and external partners, many pharmaceutical companies and wholesalers have developed and deployed integrated supply-chain security strategies to win this war. "And win it we must," according to Brian Johnson, the senior director of supply chain security at Pfizer, "not just for the good of the businesses that drug companies support but—more importantly—for the safety of the patients who depend upon drug products."[33]

Big Data and Analytics

In the new value-based healthcare system, financial reimbursement for providers is linked to quality outcome measures. Organizations, providers, and payers recognize that their approach to improving the Triple Aim measures in HEDIS, MACRA, QPP, Medicare Stars ratings, and other quality measures—and addressing quality care gaps—must be more deliberate and strategic to ensure success, remain competitive, and maximize reimbursements. Optimizing MAB will be critical to meet many of these new expectations, and the use of big data and clinical and business analytics tools will be foundational.

Analytic tools have also become a top priority for health systems and organizations looking for real-time, actionable surveillance data to reduce costs and optimize care. As organizations continue the transformation to value-based care and population health management, enterprise intelligence resources will complement electronic health records to provide leaders and clinicians with a comprehensive picture of what's happening within their organizations, down to individual providers' panels of patients. This will enable providers, organizations, and health systems to react quickly to enhance clinical outcomes, efficiency, safety, and affordability.[34]

As more clinical information becomes available through electronic medical records, and with reimbursements increasingly tied to clinical outcomes, organizations are accelerating the use of big data and analysis to do the following.

- Access real-time data about their patients, stratify risk, and set up population health management initiatives for success
- Tailor patient registries to leverage data to focus care management programs on the patients who will benefit the most
- Provide insights and information to improve outcomes and effectiveness of care

There are three types of analytics that are frequently used to transform big data into usable information in healthcare.

1. *Descriptive analytics*: This gives insight from historical data, with reporting and scorecards to yield useful information. This type of analysis uses data aggregation and data mining methods to organize data and make it possible to identify patterns and relationships that may otherwise be invisible. Querying, reporting, and data visualization may be applied to yield more insight and provide information about what happened.[35] For example, this can be used to track and trend data of diabetic patients who had a particular intervention.

2. *Predictive analytics*: This is used to identify future probabilities and trends, and tries to provide information about what might happen in the future.[36] Predictive analytics is now critical in understanding a patient or population risk relative to the disease or comorbidities to determine future costs and needs. For example, when an organization is looking at the probability of patients most likely to be readmitted after a heart attack, they will take into account predictors such as age, medication adherence, and previous admissions. They then target these patients with additional interventions to reduce the likelihood of a readmission, lower their risk, and avoid unwarranted costs.

3. *Prescriptive analytics*: This is used to try to identify the best outcomes of events, given the parameters, and to recommend decision options to best take advantage of a future opportunity or mitigate a future risk. Prescriptive analytics asks: How should we respond to those potential future events? Take, for example, Google's new self-driving car. During every trip, it makes multiple decisions about what to do based on predictions of future outcomes.

How are organizations using these types of data analytics and big data to ensure the success of MAB to optimize patient health outcomes?

Adherence

Many organizations currently use analytics to turn patients' medication claims and medical data into actionable insights and to generate scorecards and reports at an organizational and provider level. This helps providers and organizations know how they are doing compared to benchmark data, know where their variations are, and see how well they are doing over time. These scorecards and reports are very beneficial in giving teams insight into how adherent their members are.

Companies like SCIO Health Analytics are developing powerful analytic tools to help determine the reasons behind a patient's nonadherent behavior. Then, using data and advanced analytics, they move toward more sophisticated adherent solutions, including developing "personas" (representations of patients based on data analysis), to help understand what motivates them to comply with medication regimens, identify cohorts of patients who should receive tailored adherence programs, and then fine-tune adherence efforts.[37]

Companies like AllazoHealth, Optum, and RxAnte are taking adherence one step further. These and many other companies are working with organizations to address the problem of medication nonadherence through predictive analytics and personalized interventions. For example, the Accountable Care Coalition of Greater New York and AllazoHealth launched a pilot program aimed at improving adherence to medication regimens and reducing medical costs for Medicare beneficiaries who have hypertension, epilepsy, heart failure, diabetes, or hyperlipidemia. On an individual basis, annual spending for nonadherent patients with hypertension and diabetes is almost $4,000 greater than for patients who adhere to their prescriptions.[38]

AllazoHealth has also used predictive analytics to anticipate which patients were at risk of not taking their medications and predicted which medication adherence interventions would best influence individual patients' behavior.[39] RxAnte has partnered with Envision Insurance, a national provider of Medicare Part D plans and a division of EnvisionRxOptions, to improve medication adherence in key CMS Star rating therapy areas. This has been done using data from large populations of patients to predict the likelihood of individual patients to adhere to their prescribed medication therapies.

Applying these predictions, Envision and RxAnte have developed customized interventions and outreach programs for each member, which improves health outcomes and better controls costs for members, the plans, and the federal government. So far, the RxAnte and Envision relationship has yielded improvements in medication adherence rates faster than the national industry average. In the future, they hope to see further improvements in patient health outcomes and Envision's Star measures by also improving the behaviors of Part D members with high blood pressure, cholesterol, and diabetes medications.[40]

In 2017, OptumRx and Walgreens will be partnering to create a new pharmacy solution to meet consumers' changing prescription medication needs and to help employers, health plans, and their members achieve better health outcomes and greater cost savings. Through a more convenient, accessible, and connected pharmacy experience, the companies will collaborate to deliver members enrolled in the program integrated pharmacy care that will produce higher treatment adherence rates and better patient outcomes. It will also connect members to clinical guidance that addresses specific disease classes, such as diabetes; increase drug adherence; and enable OptumRx and Walgreens systems to better connect health data and analytics to ensure their members receive the most effective prescription medications at the best possible costs.[41]

Reconciliation

In a study published in the *American Journal of Managed Care*, more than 75% of patients experienced a medication reconciliation discrepancy when their EHR data was compared to their pharmacy claims data. With pharmacies' data systems becoming more integrated into the EHRs ecosystem, pharmacists are now having access to patient's holistic information, which enables them to help patients maintain an up-to-date medication list, while having the information at hand to help monitor a patient's chronic conditions more effectively.[42]

In addition, the rise of erescribing networks like Express Scripts and Surescripts are helping to smooth the process of exchanging up-to-the-minute medication data, are helping to create the most up-to-date medication lists, and may be cutting down the number of related adverse events.[43] For example, data from a network suggests hospitals that use Surescripts to develop medication lists might be preventing between three and 26 adverse drug events per person per year, while saving more than a million dollars in unnecessary costs.[44]

Walgreens is also addressing medication reconciliation using a loopback technology, which is able to provide patients' medication history to hospitals at admission to facilitate the medication reconciliation process, and then send that reconciled medication list back for use in the community pharmacy post-discharge. Joel Wright, group vice president of enterprise specialty at Walgreens, said, "Right then we clean up that patient's outpatient profile and close prescriptions the patient should no longer be on. That way the prescriptions don't get filled in error, and it helps reduce the chance of patients being confused about which medication they should really take or not take."[45]

According to Walgreens, within the first six months after implementing its WellTransitions program at five hospitals, the patients in this program had a 9.4% unadjusted rate of 30-day readmission, compared to a 14.3% 30-day readmission rate for patients eligible for, but not participating in, the program.[46]

Engagement

In this new value-based, patient-centric healthcare system, quality is measured both clinically and experientially, making patient satisfaction a critical component for organizational performance and reimbursement. Analytics can help sort through the vast amount of patient data, from which key satisfaction drivers can be discerned, such as co-pay issues, accurate estimates of self-pay costs, precise and timely billing, key clinical opportunities to improve care, and many other ways to make healthcare a better experience.[47]

Analytics can also be used to further improve patient engagement by comparing the usage rates for the many programs and apps that are available, along with monitoring the effect they have on individual and population health, inpatient stay, and emergency department visits. Armed with this data, healthcare organizations can then determine which interventions are the most effective and worth greater investment, as well as those that are no longer worthy of continued investment—freeing up the budget to develop new options or enhance existing programs.

IBM Watson Health is now focusing on improving patient engagement with the launch of a new population management tool. This tool will aggregate patient data from multiple sources—including wearable devices like the Fitbit, smart scales, and Apple's HealthKit and ResearchKit offerings—into the cloud. Providers can view and incorporate this data into the patient's overall care plan. This tool will leverage wearable technology, encourage patients to use them daily to track their conditions, and potentially give patients and providers clearer insights into patients' conditions. Since providers generally see their patients quarterly or less, using tools like this can provide insights on a much more frequent basis into what is happening with their patients, which could be transformative.[48]

Affordability

Lowering the cost structure of an organization will support lowering the cost of healthcare for all. Big data and analytics can support this by improving efficiencies, providing evidence of less expensive medications to achieve effective outcomes, supporting more effective medication selection by identifying side effects costs of medications post release, and tracking/trending costs and other data.

- *Efficiencies*: Organizations are using big data analytics to batch and tailor treatment schedules to accommodate myriad treatment protocols while smoothing out the traffic flow in their clinics. This has led to a significant reduction in drug wastage, pharmacy orders being filled in a timelier manner, less waiting time for patients, and increased utilization of facilities.

- *Less expensive medications*: Doctors Wanzhu Tu and J. Howard Pratt—co-authors of "Triamterene Enhances the Blood Pressure Lowering Effect of Hydrochlorothiazide in Patients with Hypertension," a 2016 study published in the Journal of General Internal Medicine—used big data to discover that a drug commonly prescribed to conserve potassium in the blood also significantly lowers blood pressure when taken in conjunction with a diuretic frequently prescribed to patients with hypertension. The combination of the two drugs, both available as generics, has been shown to consistently amplify blood pressure reduction in patients with or without the presence of other antihypertensive agents such as ACE inhibitors and calcium channel blockers.

According to Dr. Tu, "It is unlikely that a large clinical trial would be conducted to reexamine the blood pressure effect of triamterene, a drug that has been on the market since 1965. Yet smaller clinical trials simply do not provide sufficient power to determine the drug's effect. Observational studies based on big data, like ours, provide a viable alternative."[49]

- *Side effects*: Memorial Hermann, a healthcare organization in Houston, evaluated the current system of adverse event reporting and applied sophisticated analytics to the reporting of post-marketing side effects of new anticoagulants Eliquis (apixaban), Xarelto (rivaroxaban), and Pradaxa (dabigatran) and the true cost to their healthcare system. The outcome of their study showed that Eliquis offered a significant annual downstream cost savings over both Pradaxa and Xarelto. When adverse events are factored into their true cost, there is an estimated savings of nearly $12 million gained by switching from Xarelto to Eliquis and an estimated savings of nearly $20 million by switching from Pradaxa to Eliquis. Other organizations are now leveraging big data to do these post-marketing side effect studies and examine associated costs as a component of the review for formulary consideration.

- *Costs and other data*: Cardinal Health's Drug Cost Opportunity Analytics tool is a web-based dashboard that enables pharmacy leaders to rapidly identify top medication cost drivers and trends, as well as benchmark performances, with drill-down capabilities to the physician level. Health systems can compare their hospitals' or care delivery systems' performances against others in the system, or with other similar facilities, based on many different factors.

This dashboard provides performance metrics that identify areas requiring attention, with alerts that can be customized based on user preference and drug cost benchmarking capabilities to the DRG level, with drill-down capabilities to the National Drug Code and physician levels.[50] Its Antibiotic Analytics module also provides actionable data and insights for pharmacy leaders by tracking and trending antibiotic use and susceptibility, with drill-down capabilities to trend antimicrobial utilization, top drugs, IV-to-PO percentages, top antimicrobial opportunities, organism trends, and more.[51]

Safe Medication Use and Safety

Organizations are now using big data and analytics to determine the true cost of adverse events related to certain medications, because health systems and hospitals are making decisions about formulary drug choices without effective resources to analyze the most current post-approval drug side effect data. "In many cases, warning signs from emerging data regarding drug side effects may be overlooked, thereby risking patient safety and increasing overall cost of care," writes Patti Romeril, PharmD, in *H&HN*. In this new era of value-based payment models, organizations and providers are implementing analysis of real-world adverse events to determine the true costs and risks of drug choices.[52]

Memorial Hermann is now reviewing and responding to adverse events data and analytics, which it believes will help improve outcomes and decrease avoidable adverse events-related medical costs, such as readmissions. It also predicts that in the future, health plans and payers, including Medicare, will require provider formularies to demonstrate a systematic review of side effects—including what that data means in terms of costs, safety, and outcomes—from a broad patient population, not just an individual organization's internal tracking.[53] So organizations are embracing big data and the algorithms that make the data actionable as part of the strategy for the future management and prevention of adverse drug events.

Health Information Technology Systems (HITS)

MAB supports providers and healthcare teams as they work to improve the quality of patient care, outcomes, the health of communities, and organizational performance and to reduce healthcare costs. Now, through the advancements in health information technology systems (HITS), we can further optimize MAB and create safer, higher quality, more coordinated, more efficient, less costly care, and secure care for everyone.

HITS are the electronic systems that health care professionals and team members—and, increasingly, patients—use to store, share, and analyze health information.[54] The systems make it possible for healthcare providers to more effectively and securely manage patient care and share patients' health information between providers. It includes EHRs with computerized physician order entry (CPOE) and clinical decision support (CDS), pharmacy information management systems (PIMS), and medication/patient safety systems, to name a few. These HITS can support the optimization of MAB. Examples of two HITS follow.

1. EHRs with CPOE and CDS

An electronic health record (EHR) is a digital version of a patient's paper chart. They are real-time records that make a patient's information available instantly and securely to authorized users. EHRs have been built to collect extensive clinical data, including the patient's medical history, diagnoses, medications, treatment plans, immunization dates, allergies, radiology images, and laboratory and test results. EHRs use evidence-based tools that leverage patient information and data to support providers in making important decisions about a patient's care. EHRs also help automate and streamline provider workflow to improve efficiencies and effectiveness.[55]

Another key feature of an EHR is that health information can be shared with other providers across more than one healthcare organization—the laboratories, provider practices, medical imaging facilities, pharmacies, emergency facilities, and school and workplace clinics involved in a patient's care.[56] The adoption of EHRs has increased the volume of data available for measuring performance and increased organizational capacities for continuous, quality improvement.

CPOE is the process of a healthcare provider entering medication orders or other instructions electronically into an EHR instead of using paper charts. A primary benefit of CPOE is that it can help reduce errors related to poor handwriting or inaccurate transcription of the orders.

CDS encompasses a variety of tools including, but not limited to, the following: computerized alerts and reminders for providers and patients, clinical guidelines, condition-specific order sets, focused patient data reports and summaries, dose lists, just-in-time advice, documentation templates, diagnostic support, and contextually relevant reference information that can be deployed on a variety of platforms.[57] CDS is not intended to replace clinician judgment, but rather is a compilation of tools to assist healthcare team members in making timely, informed, higher quality decisions.[58]

Most EHRs now come equipped with CPOE and CDS, resulting in improvements in healthcare quality, care coordination and patient participation, medical practice efficiencies and cost savings, and diagnosis and patient outcomes—all while meeting the CMS meaningful use standards one and two.[59] So how can EHRs specifically help providers leverage MAB to improve patient health outcomes?

Adherence

- *Meaningful use and certified EHR adoption*: Innovations in health IT and the increased adoption of certified EHRs have presented an opportunity to improve patients' adherence to their medications. The Health Information Technology for Economic and Clinical Health Act was established to incentivize eligible hospitals and providers to adopt and meaningfully use certified EHRs. "Meaningful use" refers to healthcare providers using EHR technologies in ways that measurably improve healthcare quality and efficiency. Under this incentive program, CMS has developed objectives and measures that hospitals and healthcare professionals must meet in order to receive payments.

The Office of the National Coordinator for Health Information Technology (ONC) has established the standards and certification criteria to ensure EHR technology is capable of meeting certain minimum requirements necessary to support these actions by providers. Within the CMS objectives is support for medication adherence, including exchanging key clinical information among providers, providing patients with electronic access to their health information (including medication lists), generating and transmitting electronic prescriptions, enabling automated clinical decision support, and implementing drug formulary checks.[60]

- *Electronic prescribing*: ePrescribing is the electronic generation, transmission, and filling of a prescription and provides healthcare professionals opportunities to monitor a patient's medication regimen in real time. Between 2008 and 2010, federal incentives resulted in 89,000-94,000 more new ePrescribers than there would have been otherwise.[61] In 2011, the "National Progress Report on ePrescribing and Interoperable Health Care" found that in 2008, one in 10 office-based physicians used ePrescribing, and three years later, one in two physicians used ePrescribing.

  ePrescribing has contributed to improving medication adherence by facilitating provider-patient communications through automated triggers to notify providers and team members when a patient does not pick up medications, and by triggering potential interventions to avoid gaps in medication usage.[62] ePrescribing has also shown an increase in medication first fill prescriptions by

10%, which can improve primary nonadherence and potentially save the healthcare system $140 billion to $240 billion over the next 10 years.[63]

Reconciliation

EHRs can contribute to improving medication management by maintaining a complete medication list for patients and caregivers that is updated at each point of contact. An active reconciled medication list serves multiple purposes, including:

- Avoiding inadvertent inconsistencies during transitions in care, from the time of admission to transfer and all the way through to the discharge process
- Meeting the requirement of the Medicare Electronic Health Record Incentive Program that says eligible providers must maintain an active medication list and gives the option of reconciliation during transitions of care
- Minimizing drug interactions, duplications, and omissions
- Improving care coordination by distributing the medication list to key providers and support team members

The ONC has provided grant funds that support the expansion of health IT innovations that facilitate the secure electronic exchange of medication lists.[64]

Engagement

Providers and patients who share access to electronic health information can collaborate in informed decision making. Patient participation is especially important in managing and treating chronic conditions such as asthma, diabetes, and obesity. EHRs can foster patient participation and help providers in the following ways:

- Ensure high-quality care when providers give patients full and accurate information about all of their medical evaluations. Providers can also offer follow-up information after an office visit or a hospital stay, such as self-care instructions, reminders for other follow-up care, and links to web resources.

- Create communication opportunities with their patients by managing appointment schedules electronically and exchanging secure e-mails with patients. EHRs can foster ongoing communication between patients and providers, which may help providers identify symptoms earlier and be more proactive in reaching out to patients.[65]

Affordability

The ePrescribing component of the EHRs has been found to increase efficiency for many providers, help to save on healthcare costs, and is cheaper for doctors and pharmacies, because EHRs have most or all of a patient's health information in one place. This facilitates the prescription ordering process, reduces duplications and errors, and makes the ordering process more efficient and effective.

Safe Medication Use and Safety

Qualified and certified EHRs not only keep a record of a patient's medical history, medications, and allergies, they also automatically check for interactions and problems whenever a new medication is prescribed and alert the provider to potential interactions or conflicts. EHRs also:

- Build in safeguards to improve provider prescribing and prevent adverse events, dosage errors, incorrect calculations, and wrong medication selections
- Make it easier to consider all aspects of the patient's condition and relevant information (such as labs) when prescribing therapies
- Support the selection of the most clinically effective and cost-effective medications for patients
- Expose potential safety problems when they occur, helping providers avoid more serious consequences for patients[66]

2. PIMS

A pharmacy information management system is a complex computer system that has been designed to meet the needs of a pharmacy department with the following basic functions (not all inclusive): inpatient and outpatient order entry; clinical monitoring and screening; dispensing processes; drug utilization review database access; inventory and purchasing management; manufacturing and compounding; online refilling processes; pricing, charging, and billing; reporting (utilization, workload, and financial); secure login functionality; and interconnectivity with other systems within the enterprise, such as an EMR, CPOE, and barcode technology.[67]

Today, PIMS must be a fully integrated solution for organizations to ensure safe, timely, effective, efficient, patient-centered, and compliant prescription management, from the time the medication is prescribed to the administration or dispensing of the medication to the patient. The system should also be able to effectively manage the inventory, streamline and automate the daily workflows of the pharmacy team, and be seamlessly integrated into the organization's CPOE, ePrescribing, EHRs, medication reconciliation, and medication formulary processes. To see a comprehensive list of features, functionalities, and workflow of a pharmacy system (McKesson), read "A day in the life of a prescription" at the McKesson Pharmacy Systems and Automation website, http://betterpharmacytech.com/about-us/pms/.

Below are some of the benefits.[68,69]

- Drug interactions and duplications are recorded, including appropriate dosages based on the patient's age, weight, and other physiologic factors, as well as allergies and other possible medication-related information.
- CPOE and decision support tools incorporated into the pharmacy review process include medication reconciliation, medication synchronization, ePrescribing, electronic medication administration record, and medication formulary.

- Drug database access includes access to a national database for item/product facts and comparison and drug utilization review checks (includes daily/weekly screening and updates).
- Inventory management maintains counts of medications and provides alerts when levels fall below a specific number.
- Access to or integration with a patient's EHR enables pharmacies to develop a comprehensive patient profile with access to clinical information, such as lab results, medication history, allergies, and physiological parameters.
- From the time a prescription order is placed, the system effectively manages the process from administration to dispensing of medication to patients. This allows for easy tracking of the prescriber and the date and time drug was dispensed.
- Report generation includes inventory reports, billing for hospitals or retail pharmacy claims, and other charges related to the charge master.
- It connects with other systems within the enterprise, such as an EMR, CPOE, barcode technology, clinical information systems (to receive prescription orders), and financial information system (for billing and charging).

PIMS should also have solid internal controls pertaining to procurement, charge description master maintenance, tracking systems, traceability, storage, drug shortages, disposal and segregation of duties, pharmacy revenue cycle, wasted and expired drugs, and physical security. These control mechanisms can provide a basis for consistent quality, better financial performance, lower risk, and improved regulatory compliance when implemented appropriately and adhered to during day-to-day operations.[70]

With this in mind, how can pharmacy teams leverage the pharmacy information management system to help them ensure the success, scalability, and sustainability of MAB to improve patient health outcomes?

Adherence

CDS and monitoring tools in PIMS can help pharmacy team members address and improve timely adherence at the point of service. Some of these CDS tools can automatically identify patients who appear to be nonadherent to their medications based on algorithms built within the system.

For example, one organization's PIMS would automatically identify a patient who had not had a diabetes lab test in the last 12 months and had a medication adherence measure of less than 80%. The pharmacist would meet with the identified patient to address the lab screening test and the potential medication nonadherence behavior, and would work with the patient to identify the possible adherence challenges and offer targeted solutions or referrals as needed. A pharmacist who discovers that a patients is getting medications from multiple pharmacies would help consolidate, when possible.

Another example is the McKesson medication adherence and clinical performance technology solutions package, which is part of its PIMS. These solutions enable qualified pharmacy team members to collect, monitor, and analyze data on patient medication histories and adherence behaviors. The information can be provided on a customizable dashboard for immediate action to overcome any adherence barrier and is complemented with solutions that are high-touch services—such as behavioral coaching, patient education, refill reminder, medication reconciliation, medication synchronization, medication therapy management, financial assistance, flexible co-pays, and customer loyalty programs.[71]

PIMS can also support activities to improve medication adherence such as ePrescribing, text messaging, customized letters, interactive voice response calls informing patients that their prescriptions are ready for pickup, phone calls or email messages, and medication synchronization tools to group a patient's scripts so that they are filled on the same schedule.

Reconciliation

PIMS now have CDS to reconcile medications and check for drug interactions and duplications; drug allergies, drug versus gender and appropriate drug dosages; appropriate dosages based on patient's age, weight, and other physiologic factors as well as other possible medication-related complications. Also, with interfaces with other pharmacies and even the patient's EHRs, pharmacists are able to get and store a complete and accurate list of the patient's medication in the pharmacy system. This enables them to provide patients and providers with the most up-to-date medication lists to prevent any adverse outcomes and medication-related hospitalizations.

Engagement

As pharmacists increasingly focus on providing clinical services and engaging patients around appropriate medication management to improve patient care and organizational performance (as reflected in Medicare Stars ratings, HEDIS, MIPS, and other Triple Aim measures), they need technology and decision support tools to help them with their efforts. Many of these tools have been built into PIMS to help pharmacists and pharmacy team members more effectively engage patients as they document their interactions with the patients, build relationships, and leverage the information collected for continuity of care. Additional CDS tools being built into the pharmacy systems include:

- The medication synchronization tools: Med Sync programs are becoming more popular, which many pharmacy systems are now able to do.
- Patient's preferred method of contact: Many pharmacy systems give pharmacies the flexibility to select a patient's preferred contact method for pickup reminders, special programs, and value-added services (with the patient's permission).

- Telepharmacy: These tools allow pharmacists to engage patients in rural and widespread areas, remotely verify their prescriptions and privately counsel them.

- Appointment-based pharmacy services: This service addresses polypharmacy challenges, MTM services, and immunization services. These appointments allow the pharmacist to address patient issues in one scheduled appointment, instead of multiple unscheduled and hurried interactions, and require the right technology in their pharmacy systems to support their activities. With the right tools in PIMS, pharmacists can build new models of care to support, engage, and connect with patients; build the patient-pharmacist relationship; and improve performance.[72]

- Getting prescriptions from one location/pharmacy: A study published in the *Journal of the American Geriatrics Society* discovered that patients who get their medications at multiple pharmacies have a small but statistically significant increase in drug-drug interactions compared to patients who got their medications from a single source.[73] Most patients, however, are not aware of this issue. So it is important for pharmacists to engage patients about their medication-taking behaviors, including where they get their prescriptions. While it may not always be possible for patients to get their medications from one source, due to their benefits, pharmacists can reduce adverse outcomes by remaining engaged with patients, reconciling their medication lists often, and manually entering patients' medications filled by other locations (for example, mail order) into their systems for screening and review purposes.

Affordability

PIMS can support drug use management strategies to help organizations, pharmacies, and patients reduce overall costs by implementing the following:

- Send out alerts when less expensive effective options are available.

- Utilize data mining for patients who qualify for MTM services, are on brand medications when a generic is available, are on duplicate medications, or have opportunities to be switched to a preferred medication.
- Use the workflow and workload balancing tools in PIMS to leverage pharmacy systems to support agile staffing, increase efficiencies, increase clinical offerings, and reduce costs. Many pharmacies are challenged with insufficient distribution of the workload and prescription volumes, with some locations filling many more than others due to pharmacy size and location. With the use of PIMS and cloud-based queues, pharmacy staff can support the medication verification process, drug use management activities, and some clinical services from a centralized location or from multiple locations to effectively and efficiently spread the workload and reduce overall costs and wasted time.[74]
- Leverage patient savings programs that can be accessed directly from PIMS to help enroll patients in internal or external medication financial assistant programs.

Safe Medication Use and Safety

Pharmacy systems are critical in helping pharmacy team members eliminate errors from the data entry process, validation process, verification process, and filling process to the point-of-sales dispensing process through alerts, hard-stops, and flags. These systems also need to help the team by accomplishing the following:

- Addressing known drug interactions, duplications, and contraindications
- Having ongoing drug utilization reviews
- Hard-stopping prescriptions (not letting it be filled until verified by a qualified pharmacy team member) that have significant interactions or a high likelihood of causing adverse outcomes
- Having a double-check mandatory system for medications with narrow therapeutic windows and specialty medications

- Processing ePrescriptions efficiently and in a timely manner
- Keeping electronic prescription files for audits, recalls, and other safety processes
- Having the ability to translate directions into multiple languages
- Using barcode scanning for accuracy
- Verifying medications using visual verification and color images

Organizations are also leveraging the prescription drug monitoring programs (PDMPs) in addition to PIMS, as there is evidence that PDMPs can improve patient safety and care while preventing abuse and overdose deaths. These programs are in every state except Missouri, citing privacy concerns, and the District of Columbia. According to the assistant attorney general of the Office of Justice Programs, the "misuse of prescription drugs is a national problem that requires the cooperative efforts of all medical, health, pharmaceutical, law enforcement agencies, and other partners to solve."[75]

Medication Management Apps—Linking Patients' Devices to Better Engagement and Outcomes

One of the purposes of medication management apps is to empower patients with daily motivational tips and keep them on track with reminders to take their medications at specific times as directed. Some key features to look for in an app include security to protect patient information, reminder alerts that can be programed, the space and flexibility to put in various forms of medications (inhalers, liquids, pills), and availability for the smartphone or tablet being used. Additional features that may be helpful (usually for a fee) include the ability to track missed doses, alerts about side effects if too much medication is taken (especially for medications with strict dose limits), the ability to share information with healthcare providers and family caregivers, reminders for more complicated medication schedules, a searchable medication database, and online accessibility.[76]

With the number of apps and features growing, it can be tough to select an app that will help patients address their own Medication

A.R.E.A.S. challenges. One new concept that is being investigated by some community pharmacies is the idea of an A.R.E.A.S. Genius Bar (MAB Bar), a concept derived from the Ochsner Health System's Genius Bar (which got the concept from Apple).[77]

A MAB Bar would be set up in the pharmacy and staffed by a technician or clerk. Based on the consultation with the pharmacist, patients would be given a "script" with their own Medication A.R.E.A.S. challenges. That would be given to the technician at the MAB Bar, who would then inform the patients about the mobile apps appropriate for them. The MAB Bar would also have wearable devices that are Bluetooth-enabled such as a blood glucose monitor, a wireless weight scale, or a wireless blood pressure monitor. The technician would then involve patients in setting up the apps and train them on how to use them.

As Benjamin Franklin said, "Tell me and I forget, teach me and I may remember, involve me and I learn."[78] The value of these medication apps, coupled with wearable devices and optimized with training from the technician, will lead to greater patient engagement, better outcomes, and better health in the long run.[79]

A Solid Compliance Infrastructure

The FDA is the US government agency charged with ensuring the safety and efficacy of the medicines available to Americans. The government's control over medicines has grown significantly, and now medications are among the most regulated products in the country.[80] As a result, organizations, health systems, and pharmacies are building, or have built, solid compliance infrastructures and controls to accomplish the following:

- Comply with the significant number of state and federal regulations
- Monitor and respond to the frequent audits from the various agencies
- Minimize or eliminate the fines for noncompliance

- Prevent diversion, fraud, waste, and abuse and have a safe distribution plan
- Set up policies, procedures, and training programs to comply with the necessary regulations
- Keep track of any changes to the laws and regulations

Organizations, health systems, and pharmacies that have effective compliance infrastructures and controls in place will minimize risk and contribute to the organizations' focus and strategies like MAB. Pharmacies in particular have the following in place (not all inclusive):

- Compliance training tools: All pharmacies that work with PBMs and third-party payers, such as CMS, must have their staff participate in annual compliance training around regulations pertaining to CMS Medicare Parts C and D; fraud, waste and abuse; internal and external audits and controls; and other pertinent regulations to minimize risks and potential loss of licensure. These trainings are usually web-based and are tracked to ensure all employees participate.[81]
- Internal controls and audits: CMS has developed a self-audit tool called "Pharmacy Auditing and Dispensing: The Self-Audit Control Practices to Improve Medicaid Program Integrity and Quality Patient Care Checklist." This self-audit consists of 50 steps to help pharmacies identify potential audit triggers. The audit includes detailed information regarding each step and is divided into four sections: prescribing practices, controlled substances management, invoice management, and billing practices. These four sections can be used separately or together to meet the needs of the pharmacy practice.
- Pharmacy compliance audits: Pharmacy audits assess how compliant a pharmacy is with its procedures stipulated by regulatory or contractual arrangements. There are two types of audits that can impact MAB:

- □ Third-party provider audits: Pharmacies that contract with PBMs and third-party payers are subject to audits of their pharmacy's records, including hard-copy prescriptions, signature logs, computerized records of refills, and invoice records.
- □ Regulatory agency audits: Pharmacies are subject to audits conducted by state or federal licensing agencies such as the DEA and State Board of Pharmacy.[82]

Some Laws, Policies, and Regulations That Will Support MAB Rx Strategy:

- *The Drug Quality and Security Act*: To protect the increasingly complex supply chain, the Drug Quality and Security Act was signed into law in 2013. Title II of the act, called the Drug Supply Chain Security Act, outlines steps to build an electronic, interoperable system to identify and trace certain prescription drugs as they are distributed in the United States. The law requires the FDA to develop standards, guidance documents, and pilot programs and to conduct public meetings, in addition to other efforts necessary to support efficient and effective implementation. This law will help the FDA protect consumers from exposure to harmful drugs.[83]

- *The New Opioid Regulations & Guidelines*: The FDA is deeply concerned about the growing epidemic of opioid abuse, dependence, and overdose (see discussion in Chapter 5). In response to this crisis, the agency has developed a comprehensive action plan to take steps toward reducing the impact of opioid abuse on American families and communities. It will work in cooperation with its sister agencies and stakeholders as it reexamines the risk-benefit paradigm, seeks improved treatment of both addiction and pain, and acquires new data for opioids.[84]

  PCPs account for roughly half of all opioid prescriptions, and new guidelines are aimed at those clinicians prescribing opioids to manage chronic pain (not for opioid use in treating patients with active cancer, palliative care or end-of-life care). To develop the guidelines, the CDC updated a 2014 systemic review of the effectiveness and risks of opioids and did a supplemental review of their benefits and harms, values and preferences, and costs. The agency also consulted with experts and listened to comments from the public and other partners. There are 12 recommendations in all. Three core principles will contribute to improving patient care:

1. Nonopioid therapy is preferred for chronic pain outside of active cancer, palliative care, and end-of-life care.
2. When opioids are used, the lowest possible effective dosage should be prescribed to reduce risks of opioid use disorder and overdose.
3. Providers should always exercise caution when prescribing opioids and monitor all patients closely.[85]

The CDC has created tools and materials to improve communication between providers and patients about the risks and benefits of opioid therapy for chronic pain; to improve the safety and effectiveness of pain treatment; and to reduce the risks associated with long-term opioid therapy, including opioid use disorder, overdose, and death.[86]

Cybersecurity

Pharmacies are just as vulnerable to physical attacks and cyberattacks as large businesses are. Pharmacies are attractive to thieves because of the drugs they stock and the confidential information they house that can aid identity theft. While pharmacies are not likely to become less of a magnet for thieves anytime soon, there are steps pharmacy owners can take to curb or prevent attacks, including: installing internal and external digital cameras, shredding documents that contain confidential information, reporting suspicious activities to the police, being vigilant against social engineering attacks, and quickly addressing issues with disgruntled employees. Pharmacies should also change their business patterns when possible and be aware of where the exits, entrances, and cameras are.[87]

Chapter 10:
Building the Most Effective Teams and Leaders to Enable the MAB Rx Locally and Globally

"We need to develop and disseminate an entirely new paradigm and practice of collaboration that supersedes the traditional silos that have divided organizations, companies, governments, departments, and teams for decades and replace them with networks of partnerships working together to create a globally healthier society for all."
Elizabeth Oyekan, adapted from a quote by Simon Mainwaring[1]

"There is a desire in each of us to invest in things that matter, and to have the organizations in which we work be successful. ...Our task is to create organizations we believe in ... to be part of creating something we care about so we can endure the sacrifice, risk, and adventure that commitment entails. That's team work motivation."
Organizational development expert Peter Block[2]

Topics Covered:

- The building blocks of a high-performing and effective team
- The importance of effective leadership to optimize the MAB Rx strategy as a plan of action
- How to transform teams into an interdependent and cohesive team capable of solving complex challenges and improving performance
- Some of the key responsibilities of leaders during a project
- How leaders can support the geographic expansion and reach of clinical MAB services

This new era of value-based healthcare requires high-performing teams and effective leaders. They will be the ones to determine whether the following transpire:

- An organization will consistently provide the highest quality and most affordable care to its members.
- Patients will be compassionately cared for and treated with dignity.
- An organization will become the solution for lowering the cost of care by eliminating waste, inefficiencies, non-value-added processes, and inconsistencies in all activities.
- Through partnering with others, the healthiest communities will be built.
- Organizations will meet or exceed the expectations of what matters most to individual patients.
- Organizations will explore and act on new opportunities to improve their performance and achieve a competitive advantage.
- In the midst of challenges, organizations will adhere to their mission, vision, and core purpose.

High-performing teams and effective leaders know that strategies, initiatives, infrastructures, prescriptions, processes, technology, and innovations are just tools in the value-based healthcare system toolbox; it takes the commitment, dedication, and intelligence of people to use those tools effectively to make the difference. Effective teams and leaders can utilize tools such as MAB to deliver dramatic results across the continuum of care—from better patient outcomes, fewer healthcare errors, better healthcare costs, and increased coordination of care to creating effective innovations that will improve the health and wellbeing of patients and team members. This will lead to improved organizational performance and a competitive advantage.

According to Jon Katzenbach and Douglas Smith, authors of *The Wisdom of Teams: Creating the High-Performance Organization*, the definition of teams is "a small number of people with complementary skills who are committed to a common purpose, performance goals, and approach for which they hold themselves mutually accountable."[3] To effectively implement the MAB prescription or any other organizational strategy, organizations need to develop high-performing teams that will take strategic tools and use them to transform or optimize the care delivered to patients and populations.

So how are these high-performing teams developed? There are three core areas that help teams transition from where they currently are (even if they are already good) to becoming high performing. These include the following:

- Identifying the behavioral traits and core elements of high-performing teams and becoming more intentional about developing them
- Identifying the most important competencies that an effective team builder and leader must have to help teams become highly effective
- Leveraging the right tools to bring effective team members together to create an interdependent effective team that will consistently deliver high performance

Behavioral Traits, Skills, and Core Elements Associated with a High Performer

All potentially high-performing and effective teams are L.E.A.D.E.R.S. at heart. They are always looking for: ways to make a positive impact on behalf of the patient and organization, ways to improve the status quo, and opportunities to lead even the smallest project that will make a difference. L.E.A.D.E.R.S. is both a word and an acronym for the key traits and qualities typically found in most high-performing teams and leaders. It stands for:

- Leading with a purpose
- Engaging and communicating effectively
- Accountability and ownership

- Development of self and others
- Executing effectively
- Recognizing and acknowledging improvements, excellence, and calculated risks
- Solidifying relationships

Dr. Sam, the director of pharmacy operations in a large healthcare system from Chapter 5, and his team effectively built a multidisciplinary leadership team that contributed to the development and implementation of the MAB strategy across the continuum and within their clinical and support teams. They used the L.E.A.D.E.R.S. core elements in the following ways:

- *Leading with a purpose*: For teams and team members to become effective, they must understand, internalize, and be committed to the purpose, mission, and vision of the project or strategy they are about to embark on and determine how it is aligned with the bigger picture. They must also understand how their contributions will impact the organization's priorities, and they must share mutual accountabilities. Unless they understand, internalize, and commit, individuals will most likely not become an effective, high-performing team. As Mark Twain famously said, "The two most important days in your life are the day you are born and the day you find out why."[4] When team members understand the "why" behind what they have been asked to do, and how it fits into the bigger picture, they will find innovative ways to make the purpose, mission, and vision a reality.

- *Engage and communicate effectively*: Communication is the cornerstone of an engaged team, and when teams are engaged, they are generally more loyal, productive, and committed to the success of the organization, and they generally go above and beyond the call of duty.

  Dr. Sam's pharmacy team engaged key stakeholders, physicians, pharmacists, nurses, patients, and other leaders who played a role in the organization's medication management practices to co-design how MAB would be implemented within their healthcare system. By contributing to the initiative, the key stakeholders gained support and buy-in, a supportive rollout, and eventually the creation of a high-performing culture.

Engagement and effective communication are key skills that teams must have. They must be able to engage one another effectively and respect the contributions each member brings. One of the most common causes of strategy and project demise is a lack of communication or a fear to give constructive feedback during meetings. The inability to engage each other may be due to hierarchy (for example, manager and staff communication), being extremely busy, perceived disrespect or intimidation by other team members, lack of acknowledgment of one another, or simply a culture that does not permit healthy discussions at all levels.

It is important that team members recall both what is at stake when communication breaks down and the lives that depend on their ability to work well together. Consciously remembering this on a regular basis will make team members more likely to speak up, address the barriers to engagement, and make a concerted effort to ensure the barriers are not resurrected (and if they do begin to resurrect, establish a culture where they can be addressed quickly).

- *Accountability and ownership*: Accountabilities begin with clarity of goals, purposes, and roles. When teams are brought together, if they do not know what their core deliverables, goals, measures of success, and roles are, they will not know what takes priority, what needs to be put on the back burner, and who should do what. As George Harrison wrote in his song "Any Road," "If you don't know where you're going, any road will take you there."[5]

  When Dr. Sam's multidisciplinary team came together, the team leaders took the time to create agreed-upon goals that were simple, measurable, and clearly relevant to the team's task. They also demonstrated how the goals aligned with the bigger picture and worked on role clarification within the team (which was modified along the way). They helped the team understand the clear mutual accountability for performance. This focused the team, built trust, and motivated them to excel on core deliverables.

- *Development of self and others*: It is critical that teams develop the competencies, skills, and behaviors needed to successfully navigate through the uncertainties and challenges in healthcare today. Some of the ways to build up these skills and behaviors include seeking new experiences and opportunities; developing self-awareness and awareness in how others function based on personalities and temperaments; leveraging the strengths of team members; finding ways to continue learning; participating in mentorship and coaching programs; and continuously developing the core competencies associated with job functions, while exhibiting and maintaining strong character. When developing others, focus on the Leadership Intelligence (LQ) Pyramid (see Figure 10.1) of hiring the right team members with L.E.A.D.E.R.S. skills; training them; providing meaningful experiences; providing accountability and feedback; and, when possible, promoting them.

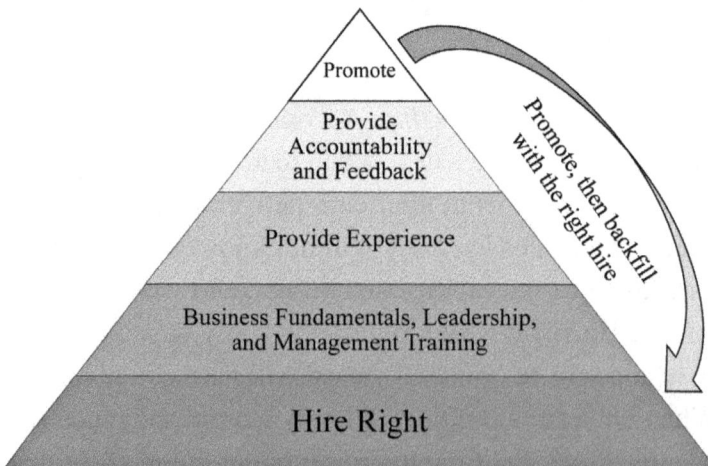

Figure 10.1: The LQ Pyramid for developing others

The clinical pharmacists and other team members for Dr. Sam's new clinical MAB services were selected based on their L.E.A.D.E.R.S. skills and the clinical competencies required for the role. They also showed an aptitude for continuously learning and improving, were compassionate and credible, and had a willingness to work at the highest scope of practice to make MAB a reality for their patients and populations.

To support and sustain these new clinical teams, the training department developed the following:

- Experiential, didactic, and/or modular training programs with these components: disease management, change management, continuous improvement, population management strategies, process workflows, teamwork, rounding skills, journal clubs, and other skills, tools, and competencies needed for the new environment
- Experiential learning with physicians and other providers, which was updated every six months
- Other core skills training to help team members learn how to set goals, manage expectations, focus on core purpose, use quality measures for effective care management, use performance reports for continuous improvement, execute strategies to get results, and have effective communication skills

- *Executing effectively*: Getting teams and team members to focus their energies and implement the important goals, projects, tasks, and initiatives that ultimately matter most to patients and the organization remain enormous challenges for organizations today. Why is this so? According to Chris McChesney, coauthor of *The 4 Disciplines of Execution: Achieving Your Wildly Important Goals*, the fundamental reason why execution is so difficult is because it requires people to change their behavior and to implement these changes in a new healthcare environment that's already swirling with other urgent priorities.[6]

To execute effectively, teams must have clarity of purpose, be willing to engage their members in developing mutually accountable measures of success, and create a plan and process with interdependent teams and stakeholders. Execution also involves the development of a rhythm of accountability, displaying and communicating early wins, celebrating successes, learning from failures, and conducting post-project reviews without blame.

- *Recognizing and acknowledging improvements, excellence, and calculated risks*: In many organizations, the pace of change and focus on multiple priorities often prevents teams from remembering and celebrating accomplishments. When people are recognized, it is generally for big innovations or improvements. While this is very important, it is also crucial to recognize calculated risks that performed as expected, so team leaders should create a balanced environment where people can take calculated risks, fail fast, and learn from their failures to eventually achieve excellence.

   According to research on employee recognition in *Forbes*, organizations that offer regular thanks to their employees far outperform those that do not.[7] In a recent study conducted by the Jackson Organization, 26,000 employees were asked to rate their level of agreement with the following statement: "My organization recognizes excellence." Results confirmed that the return on equity for companies scoring highest in employee recognition was more than three times greater than that of low-scoring companies.[8]

   It is also important to understand how people and employees want to be recognized. This varies from person to person. Some people like to be recognized publicly, while others prefer private acknowledgment. Taking time to understand how people want to be recognized will have an enormously positive impact on performance, productivity, and ultimately the bottom line. Using the MAB Prescription Strategy project, the medical group and health plan leaders recognized the teams quarterly for the outcomes achieved. They listened and understood the challenges that the teams faced, and acted as barrier "busters" for the teams and programs so the teams could focus on progress.

- *Solidifying relationships*: What are the fundamental relationships that need to be developed, fostered, and solidified to build a positive work environment for teams to flourish and promote excellence? While it is important to develop good relationships with everyone, there are four types of professional relationships we must focus on, build, manage, strengthen, and solidify. These include relationships with team members and subordinates, peers across departments and silos, manager(s), and customers. Solidifying these core relationships will make the work more rewarding and effective.

Important Competencies for the Effective Team Builder and Leader
In this value-based healthcare system, leaders and managers are going to need new or additional competencies and skills to effectively navigate the ongoing changes and to help team members come together to become high-performing teams. According to key experts from Integrated Healthcare Strategies and Arthur J. Gallagher & Co, there are four essential competency clusters to ensure leadership success in this new healthcare era. These include inspiring and persuasive leadership, exceptional people skills, a focus on execution and results, and personal character.[9]

- *Inspiring and persuasive leadership*: An effective team builder and leader must be able to lead with a vision aligned with the mission of the organization and inspire others to follow. This person must also be a champion of change, inspire trust and commitment, coach and mentor others, be innovative and creative, and create a sense of urgency to act.[10]
- *Exceptional people skills*: An effective team builder and leader must be able to embrace collaboration, have a keen understanding

of people (their strengths and capabilities), develop leaders, shape the culture, be an excellent negotiator, respect providers and team members, and effectively communicate and engage teams and team members. They must also ensure that teams and team members have the knowledge to accomplish their tasks/projects/initiatives, manage egos and the team's need for attention and recognition, be empathetic and caring, and internalize the L.E.A.D.E.R.S. elements as core competencies.

- *Focus on execution and results*: An effective team builder and leader must be focused, help others focus and be engaged, create shared and mutually accountable goals and measures, be an architect of change, be tenacious, and be financially astute. A leader must also create an environment that promotes problem solving and allows team members to view mistakes as opportunities for improving team process and results. He or she must not be afraid to course-correct, make difficult decisions, and establish standards of performance that are constantly being met and improving at all times. A leader also provides proactive and ongoing feedback to help teams stay on track, recognizes expected core behaviors, and remains flexible and adaptable to changing situations.[11]
- *Personal character*: An effective team builder and leader must have integrity, be curious and eager to learn, be accountable and courageous, be humble and modest, have self-awareness of his or her leadership style and techniques, be emotionally intelligent, and be comfortable with oneself.[12]

Team builders and leaders with these skills and competencies are definitely worth their weight in gold (or perhaps even platinum).

Transforming Team Members into High-Performing Teams

Team members bring their expertise to the table when they first come together. However, to form a team that is greater than the sum of each member's area of expertise—one that will solve complex and new challenges—these members must go from independence to interdependence and must go through the stages of team development. They must also adopt the L.E.A.D.E.R.S. behavioral traits and core elements.

Independence to Interdependence

According to the Center for Creative Leadership, independent leadership can be characterized by knowledge and expertise—a depth of understanding and proficiency in a particular functional area. However, this type of leadership can sometimes lead to decentralized decision making, high demand for individual responsibility, a reliance on that person's expertise, and a focus on individual performance.[13] While these attributes are very important, an organization with primarily independent team members and leaders may not adjust well when there is a collective demand for more fully integrated services across the various disciplines and areas of expert knowledge.

As healthcare becomes more complex, beyond the scope of any one department or entity, independent leadership must be coupled with interdependent leadership.[14] Interdependent leadership requires mutual inquiry and learning. It is a highly developed stage of leadership culture that has the capacity to create commitment, leverage, alignment, and direction in a variety of challenging contexts. It is highly valuable in situations that demand collaboration across departments, silos, and systems, in which outcomes are more evolving and less linear.[15] These same principles of independent and interdependent leadership also apply to teams and team members. Figure 10.2 (adapted from *The Center for Creative Leadership Handbook*) shows how independent and interdependent teams approach certain situations.[16]

For more information about understanding and incorporating the elements of interdependent leadership and culture into the fabric of the team, go to http://www.ccl.org/Leadership/index.aspx and http://www.teachinghorse.com.

Stages of Team Development

Organizations striving for a competitive advantage are increasingly building and incorporating the use of interdependent high-performance teams to execute complex business strategies. They are doing this by training team members on the stages of team development: the forming-storming-norming-performing stages.[17] These four stages of team development build the cohesiveness of a team, which makes them more cooperative and effective in achieving the goals they set for themselves.

Approach	Independent Teams	Interdependent Teams
How direction of the team is decided	Based on discussion, mutual influence, and compromise	Based on shared exploration and the emergence of new perspectives
Alignment of work	Based on negotiation among self-responsible people	Based on ongoing mutual adjustment among system-responsible people
Commitment to purpose	Commitment results from evaluation of the benefits for self while benefiting the larger community	Commitment results from engagement in a developing community
Change process	Calculated risks are taken	Creative energy and possibilities to develop new solutions
Dealing with uncertainty	Resorts back to one's expertise	Develops aligned and shared leadership
Leadership style	Archiver	Collaborator

Figure 10.2: The approach independent and interdependent teams take to certain situations

The forming-storming-norming-performing stages seem obvious but are in fact difficult. They need to be addressed in order for teams to be successful. Many teams want to move to the performing stage without passing through the first three stages, but this usually does not work. The first stage, the forming stage, is relatively easy. The storming and norming stages, however, can be difficult and can sometimes cause a team to fail. The performing stage is usually effective once the storming and norming stages are complete and teams are more cohesive. For more information about these stages and how to implement them in teams, go to https://www.mindtools.com/pages/article/newLDR_86.htm and http://www.teachinghorse.com.

An Example of How Effective Leadership Worked

The CEO of Dr. Sam's company set a 5.4.3 organizational goal to be accomplished over a three-year period: 5 stars in Medicare Stars and Hospital Stars programs, 4 stars in member care experience (CAHPS measures), and a 3% profit margin. This was a huge undertaking because their baseline numbers at the time were 3 stars in the Medicare Stars program, 2 stars in the Hospital Stars program, 2 stars in the CAHPS measures, and 0.5% profit margin. Understanding these goals and the healthcare environment, Dr. Sam engaged his team and key stakeholders to adopt MAB as one of the key organizational strategies to directly and indirectly contribute to meeting the audacious 5.4.3 goals.

Dr. Sam met with the senior leaders and some of the key stakeholder's leaders to share how the MAB Rx strategy would significantly contribute to the organizational goals by improving many of the core quality measures, improving coordination of care for individual patients and the population, reducing readmissions, reducing total cost of care, and improving the patient care experience. After meaningful review and discussions, the senior leaders adopted MAB as one of the organization's key strategies. The senior leaders and the pharmacy team did the following:

- Created a sense of urgency, clarity, and importance around this strategy for the organization
- Identified key champions, including physician and senior leader sponsors
- Obtained funding for the initiative
- Worked with marketing to incorporate the communication of this initiative into the overall organizational communication strategy
- Helped remove barriers and obstacles
- Communicated early wins, recognized milestones, and built momentum and motivation to improve long-term sustainability

These were key attributes that the teams were looking for from their senior leaders as a sign of commitment to this and other organizational priorities.

The deeply interactive clinical nature of MAB required that providers throughout the organization not only understood what was at stake, but truly embraced the strategy to ensure a successful implementation. The clinical champion was in the best position to orient other peer physicians to MAB through multiple communication channels including presentations, staff meetings, and other group settings. A well-formatted document outlined the purpose of the initiative, its pros and cons, the draft rollout processes, teams the initiative would impact, and the benefits of MAB to patients and the organization.

Also in these meetings, the champions gave providers an opportunity to converse, welcomed their feedback, and informed them of venues that would be available for their suggestions for improvement. While teams reviewed their own MAB data every two weeks initially and eventually monthly, Dr. Sam and the champions had the MAB measures on the organization's vital signs scoreboard reviewed monthly and then reviewed the data with the senior leaders on quarterly bases. At these meetings, challenges, barriers, obstacles, and successes were discussed, as well as action plans to course-correct where necessary. The quarterly meetings, coupled with the recognition of milestones and early wins, built momentum in team members and motivated them to aspire for excellence while meeting the established goals.

Expanding the Geographic Reach of the MAB Rx Strategy from One Entity to Multiple Systems

To support the adoption of MAB on a larger scale, new partnerships have to be formed at a local, national, and global level. Within one year, the organization saw how the systematic implementation of MAB across the continuum of care had made a significant impact on the health outcomes of patients and on the organizational quality, service, and cost measures. Dr. Sam and the champions were then asked about the possibility of spreading the MAB Rx strategy to all the other hospitals and ambulatory service systems within the organization's network across the country.

After doing a significant amount of research and having preliminary meetings with a few key interested leaders (early adopters) from these other systems, Dr. Sam and his team found the following:

- There were a number of committed leaders and stakeholders in the network organizations ready to adopt the MAB Rx strategy.
- Many of the hospitals and clinics in the network across the country were struggling with their quality, service, and affordability measures and saw MAB as a possible strategy for improvement.
- Many of the network organizations, when they looked hard enough, identified resources (or repurposed existing resources) that could be leveraged to implement the MAB Rx strategy in key settings.
- The MAB Rx strategy offering was a consistent approach of optimizing health and healthcare in patients with chronic conditions—different from the current variation in approaches used by pharmacists and other clinicians in many of their network organizations.
- There would be an opportunity to further consolidate some of the necessary capabilities and core infrastructures that support the success of MAB—such as mail-order service, inventory management, workload balancing, drug use management strategic services, research, quality performance management, compliance services, and specialty services, potentially reducing costs even more across the network.
- A marketing strategy and the necessary tools to support this expansion would include the development of the MAB playbook and toolkit, which would contain the following:

  - The overarching MAB Rx strategy, purpose, and potential benefits
  - Performance measures and scoreboards
  - Roles of the team members
  - Infrastructures needed for support and sustainability
  - Leadership support
  - Training of BSMART to implement MAB

- Collaborate with organizations to develop MAB training tailored for specific healthcare organizations
- Facilitate the spread of MAB as a successful, consistent practice to make the Triple Aim a reality
- Collaborate in seeking reimbursement for these services under the new enhanced MTM program and, eventually, from other CMS programs like MIPS and insurance payers

Pharmacy schools

Many pharmacy schools have partnered with pharmacy organizations to develop and implement curricula strategies in medication therapy management (MTM). For example, the American Pharmacists Association and the American Association of Colleges of Pharmacy jointly developed a report that summarized the work that 18 colleges and schools of pharmacy had done to successfully incorporate MTM into their curricula.[20] Also, the American Pharmacists Association developed a certificate training program framework that is being used to develop courses to teach MTM concepts to student pharmacists.[21]

Today, most schools of pharmacy offer a variety of certificate programs in partnership with pharmacy organizations to prepare pharmacists to become MTM patient care clinicians and to address the multiple needs of patients with chronic or complex conditions. Leaders on Dr. Sam's team serve as adjunct and assistant professors on the faculty of a number of pharmacy schools to provide students with real-life examples and experiences of how MTM and MAB work, their purpose, and their benefits in the lives of patients.

Partnerships with Other Healthcare Systems

As the network of systems Dr. Sam worked for began to acquire new hospitals and healthcare services, the CEO wanted to know how Dr. Sam and his team would be able to further expand the geographic reach of the MAB Rx strategy—not just to the newly acquired pharmacies, hospitals, and clinics, but also to their partnership organizations such as the chain pharmacies and the PBM. Dr. Sam knew the newly acquired pharmacies and their partner organizations probably already had their own clinical pharmacy strategies, so he met with their leaders to understand their strategies and services. Then he proposed a joint alliance with the newly acquired pharmacies, the chain pharmacies, the PBM, and his pharmacy system.

This new alliance focused on developing a shared vision for clinical pharmacy services that would improve patient health outcomes, reduce cost of care, and improve the coordination of care for the patients in the current and new expanded health system network. At the same time, it would contribute to the 5.4.3 performance goals of the whole health system network. They worked together to develop and build a new shared clinical pharmacy services strategy that was about 70% consistent across the newly acquired pharmacies, the chain pharmacies, and Dr. Sam's existing pharmacy system, and a 30% warranted variation based on the unique situations of their practices. One of the core components of this new shared clinical pharmacy services strategy was the implementation of MAB.

Partnership with Local and National Agencies

With their collective experiences with the MAB strategy, Dr. Sam and his organization have decided to share the strategy with some of the local and national quality agencies. During 2017, they will meet with CMS as well as local healthcare systems, accountable care organizations, PBMs, hospitals, and retail pharmacies to introduce the MAB strategy and demonstrate how it will positively contribute to their strategies and programs, including:

- NQS
- CMS Quality Strategy
- New CMS Part D Enhanced Medication Therapy Management Model
- CMS Medicare Stars ratings
- The Hospital Readmissions Reduction Program
- The FDA and CDC focus on opioid and prescription drug abuse
- Patient safety goals

In the meantime, Dr. Sam has introduced the MAB Rx strategy and toolkit to many organizations that are now seeing improvement in patient health outcomes, cost reductions, and improved organizational performance—and just in time, they are moving from fee-for-service to a value-based healthcare environment.

Chapter 11:
Putting It Together: The MAB Rx Strategy—A Prescription Solution for Creating Healthcare Value

"Increasing the effectiveness of adherence interventions may have a far greater impact on the health of the population than any improvement in specific medical treatments."
R.B. Haynes[1]

Topics Covered:

- A brief review of Parts I and II
- The possibilities of leveraging MAB to address future challenges and support new trends and opportunities
- A summary of the MAB Rx strategy

This book began by looking at the good and challenging aspects of the United States' healthcare system, especially the unstainable trends such as the large numbers of uninsured people, growth in personal debt and bankruptcy from medical costs, the ever-increasing costs of healthcare, and average-to-poor quality outcomes in spite of the cost per capita spent on healthcare. And so, in 2010, the ACA was introduced to address many of these challenges. It made health insurance more accessible and affordable for lower and middle income Americans and small business employers, improved the quality and value of healthcare provided, created important new consumer protections, eliminated wasteful spending, and enforced reforms aimed at addressing and transforming the US healthcare system.

While the fate of the ACA is in the balance, it has made some important steps forward toward its goal of becoming a catalyst for extensive reform by providing strong incentives for publicly financed healthcare programs to connect provider payment to quality care and efficiency. The ACA has also made provisions to improve the quality of care by requiring the secretary of HHS to create a strategy for improving healthcare, including setting priorities and providing a plan for achieving its goals for better care, smarter spending, and healthier people and communities. As a result, the NQS was created as the first overarching strategy and policy designed to lead federal, state, and local efforts to improve the quality of care and align public and private payers in quality and safety efforts.

In 2015, the bipartisan law MACRA was passed to further support the ongoing transformation of the healthcare delivery system. MACRA was built on the principles set by the ACA, tying Medicare reimbursements to quality of care through merit-based incentive payment systems and APMs. In 2016, MACRA legislation introduced QPP to focus on improving the quality and health outcomes for Medicare beneficiaries, support the transition from fee-for-service to fee-for-value, and promote healthcare quality transformation to meet the NQS's three aims of better care, smarter spending, and healthier communities and people. In addition to the QPP, there are many other organizations and programs on this quest to transform the healthcare and care delivery systems, each having strategies, initiatives, and measures to change components of these systems.

This commitment to healthcare value and the QPP has led organizations and provider practices to put critical physical, technical, operational, and talent management infrastructures in place; adopt evidence-based practices such as care coordination and population management to augment these new infrastructures; and leverage the use of technology and analytics to identify populations for personalized interventions. These are all critical components for organizational success and business advantage in the new value-based healthcare system.

Providers and organizations are adopting a new strategy to support their efforts to achieve the NQS priorities, the quality measures aligned with MIPS and APM, and existing quality goals (such as Medicare Stars and HEDIS). The strategy is an integrated set of solutions that improves patients' adherence to their medication regimens; ensures these regimens are reconciled to reduce drug interactions, duplications, errors, and risk of hospitalizations; improves patient engagement and provider interactions; addresses medication affordability while minimizing prescription waste; and embeds practices to ensure patients use their medications safely and effectively. This integrated solution set is known as Medication A.R.E.A.S. Bundle Prescription or MAB Rx.

MCC patients have become a primary focus in healthcare because, driven by human factors such as aging and increased obesity and cardiovascular diseases, the number of these patients has risen significantly. They are now the most frequent users of healthcare in the United States and worldwide. Therefore, integrating the MAB Rx into the care delivery and care process of the MCC population would significantly improve quality and health outcomes, reduce the cost of total care, and improve the organization's performance and value as reflected in MIPS, Medicare Stars, HEDIS, ACO quality measures, and other Triple Aim measures.

Over a six-month period, Dr. Sam, key stakeholders, and team members developed the MAB Rx strategic plan for his organization, which became the gold standard for effectively treating MCC patients in the organization's nationwide network. To develop the MAB strategic plan and operationalize it in the care delivery system, Dr. Sam and his team focused on the following enablers:

- *Framework*: Using the BSMART checklist framework, MAB was integrated into existing and new care models.
- *Performance*: By identifying the patient-centered outcomes and process measures, MAB would directly and indirectly impact the continuum of care. Pilots would demonstrate the value of MAB by

showcasing early wins, increasing accountability, and continuing improvements by using MAB dashboards with the identified measures of success.

- *Infrastructure and business capabilities*: Dr. Sam and his team assessed, developed, built, and/or optimized key infrastructures and capabilities that were needed to ensure the successful implementation, support, scalability, and sustainability of MAB.
- *Collaborative alternative care delivery model*: They developed a new MAB model with key components to spread to the nationwide networks and to other like-minded organizations.
- *People*: Finally, they focused on the importance of high-performing people, teams, and effective leaders who were committed to the success of the MAB Rx strategy, optimized it, and contributed to expanding its geographic reach through internal and external partnerships and alliances.

Trends, Opportunities, and Future Challenges—the MAB Rx Strategy and the Crystal Ball

Moving forward, it's essential to identify some of the future challenges, trends, and opportunities in healthcare and see how the MAB Rx Stragegycan be leveraged in many of these instances. Some of the ongoing healthcare challenges—which might be opportunities in disguise—include the aging population, increased prevalence of chronic conditions, high-cost medications, barriers to coordination of care and patient engagement, healthcare disparities and pockets of excellence in care that are not available to all, increased co-payments and out-of-pocket costs by patients, lack of access to care in remote areas, the workforce acclimating to the new healthcare realities, and prescription medication overdoses.

Some of the new trends and opportunities in healthcare include precision medicine, the transformation from fee-for-service to pay-for-value, consumerism, new technologies, consolidations, value-based contracts, health and wellness apps, and new care delivery models.

These and other challenges, trends, and opportunities are grouped in the following categories: patients and consumers, healthcare organizations, teams and the workforce, affordability and finance, quality and safety, technology and innovation, and government and policies. MAB can directly and indirectly impact them all.

Patients and Consumers

- *Increased prevalence of chronic conditions*: With the increase in the aging population and lifestyle-induced diseases (like obesity, cardiovascular diseases, and cancer), the number of people with MCC has risen significantly. Studies have shown that if 65% of Americans achieved "six normal" ranges for blood pressure, blood sugar, waist-to-height ratio, stress management, LDL cholesterol, and tobacco toxins, the nation would save well over $600 billion in healthcare spending per year. MAB, along with diet, exercise, and behavior modification, will be the most effective way of helping patients achieve these goals,; currently only 3% to 4 % of the US population entering Medicare meet these goals.[2]

- *Barriers to coordination of care and patient engagement*: One of the priorities of the NQS and the CMS Quality Strategy includes a focus on these two barriers in an effort to improve patient health outcomes. Providers are using MAB to improve the coordination of care by engaging patients in identifying their medication adherence barriers, helping them reconcile their medications, addressing affordability and safety concerns, and coordinating these findings with other providers.

- *Increased co-payments and out-of-pocket costs*: Pharmacists and providers are seeing more patients neglecting to pick up their medications and forgoing treatment due to the cost. Pharmacists are therefore working diligently with providers to identify alternative therapies, formulary therapies, and financial assistance programs to help patients with their medication costs. In one study, 41% of the people surveyed who had health insurance reported skipping or putting off filling a prescription in the last year.[3]

Healthcare Organizations

- *Healthcare disparities and pockets of excellence in care but not available to all*: In the United States, there are pockets of excellent care, especially if patients can afford it; however, in significant parts of the country, healthcare is average to suboptimal, with disparities between ethnic groups. The causes of disparities are complex and interrelated, ranging from one's behavior, genetics, social circumstances, education, and the environment in which one lives. Often, racial and ethnic minorities receive a poorer standard of healthcare. This is detailed in the *National Healthcare Quality and Disparities Report*, which is published annually by the Agency for Healthcare Research and Quality. MAB is a strategy that can contribute to closing the disparity gap in patients with chronic conditions who are taking multiple medications.
- *New care delivery models*: To move organizations along the path to value, CMS has set the following goals: 30% of traditional Medicare payments will be tied to APMs (for example, certain bundled payments, ACOs, or medical homes) by the end of 2016, and 50% of such payments will be tied to these models by the end of 2018.[4] These new advanced APMs need clinical MAB pharmacists to help meet the new value-based quality goals.

Teams and the Workforce

- *Acclimating to the new healthcare realities*: Many providers and healthcare team members are not aware of some of the major changes happening in healthcare. Few understand the ACA's focus shift from fee-for-service to pay-for-value, and fewer understand the impact that legislation such as MACRA will have on fee-for-service organizations and practices. Providers and organizations need to become very familiar with MACRA and the focus on value if they are going to succeed in this new value-based healthcare system. They must also have their pharmacy teams implement the MAB Prescription Strategy and related services to improve patient outcomes and to perform well on the quality measures associated with MIPS and APMs under MACRA.

Affordability and Finance

- *High-cost medications*: Over the last decade, there have been significant increases in medication costs, ranging from the Ariad's leukemia drug, to Turing's drug Daraprim, to Mylan's EpiPens, and now the new high-cost biologics. However, these are not the only places we are seeing cost increases. Over 3,500 generic medications doubled in price from 2008 to 2015, and nearly 400 generics increased by over 1,000%.[5] Organizations and PBMs are working with the FDA to prioritize speed of approvals and market access to new generics, biosimilars, and competitive medications to drive competition. Formulary focus, rebates, and negotiating the best contracts are major priorities for organizations.
- *Value-based contracts*: Value-based contracts between drug manufacturers and payers are growing in number. Since 2014, payers and PBMs have reached at least a dozen "value-based" or "at-risk" deals with manufacturers, by bringing higher payment rates for improving patient outcomes. Both manufacturers and organizations need to have MAB in place to ensure that contracted medications are used optimally to achieve the desired outcomes.

Quality and Safety

- *Organizational performance*: MAB can support organizational performance by positively impacting Medicare Stars, HEDIS, MACRA, and other Triple Aim measures.
- *Opioid overdoses and deaths*: Deaths involving overdoses due to prescription opioids quadrupled in the United States between 1999 and 2015, and so have the sales of opioid prescription medications. More than 183,000 people have died from overdoses related to prescription opioids during the same time period. In 2015 alone, more than 15,000 people died from overdoses involving prescription opioids.[6]

- *HRRP*: The HRRP has penalized hospitals for higher than expected readmission rates. Inappropriate medication use is one of the top three reasons for many of the readmissions. Implementing the MAB Prescription Strategy will help organizations reduce medication-related readmissions as well as these penalties.

Technology and Innovation

- *Access to care in remote areas*: Many hospitals and healthcare systems in remote areas are now using telehealth technology to increase access and quality of healthcare. MAB pharmacists in centralized locations can use this technology to provide convenient and timely care to patients in rural areas, helping to improve patient outcomes and organizational performance.
- *Mobile apps*: Consumers are now using mobile apps with their providers or care managers, or sometimes on their own, to optimize MAB. Many apps do one or more of the following to support MAB: remind patients to take their medications as scheduled, notify patients if there are any drug interactions or duplications on their medication lists, remind them when to pick up their refills, locate the best prices for patients who do not have insurance, and provide information about side effect management.
- *Precision medicine*: Most medications are designed for the "average patient," which results in successful outcomes for some patients but not for others. Precision medicine is an innovative approach that takes into account individual differences in people's lifestyles, environments, and genetics when determining which therapies to use. This enables providers to target specific treatments to the illnesses they are treating. For example, patients with certain types of cancer usually undergo molecular testing as part of their care; this enables physicians to select treatments that improve chances of survival and reduce exposure to adverse effects.[7]

Government and Policies

- *The Affordable Care Act* (see Chapter 2)
- *The Drug Quality Security Act* (see Chapter 9)
- *The 21st Century Cures Act*: This landmark bipartisan legislation passed at the end of 2016. It has a number of components that MAB will be needed for, to support clinical practice and ensure no unintended consequences result.[8] Some key parts of the legislation that MAB can contribute to include (not all inclusive):
  - Readmissions: There are new provisions that allow hospitals serving predominantly poor patients to compare their readmission rates against similar hospitals rather than all hospitals to address issues such as socioeconomic and social determinants of health for which these hospitals are being penalized for. The MAB Rx implemented in all practice settings will continue to help reduce medication-related admissions and readmissions even in hospitals that serve predominantly poor patients with socioeconomic and social determinants of health issues.
  - Opioid abuse: About $1 billion has been slated to fight the opioid abuse epidemic and improve safe medication use practices.
  - Mental illness: States are required to use at least 10% of their mental health block grants on early intervention for psychosis, which includes appropriate medication management to ensure success.
  - Patient engagement: The FDA will now be required to include a statement regarding any patient experience data that was used at the time of a drug's approval. The agency will also be allowed to request timely feedback and information from patients regarding their disease or treatments by eliminating the need to go through the Paperwork Reduction Act clearance process.
  - Ensuring safe medication use and practices through:
    - Enhanced practices, such as infusion medications given in providers' offices

- Changes in the drug approval process. The FDA will have more leniency in regards to the kind of evidence it can consider in the approval process—for example, the use of "real world evidence" for the approval of new indications for certain FDA-approved drugs, rather than full clinical trial data.
- Shortening the required times for drug development and medical research, to speed cures coming to market
- The approval of drug companies to promote off-label uses to insurance companies, which allows them to expand their markets
- New cures for cancer and Alzheimer's (and other brain diseases) and the focus on precision medicine (including pharmacogenomics) will need MAB for success.

The president of the National Association of Chain Drug Stores noted in a letter a year prior to the passage of the bill, "Pharmacies and pharmacists in every community stand ready to help foster access to promising cures and treatments that can save and improve patients' lives, and those of their loved ones" through many of the provisions in the 21st Century Cures Act.[9]

The MAB Rx—Strategies for Doing It Right

The primary goal of every organization in this new era of value-based healthcare is best articulated by Professor Michael Porter: "Achieving high value for patients must become the overarching goal of health care delivery, with value defined as the health outcomes achieved per dollar spent. This goal is what matters for patients and unites the interests of all actors in the system."[10]

Organizations are working diligently to make this goal a reality by aiming to have in place the 7Rs: the right people; right/most effective care delivery model(s) aligned with mission, vision, and strengths of the organization; right culture; right processes and systems; right measures and metrics; right innovations and infrastructures; and right partnerships and collaborations. They should also be on the lookout for the right overarching enabling strategies that can be leveraged by these 7Rs to achieve high value, give them a competitive advantage, and optimize their chances of providing better care, smarter spending, and healthier communities.

The last six chapters have demonstrated that the MAB Prescription Strategy is one of these overarching enabling strategies. It will contribute to creating high value in organizations by enabling the 7Rs using the following five strategic anchors (see Figure 11.1):

- *Strategic Anchor 1—Engaged People*: Activate and engage healthcare consumers to become contributors to their health and healthcare while developing highly effective and high-performing healthcare teams to ensure the success of MAB.
- *Strategic Anchor 2—Care Delivery Transformation*: Create new MAB APMs and/or integrate clinical MAB services into the current and new models of care, to optimize the health outcomes of MCC patients and reduce healthcare disparities.
- *Strategic Anchor 3—Performance Outcomes*: Optimize MAB's impact on the following regulatory and quality measures: Medicare Stars, HEDIS, MIPS, APMs, HRRP, and others. Also, demonstrate a reduction in the total cost of care by reducing the progression of diseases, eliminating waste, effectively using drug management programs, creating value-based contracts, preventing adverse outcomes and readmissions, and reducing penalties and/or increasing bonuses from improved quality outcomes.
- *Strategic Anchor 4—Solid Infrastructures and Business Capabilities*: Develop/build/optimize/consolidate infrastructures and business capabilities to successfully implement, support, scale, spread, and sustain clinical MAB services.
- *Strategic Anchor 5—Effective Leadership*: Provide MAB sponsorship, focus on talent and culture management, build internal and external partnerships and alliances to optimize health outcomes in MCC patients globally, and expand geographic reach.

Organizations that identify overarching enabling strategies like the MAB Rx and execute them successfully to achieve high value for patients will have a competitive advantage in this new value-based healthcare environment. And when value in healthcare improves, patients, providers, teams, payers, and suppliers will all benefit, and there will be increased economic sustainability in the healthcare system.[11]

Appendix A:
Payment Options for MIPS and AAPMs

Clinicians must choose one of these two models in 2017 and will receive their first payments under the new framework in 2019. Due to the complexity of implementation, CMS is offering eligible clinicians five options to comply with the new payment methods for the first performance period beginning January 1, 2017 (see figure). According to CMS Acting Administrator Andy Slavitt, "Choosing one of these options would ensure you do not receive a negative payment adjustment in 2019" (https://blog.cms.gov/2016/09/08/qualitypaymentprogram-pickyourpace/). These options—with more details at the QPP website (https://qpp.cms.gov)—are:

1. *Opt to not participate in the QPP*: A provider who chooses not to submit any 2017 data will receive a negative 4% payment adjustment in 2019.
2. *Test the QPP*: Eligible clinicians who submit a minimum amount of 2017 data to the payment program (for example, one quality measure or one improvement activity, or four or more required Advanced Care Information measures) will avoid a negative payment adjustment. This option is designed to ensure the system is working and that eligible clinicians are prepared for broader participation in 2018 and 2019.
3. *Participate for part of the calendar year*: Eligible clinicians who choose to submit 90 days of 2017 quality data (from the list of quality measures and improvement activities) will earn a neutral or small positive payment adjustment. They can start the data collection anytime between January 1 and October 2, 2017.
4. *Participate for the full calendar year*: Practices that were ready on January 1, 2017, were able to choose to submit information for the full calendar year. This meant the first performance period began on the first day of the year. Practices that chose this option could

on the first day of the year. Practices that chose this option could qualify for a moderate positive payment adjustment.

5. *Participate in an Advanced APM in 2017*: Instead of reporting quality data and other information, the law allows eligible clinicians to participate in the payment program by joining an AAPM in 2017. If eligible clinicians receive 25% of Medicare-covered professional services or see 20% of their Medicare patients through an AAPM in 2017, they will earn a 5% incentive payment in 2019. The size of a provider's or organization's payment adjustment will depend both on how much data is submitted and their quality results.

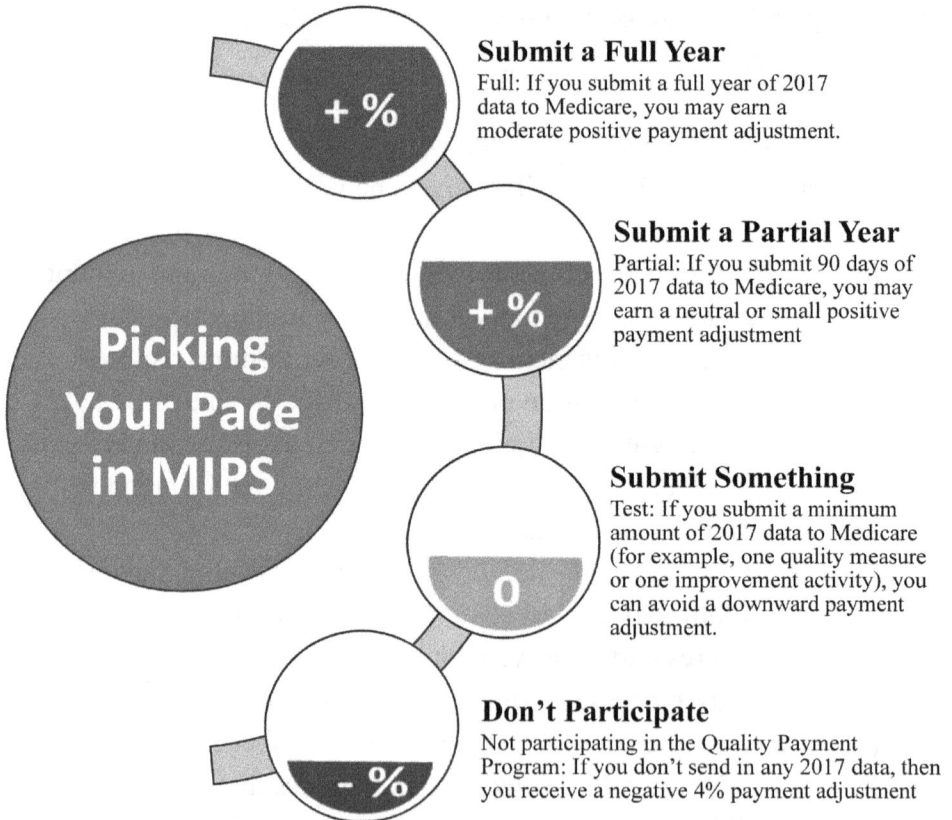

Submit a Full Year
Full: If you submit a full year of 2017 data to Medicare, you may earn a moderate positive payment adjustment.

+ %

Submit a Partial Year
Partial: If you submit 90 days of 2017 data to Medicare, you may earn a neutral or small positive payment adjustment

+ %

Picking Your Pace in MIPS

Submit Something
Test: If you submit a minimum amount of 2017 data to Medicare (for example, one quality measure or one improvement activity), you can avoid a downward payment adjustment.

0

Don't Participate
Not participating in the Quality Payment Program: If you don't send in any 2017 data, then you receive a negative 4% payment adjustment

- %

Picking your pace in MIPS: The payment adjustment options

Appendix B:
Components of MIPS and a Timeline

Below is a summary of the four performance categories and proposed weights. (See https://qpp.cms.gov, https://qpp.cms.gov/measures/performance, and http://www.saignite.com/resources/faq-about-merit-based-incentive-payment-mips#.)

1. **Quality**: The MIPS quality measures will be used to incentivize clinicians to report on specific quality measures and account for 60% of the MIPS score in the first year. For this category, clinicians can choose six measures to report from the QPP website (https://qpp.cms.gov/measures/quality).

   Additionally, MIPS will calculate two population measures based on claims data for individual physicians and small groups (less than nine clinicians) and three population measures for groups with 10 clinicians or more. Clinicians will receive 3 to 10 points on each quality measure based on performance against benchmarks (https://www.cms.gov/Medicare/Quality-Initiatives-Patient-Assessment-Instruments/Value-Based-Programs/MACRA-MIPS-and-APMs/Quality-Payment-Program-Long-Version-Executive-Deck.pdf). The proposal is looking to align with the private sector to reduce the reporting burden by including the core quality measures that private payers already use for their clinicians.

   When choosing the six quality measures, clinicians will need to choose one cross-cutting measure, which includes activities that any physician, no matter which specialty, should be able to perform, such as smoking cessation counseling, checking and controlling blood pressure, or surveying patients on their care experience. Another one of the six measures must be an outcomes measure—for example, diabetes HbA1c control, specific surgical complications, patient-reported function after a procedure, or a high-priority measure. High-priority measures are those related to patient outcomes, appropriate use, patient safety, efficiency, patient experience, or care coordination. There will be about 300 measures to choose from, giving clinicians the flexibility to choose measures most meaningful to their practices. The 300 measures will replace the PQRS measures.

2. **Resource use/efficiency/cost**: This category replaces the Value-Based Modifier Program and will not have any reporting requirements or scores associated with it in 2017 (see https://qpp.cms.gov/docs/Quality_Payment_Program_Overview_Fact_Sheet.pdf). In 2018, that will change. MIPS will calculate scores based on Medicare claims, including all Part A and B costs and Part D drugs, and will focus on how clinicians manage expenditures within their practices, including the costs for specific care episodes. For cost measures, clinicians that deliver more efficient, high-quality care achieve better performance, so clinicians scoring the highest points would have the most efficient resource use. Each cost measure would be worth up to 10 points, and the clinician's cost score would be calculated based on the average score of all the cost measures that can be attributed to the clinician (https://qpp.cms.gov/learn/qpp).

3. **Advancing Care Information (ACI)**: This category focuses on interoperability and the use of the EHR to promote patient engagement and electronic exchange of information; to improve quality, safety, and efficiency; and to reduce health disparities. This category accounts for 25% of the MIPS score in 2017 and replaces the Medicare EHR Incentive Program also known as Meaningful Use. In this category, clinicians must use certified EHR technology and can report from two customizable sets of measures that reflect how they use EHR technology in their day-to-day practice. While CMS will offer several methods for reporting the quality measures, clinicians may choose only one method to report all measures. The ACI score will be made up of a base score and a performance score for a maximum score of 100 points.

4. **Improvement activities (IA)**: This is a new category and accounts

for 15% of the MIPS score in 2017. MIPS would reward IA that contribute to advancing patient care, safety, and care coordination such as expanded practice access, population management, care coordination, beneficiary engagement, patient safety, participation in APMs, and participation in the certified quality reporting system. In addition, clinicians will earn at least half (7.5%) of the IA score in this category for participating in Advanced APMs. CMS proposes more than 90 activities (which will be updated annually) that clinicians may choose from in the following nine subcategories:

- Achieving health equity
- Beneficiary engagement (for example, self-management training)
- Care coordination (for example, telehealth)
- Emergency preparedness and response
- Expanded practice access (for example, same-day appointments)
- Integrated behavioral and mental health
- Participation in APMs, including a medical home model
- Patient safety and practice assessment (for example, use of clinical checklists)
- Population management (for example, monitoring population health)

The maximum total points in this category would be 60 points. Activities will be categorized into the following:

- High-weighted activities supporting the patient-centered medical home, the transformation of clinical practice, or a public health priority will be worth 20 points.
- Medium-weighted activities will be worth 10 points.

For a list of high- and medium-weighted activities, go to: http://www.telligen.com/sites/default/files/documents/CPIA%20Subcategories.pdf

Clinicians who are not patient-facing (for example, pathologists or radiologists) will only need to report on one activity (see https://www.cms.gov/Medicare/Quality-Initiatives-Patient-Assessment-Instruments/Value-Based-Programs/MACRA-MIPS-and-APMs/Quality-Payment-Program-MIPS-NPRM-Slides.pdf).

Summary of the Four MIPS Performance Categories from CMS			
Quality	Resource Use/Cost /Efficiency	Improvement Activities (IA)	Advancing Care Information
Clinicians must select: Up to six measures from individual measures or a specialty measure set that reflect their practice—one cross-cutting measure and one outcomes measure or high-priority measure. **Groups using the web interface:** Report 15 quality measures for a full year. Key changes from the PQRS program include: The quality requirements have been reduced from nine measures to six measures with no domain requirement. Population measures are automatically calculated. There is a major emphasis on outcomes.	CMS will compare resources used to treat similar care episodes and clinical condition groups across practices (can be risk-adjusted to reflect external factors). All available resource use measures will be assessed as applicable to the clinician. CMS calculates based on claims, so there are no reporting requirements for clinicians. Key changes from current Value-Modifier Program: Adding 40+ episode- specific measures to address specialty concerns.	Clinicians can choose the activities best suited for their practice. Attest to completing up to four IA activities (from 90+ proposed activities) with additional credit for more activities. Examples include care coordination, shared decision making, safety checklists, expanding practice access. **Groups with fewer than 15 participants or in a rural or health professional shortage areas** can attest to completing up to two activities. Full credit for patient-centered medical home. Minimum of half credit for APM participation. Key changes from current program: Not applicable (new category).	Clinicians will report up to nine key measures of patient engagement and information exchange from these five CMS objectives: Protection of patient health information (security risk analysis) Electronic prescribing Provide patient electronic access Coordination of care through patient engagement Health information exchange (send summary of care and request/accept summary of care) **For bonus credit, clinicians can:** Report public health and clinical data registry reporting measures Use certified EHR technology to complete certain improvement activities in the improvement activities performance category Clinicians may not need to submit Advancing Care Information if these measures do not apply to their practices. Key changes from current program (EHR/MU Incentive): Dropped "all or nothing" threshold for measurement Removed redundant measures to alleviate reporting burden Eliminated clinical provider order entry and clinical decision support objectives Reduced the number of required public health registries to which clinicians must report
Year 1 weight: 60%	Year 1 weight: 0%	Year 1 weight: 15%	Year 1 weight: 25%

Timeline for MIPS

Performance and payment cycle for MIPS and AAPM providers and practices

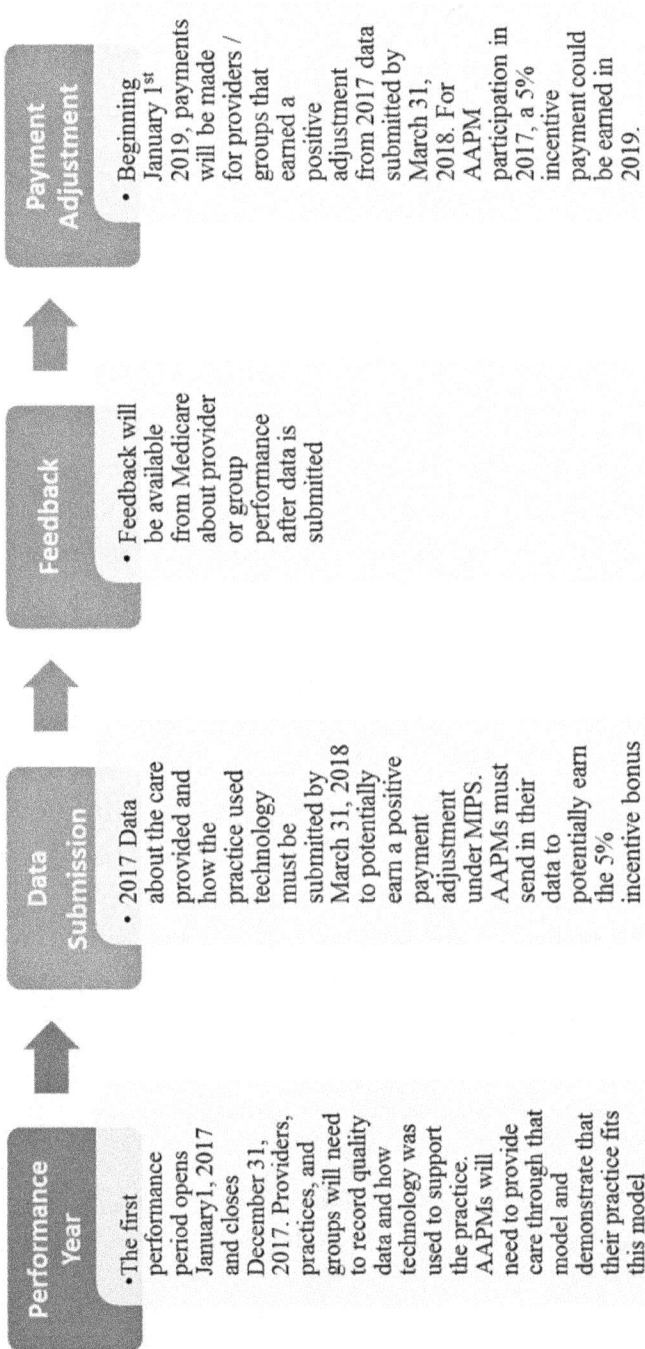

Performance Year

- The first performance period opens January 1, 2017 and closes December 31, 2017. Providers, practices, and groups will need to record quality data and how technology was used to support the practice. AAPMs will need to provide care through that model and demonstrate that their practice fits this model

Data Submission

- 2017 Data about the care provided and how the practice used technology must be submitted by March 31, 2018 to potentially earn a positive payment adjustment under MIPS. AAPMs must send in their data to potentially earn the 5% incentive bonus

Feedback

- Feedback will be available from Medicare about provider or group performance after data is submitted

Payment Adjustment

- Beginning January 1st 2019, payments will be made for providers / groups that earned a positive adjustment from 2017 data submitted by March 31, 2018. For AAPM participation in 2017, a 5% incentive payment could be earned in 2019.

Appendix C:
Resources and Websites on MACRA

Below are some resources and websites that can help educate organizations and providers about MACRA and how to implement it, including training and advocacy:

- Transforming Clinical Practice Initiative: https://innovation.cms.gov/initiatives/Transforming-Clinical-Practices/
- Quality Improvement Organizations: http://qioprogram.org/contact-zones?map=qin
- American Academy of Family Physicians: http://www.aafp.org/practice-management/payment/medicare-payment.html
- American College of Physicians: https://www.acponline.org/practice-resources/business-resources/payment/medicare/macra
- American Hospital Association: http://www.aha.org/advocacy-issues/physician/index.shtml
- American Medical Association: https://www.ama-assn.org/practice-management/understanding-medicare-payment-reform-macra
- Centers for Medicare and Medicaid Services: https://www.cms.gov/Medicare/Quality-Initiatives-Patient-Assessment-Instruments/Value-Based-Programs/MACRA-MIPS-and-APMs/MACRA-MIPS-and-APMs.html and https://www.cms.gov/Medicare/Quality-Initiatives-Patient-Assessment-Instruments/Value-Based-Programs/MACRA-MIPS-and-APMs/Final-MDP.pdf
- Patient-Centered Primary Care Collaborative: https://www.pcpcc.org/2016/06/17/implementing-macra
- Healthcare Dive: http://www.healthcaredive.com/news/macra-rule-summary/430788/
- Quality Payment Program: https://qpp.cms.gov/
- Brookings: https://www.brookings.edu/research/how-the-money-flows-under-macra/
- Documents:

- □ CMS Final Rule, published on October 14, 2016: https://www.federalregister.gov/documents/2016/11/04/2016-25240/medicare-program-merit-based-incentive-payment-system-mips-and-alternative-payment-model-apm
- □ Executive Summary: https://qpp.cms.gov/docs/QPP_Executive_Summary_of_Final_Rule.pdf
- □ QPP Fact Sheet: https://qpp.cms.gov/docs/Quality_Payment_Program_Overview_Fact_Sheet.pdf
- □ Learn about improvement activities and APMs: https://qpp.cms.gov/docs/QPP_APMs_and_Improvement_Activities.pdf

Appendix D:
The NQS Six Priorities and Associated Long-Term Goals

1. *Making care safer by reducing harm caused in the delivery of care*
   Long-term goals:
   - Reduce preventable hospital admissions and readmissions.
   - Reduce the incidence of adverse healthcare-associated conditions.
   - Reduce harm from inappropriate or unnecessary care.

2. *Ensuring each patient and family member is engaged as a partner in his or her care*
   Long-term goals:
   - Improve patient, family, and caregiver experience of care related to quality, safety, and access across settings.
   - In partnership with patients, families, and caregivers, develop culturally sensitive and understandable care plans by using a shared decision-making process.
   - Enable patients, their families, and caregivers to navigate, coordinate, and manage their care appropriately and effectively.

3. *Promoting effective communication and coordination of care*
   Long-term goals:
   - Improve the quality of care transitions and communications across care settings.
   - Improve the quality of life for patients with chronic illnesses and disabilities by following a current care plan that anticipates and addresses pain and symptom management, psychosocial needs, and functional status.
   - Establish shared accountability and integration of communities and healthcare systems to improve quality of care and reduce health disparities.

4. *Promoting the most effective prevention and treatment practices for the leading causes of mortality, starting with cardiovascular disease*

   Long-term goals:
   - Promote cardiovascular health through community interventions resulting in improving social, economic, and environmental factors.
   - Promote cardiovascular health through interventions resulting in adoption of healthier lifestyle behaviors across the lifespan.
   - Promote cardiovascular health through receipt of effective clinical preventive services across the lifespan in clinical and community settings.

5. *Working with communities to promote wide use of best practices to enable healthy living*

   Long-term goals:
   - Promote healthy living and well-being through community interventions resulting in improvement of social, economic, and environmental factors.
   - Promote healthy living and well-being through interventions resulting in adoption of the most important healthy lifestyle behaviors across the lifespan.
   - Promote healthy living and well-being through receipt of effective clinical preventive services across the lifespan in clinical and community settings.

6. *Making quality care more affordable for individuals, families, employers, and governments by developing and spreading new healthcare delivery models*

   Long-term goals:
   - Ensure affordable and accessible high-quality healthcare for people, families, employers, and governments.
   - Support and enable communities to ensure accessible, high-quality care while reducing waste and fraud (see http://www.ahrq.gov/workingforquality/nqs/nqs2011annlrpt.pdf).

Glossary of Abbreviations

AAFP	Academy of Family Physicians
AAPM	Advanced Alternative Payment Model
ABC	Administrative, Benefits Management, and Clinical Services
ACA	Affordable Care Act
ACCORD	Action to Control Cardiovascular Risk in Diabetes
ACEI	ACE (Angiotensin-Converting Enzyme) Inhibitors
ACI	Advancing Care Information
ACO	Accountable Care Organizations
ADE	Adverse Drug Events
AHA	American Hospital Association
AHIP	America's Health Insurance Plans
AHRQ	Agency for Healthcare Research and Quality
AIDS	Acquired Immune Deficiency Syndrome
AIR	American Institutes for Research
AMA	American Medical Association
APM	Alternative Payment Models
ARB	Angiotensin Receptor Blocker
ASC	Ambulatory Surgery Centers
BMI	Body Mass Index
BMQ	Beliefs about Medications Questionnaire
BP	Blood Pressure
BPCI	Bundled Payments for Care Improvement
BPMH	Best Possible Medication History
BREAM	Beliefs and Motivation, Relationships, Experiences, Affordability, Medication Related Challenges
CABG	Coronary Artery Bypass Graft
CAHPS	Consumer Assessment of Healthcare Providers and Systems

CCC	Communication and Care Coordination
CDC	Centers for Disease Control and Prevention
CDS	Clinical Decision Support
CEC	Comprehensive ESRD Care
CHIP	Children's Health Insurance Program
CJR	Care for Joint Replacement
CM	Care Manager
CMMI	Centers for Medicare and Medicaid Innovation
CMR	Comprehensive Medication Reviews
CMS	Centers for Medicare and Medicaid Services
COPD	Chronic Obstructive Pulmonary Disease
CPC+	Comprehensive Primary Care Plus
CPH	Community/Population Health
CPOE	Computerized Physician Order Entry
DoD	Department of Defense
DQSA	Drug Quality and Security Act
DRG	Diagnosis-Related Group
ECC	Effective Clinical Care
ECHO	Economic, Clinical, and Humanistic Outcomes
ECR	Efficiency and Cost Reduction
EFEP	Engage, Focus, Evoke, Plan
EHR	Electronic Health Record
EMTALA	Emergency Medical Treatment and Labor Act
ESCO	ESRD Seamless Care Organization
ESRD	End-Stage Renal Disease
FDA	Federal Drug Agency
FFS	Fee for Service
FRAMME	Forgetfulness, Relationships, Affordability, Motivation (lack of), Medication-Related Challenges, Experiences

HAC	Hospital Acquired Conditions
HCAHPS	Hospital Consumer Assessment of Healthcare Providers and Systems
HCPLAN	Health Care Payment Learning and Action Network
HCTZ	Hydrochlorothiazide
HEDIS	Healthcare Effectiveness Data and Information Set
HgA1c/HbA1c	Glycated Hemoglobin (diabetes marker)
HHS	Health and Human Services
HIPAA	Health Insurance Portability and Accountability
HITS	Health Information Technology System
HIV	Human Immune Virus
HOPE	Heart Outcomes Prevention Evaluations
HOS	Hours of Service
HRRP	Hospital Readmissions Reduction Program
HRSA	Health Resources and Services Administration
HTN	Hypertension
IA	Improvement Activities
ICHOM	International Consortium for Healthcare Outcome Measurement
IDN	Integrated Delivery Network
IFHP	International Federation of Health Plans
IHI	Institute for Healthcare Improvement
IMPACT	Improving Medicare Post-Acute Care Transformation
IOM	Institute of Medicine
IPU	Integrated Practice Units
IQR	Inpatient Quality Reporting
ISMP	Institute of for Safe Medication Practices
ISQua	International Society of Quality
IVD	Ischemic Vascular Disease
JAMA	Journal of the American Medical Association

LDL	Low Density Lipoprotein
LDL-C	Low Density Lipoprotein Cholesterol
LDO	Large Dialysis Organization
LVSD	Left Ventricular Systolic Dysfunction
MA	Medicare Advantage
MAB	Medication A.R.E.A.S. Bundle
MACRA	Medicare Access and CHIP Reauthorization Act
MAP	Measure Applications Partnership
MCC	Multiple Chronic Conditions
MCP	MAB Clinical Pharmacists
MDP	Measurement Development Plan
MedRec	Medication Reconciliation
MI	Motivational Interviewing
MIPS	Merit-Based Incentive Payment System
MPC	Measurement Policy Council
MPR	Medication Possession Ratio
MPS	Medication Process Stages
MS	Multiple Sclerosis
MSSP	Medicare Share Savings Program
MTM	Medication Therapy Management
NCQA	National Committee for Quality Assurance
NEJM	New England Journal of Medicine
NQF	National Quality Forum
NQS	National Quality Strategy
OCP	Outpatient Clinical Pharmacists
OECD	Organization for Economic Cooperation and Development
ONC	Office of the National Coordinator for Health Information Technology
OPCS	Outpatient Pharmacy Clinical Services
OQR	Outpatient Quality Reporting

PBM	Pharmacy Benefit Management
PCEO	Person and Caregiver-Centered Experience and Outcomes
PCMH	Primary Care Medical Home
PCOR	Patient-Centered Outcomes Research
PCORI	Patient-Centered Outcomes Research Institute
PCP	Primary Care Physician
PCPCC	Patient-Centered Primary Care Collaborative
PDC	Proportion of Days Covered
PDMP	Prescription Drug Monitoring Program
PFPM	Physician-Focused Payment Models
PhRMA	Pharmaceutical Research and Manufacturers of America
PIMS	Pharmacy Information Management Systems
PMPM	Per Member Per Month
PMPY	Per Member Per Year
PQA	Pharmacy Quality Alliance
PQRS	Physician Quality Reporting System
PS	Patient Safety
QP	Qualifying Participants
QPP	Quality Payment Program
RULE	**Resist** the "righting reflex," **Understand** your patient's motivation, **Listen** to and understand the patient, and **Empower** and support the patient
SWOT	Strengths, Weaknesses, Opportunities, and Treats
	TJC The Joint Commission
TPS	Toyota Production System
US	United States

VBM	Value-Based Modifier
VBP	Value- Based Purchasing
VIPPS	Verified Internet Pharmacy Practice Site
WHO	World Health Organization

Notes

[1] "The IHI Triple Aim," Institute for Healthcare Improvement, accessed December 8, 2016, http://www.ihi.org/engage/initiatives/tripleaim/pages/default.aspx.

Preface

[2] "The Growing Crisis of Chronic Disease in the United States," Partnership to Fight Chronic Disease, accessed December 12, 2016, http://www.fightchronicdisease.org/sites/default/files/docs/GrowingCrisisofChronicDiseaseintheUSfactsheet_81009.pdf.

Chapter 1

[1] Dan Munro, "Top 10 Quotes From Harvard's Forum On Healthcare Innovation," *Forbes*, July 9, 2013, http://www.forbes.com/sites/danmunro/2013/07/09/top-10-quotes-from-harvards-first-forum-on-healthcare-innovation/#31f45f71198a.
[2] "Most Republicans Think the U.S. Health Care System Is the Best in the World. Democrats Disagree," Harvard T.H. Chan School of Public Health, March 20, 2008, https://www.hsph.harvard.edu/news/press-releases/republicans-democrats-disagree-us-health-care-system/.
[3] Jeff Goldsmith, "U.S. Health System Performance Has Gotten Better, Not Worse," *H&HN*, March 14, 2016, http://www.hhnmag.com/articles/7018-us-health-system-performance-has-gotten-better-not-worse.
[4] "Cancer Facts & Figures 2015," American Cancer Society, accessed August 30, 2016, http://www.cancer.org/acs/groups/content/@editorial/documents/document/acspc-044552.pdf.
[5] Jeff Goldsmith, "U.S. Health System Performance Has Gotten Better, Not Worse."
[6] Ibid.

[7] Ibid.

[8] Ibid.

[9] "Medical Cost Trend: Behind the Numbers 2017," PWC Health, June 26, 2016, http://pwchealth.com/cgi-local/hregister.cgi/reg/pwc-hri-medical-cost-trend-2017.pdf.

[10] "American Health Coverage Continues to Rise," accessed August 30, 2016, Obamacare Facts, http://obamacarefacts.com/sign-ups/obamacare-enrollment-numbers/.

[11] "Drug Supply Chain Integrity," FDA, accessed August 30, 2016, http://www.fda.gov/Drugs/DrugSafety/DrugIntegrityandSupplyChainSecurity/.

[12] Maria Evans, "What Are the Benefits of the United States Health Care System," http://www.ehow.com/list_7411670_benefits-states-health-care-system_.html.

[13] "EMTALA," American College of Emergency Physicians, 2014, https://www.acep.org/news-media-top-banner/emtala/.

[14] "10 Reasons Why The US Health Care System Is The Envy Of The World," *Business Insider*, accessed August 30, 2016, http://www.businessinsider.com/10-reasons-why-the-us-health-care-system-is-the-envy-of-the-world-2010-3#1-most-preemptive-cancer-screening-1.

[15] Ibid.

[16] Ibid.

[17] Ibid.

[18] Ibid.

[19] Ibid.

[20] "Health Care Facts: Why We Need Health Care Reform," Obamacare Facts, accessed November 30, 2016, http://obamacarefacts.com/healthcare-facts/.

[21] "2017 AHA Environmental Scan," *H&HN*, 2016, http://www.hhnmag.com/ext/resources/inc-hhn/pdfs/PartnerArticles/2016/EnviroScan_2017.pdf.

[22] "What Is Driving U.S. Health Care Spending? America's Unsustainable Health Care Cost Growth," Bipartisan Policy Center, September 2012, http://bipartisanpolicy.org/wp-content/uploads/

sites/default/files/BPC%20Health%20Care%20Cost%20Drivers%20
Brief%20Sept%202012.pdf.

[23] Srimoyee Bose, "Determinants of Per Capita State-Level Health
Expenditures in the United States: A Spatial Panel Analysis," *The
Journal of Regional Analysis & Policy* No. 1 (2015): 93-107, http://
www.jrap-journal.org/pastvolumes/2010/v45/jrap_v45_n1_a8_bose.pdf.

[24] "What Is Driving U.S. Healthcare Spending? America's
Unsustainable Health Care Cost Growth," Bipartisan Policy Center,
September 2012, http://bipartisanpolicy.org/wp-content/uploads/
sites/default/files/BPC%20Health%20Care%20Cost%20Drivers%20
Brief%20Sept%202012.pdf.

[25] Ibid.

[26] "IOM Report: Estimated $750B Wasted Annually In Health Care
System," *KHN*, accessed August 30, 2016, http://khn.org/morning-
breakout/iom-report/.

[27] Eric Pianin, "Taxpayers' Health Care Costs Are Rising—And So
Are the Profits of Big Pharmaceutical Companies," Business Insider,
July 30, 2015, http://www.businessinsider.com/taxpayerss-health-
care-costs-are-rising-and-so-are-the-profits-of-big-pharmaceutical-
companies-2015-7.

[28] "What Is Driving U.S. Healthcare Spending?" Bipartisan Policy Center.

[29] Amanda J. Forster, Blair G. Childs, Joseph F. Damore, Susan D.
DeVore, Eugene A. Kroch, and Danielle A. Lloyd, "Accountable
Care Strategies Lessons from the Premiere Health Care Alliance's
Accountable Care Collaborative," The Commonwealth Fund, August
2012, http://www.commonwealthfund.org/~/media/Files/Publications/
Fund%20Report/2012/Aug/1618_Forster_accountable_care_
strategies_premier.pdf.

[30] "What Is Driving U.S. Healthcare Spending?" Bipartisan Policy
Center.

[31] Dante Michael Panella, "WHEN Health Care Costs INCREASE, so
do Premiums" LinkedIn, May 29, 2015, https://www.linkedin.com/
pulse/when-health-care-costs-increase-so-do-premiums-dante-michael-
panella?redirectFromSplash=true.

[32] "Why Do We Need the Affordable Care Act?" American Public Health Association, August 2012, https://www.apha.org/~/media/files/pdf/topics/aca/why_we_need_the_aca_aug2012.ashx

[33] Theresa Tamkins, "Medical bills prompt more than 60 percent of U.S. bankruptcies," CNN, June 5, 2009, http://www.cnn.com/2009/HEALTH/06/05/bankruptcy.medical.bills/.

[34] Ibid.

[35] Amer Kaissi, "The US Healthcare System: The Good, The Bad, and The Ugly," Healthcare Hacks, September 8, 2009, http://healthcarehacks.com/the-us-healthcare-system-the-good-the-bad-and-the-ugly.

[36] Ibid.

[37] K. Davis, K. Stemikis, D. Squires, and C. Schoen, "Mirror, Mirror on the Wall, 2014 Update: How the U.S. Health Care System Compares Internationally," The Commonwealth Fund, June 2014, http://www.commonwealthfund.org/publications/fund-reports/2014/jun/mirror-mirror.

[38] Ibid.

[39] Ibid.

[40] Ibid.

Chapter 2

[1] "What Is the Patient Protection and Affordable Care Act?" Obamacare Facts, accessed December 8, 2016, http://obamacarefacts.com/affordable-care-act-facts/.

[2] "Better Care. Smarter Spending. Healthier People: Paying Providers for Value, Not Volume," CMS.gov, January 26, 2015, https://www.cms.gov/Newsroom/MediaReleaseDatabase/Fact-sheets/2015-Fact-sheets-items/2015-01-26-3.html.

[3] "Accomplishments of the Affordable Care Act: A 5th Year Anniversary Report," Families USA, March 23, 2015, The White House, https://www.whitehouse.gov/sites/default/files/docs/3-22-15_aca_anniversary_report.pdf.

[4] Caitlin Morris and Kim Bailey, "Measuring Health Care Quality: An Overview of Quality Measures," Families USA, May 2014, http://familiesusa.org/sites/default/files/product_documents/HSI%20Quality%20Measurement_Brief_final_web.pdf.

[5] Obamacare Facts website, accessed December 8, 2016 http://obamacarefacts.com/.

[6] "Remarks by the President on the Affordable Care Act," whitehouse.gov, September 26, 2013, https://www.whitehouse.gov/the-press-office/2013/09/26/remarks-president-affordable-care-act

[7] "Obamacare Myths," Obamacare.net, October 28, 2016, https://obamacare.net/obamacare-myths/.

[8] "Why Is Obamacare So Controversial?" *BBC News*, November 11, 2016, http://www.bbc.com/news/world-us-canada-24370967.

[9] "Public health insurance exchanges: Opening the door for a new generation of engaged health care consumers Insights from the Deloitte Center for Health Solutions 2015 Survey of US Health Care Consumers," Deloitte, 2015, https://www2.deloitte.com/content/dam/Deloitte/us/Documents/life-sciences-health-care/us-lshc-hix-consumer-survey.pdf.

[10] Sean Williams, "Will All 23 of Obamacare's Healthcare Cooperatives Fail?" The Motley Fool, July 23, 2016, http://www.fool.com/investing/2016/07/23/will-all-23-of-obamacares-healthcare-cooperatives.aspx.

[11] John Goodman, "Six Problems With The ACA That Aren't Going Away," Health Affairs Blog, June 25, 2015, http://healthaffairs.org/blog/2015/06/25/six-problems-with-the-aca-that-arent-going-away/.

[12] "Obamacare's Next 5 Hurdles to Clear," *Kaiser Health News*, June 26, 2015, http://khn.org/news/five-hurdles-ahead-for-obamacare/.

[13] "5 Challenges Still Facing Obamacare," NPR, June 26, 2015, http://www.npr.org/sections/health-shots/2015/06/26/417733970/5-challenges-still-facing-obamacare.

[14] "Affordable Care Act Facts," Obamacare Facts, accessed December 8, 2016, http://obamacarefacts.com/affordable-care-act-facts/.

[15] "ObamaCare Replacement Plan: 'CARE' Act Facts," Obamacare

Facts, accessed December 8, 2016, http://obamacarefacts.com/
obamacare-replacement-plan-facts/.

[16] Ibid.

[17] "Repeal ObamaCare or Defund ObamaCare?" Obamacare Facts,
accessed December 8, 2016, http://obamacarefacts.com/repeal-
obamacare/.

[18] Ibid.

[19] "What Happens if ObamaCare Is Repealed?" Obamacare Facts, June
19, 2015, http://obamacarefacts.com/2015/06/19/what-happens-if-
obamacare-is-repealed/.

[20] "ObamaCare Replacement Plan," Obamacare Facts, http://
obamacarefacts.com/obamacare-replacement-plan-facts/.

[21] Jim Collins, "Building Companies to Last," Jim Collins, 1995, http://
www.jimcollins.com/article_topics/articles/building-companies.html.

[22] Emily Rappleye, "House GOP Unveils Changes to AHCA: 3 Things
to Know," Becker's Hospital Review, March 21, 2017, http://www.
beckershospitalreview.com/hospital-management-administration/
house-gop-unveils-changes-to-ahca-3-things-to-know.html.

[23] James C. Collins, "Leadership: Building Companies to Last," *Inc.*,
May 15, 1995, http://www.inc.com/magazine/19950515/2692.html.

[24] Ibid.

Chapter 3

[1] "Administration takes first step to implement legislation modernizing
how Medicare pays physicians for quality," HHS, April 27, 2016,
http://www.hhs.gov/about/news/2016/04/27/administration-takes-
first-step-implement-legislation-modernizing-how-medicare-pays-
physicians.html.

[2] "CMS Quality Measure Development Plan: Supporting the Transition
to the Merit-based Incentive Payment System (MIPS) and Alternative
Payment Models (APMs)," CMS, May 2, 2016, https://www.cms.gov/
Medicare/Quality-Initiatives-Patient-Assessment-Instruments/Value-
Based-Programs/MACRA-MIPS-and-APMs/Final-MDP.pdf.

[3] "The Quality Payment Program Overview Fact Sheet," CMS, accessed December 7, 2016, https://qpp.cms.gov/docs/Quality_Payment_Program_Overview_Fact_Sheet.pdf.

[4] "Moving Toward a Better, Smarter Health Care System with an Engaged and Empowered Consumer at the Center," HHS, October 23, 2015, http://www.hhs.gov/healthcare/facts-and-features/fact-sheets/moving-toward-better-smarter-health-care-system.html.

[5] Ibid.

[6] Ibid.

[7] "CMS Quality Reporting Programs under the 2016 Medicare Physician Fee Schedule Proposed Rule," CMS, July 16, 2015, https://www.cms.gov/Outreach-and-Education/Outreach/NPC/Downloads/2015-07-16-PQRS-Presentation.pdf.

[8] "10 FAQs About the Merit-Based Incentive Payment System (MIPS)," Saignite.

[9] "The Merit-Based Incentive Payment System: MIPS Scoring Methodology Overview," CMS, accessed December 7, 2016, https://www.cms.gov/Medicare/Quality-Initiatives-Patient-Assessment-Instruments/Value-Based-Programs/MACRA-MIPS-and-APMs/MIPS-Scoring-Methodology-slide-deck.pdf.

[10] "Quality Payment Program Modernizing Medicare," CMS.

[11] "CMS Quality Measure Development Plan" CMS.

[12] "What's the Merit-based Incentive Payment System (MIPS)?" Quality Payment Program, accessed December 7, 2016, https://qpp.cms.gov/learn/qpp.

[13] "Medicare Shared Savings Program in the Quality Payment Program," CMS, October 27, 2015, https://www.cms.gov/Medicare/Quality-Initiatives-Patient-Assessment-Instruments/Value-Based-Programs/MACRA-MIPS-and-APMs/APMs-in-The-Quality-Payment-Program-for-Shared-Savings-Program-SSP-webinar-slides.pdf.

[14] "The Quality Payment Program Overview Fact Sheet," CMS.gov.

[15] "What's the Merit-based Incentive Payment System (MIPS)?" Quality Payment Program.

[16] "Accountable Care Organizations (ACO)," CMS, January 6, 2015,

https://www.cms.gov/Medicare/Medicare-Fee-for-Service-Payment/
ACO/index.html?redirect=/aco/.

[17] Ibid.

[18] "Defining the Medical Home A patient-centered philosophy that
drives primary care excellence," Patient-Centered Primary Care
Collaborative, accessed December 7, 2016, https://www.pcpcc.org/
about/medical-home.

[19] Joanne Conroy, "Transforming Care: HIZs, ACOs, Bundling…what
does it all mean for AMCs?" AAMC, accessed December 7, 2016,
https://members.aamc.org/eweb/upload/OSR%20Conroy%20ANN11-
059.pdf.

[20] "Bundled Payments for Care Improvement (BPCI) Initiative:
General Information," CMS.gov, November 28, 2016, https://
innovation.cms.gov/initiatives/bundled-payments/.

[21] Virgil Thomas, "Value Based Payment Goals," Eden Alternative,
January 27, 2015, http://www.edenalt.org/value-based-payment-goals/.

[22] "Medicare Alternative Payment Models," AMA, accessed December
7, 2016, http://www.ama-assn.org/ama/pub/advocacy/topics/medicare-
alternative-payment-models.page.

[23] "Next Generation ACO Model," CMS.gov, accessed December 7,
2016, https://innovation.cms.gov/initiatives/Next-Generation-ACO-
Model/.

[24] "CMS Welcomes New Medicare Shared Savings Program (Shared
Savings Program) Participants," CMS, January 11, 2016, https://www.
cms.gov/Newsroom/MediaReleaseDatabase/Fact-sheets/2016-Fact-
sheets-items/2016-01-11-2.html.

[25] "Accountable Care Organizations: What Providers Need to Know,"
CMS, March 2016, https://www.cms.gov/Medicare/Medicare-Fee-for-
Service-Payment/sharedsavingsprogram/Downloads/ACO_Providers_
Factsheet_ICN907406.pdf.

[26] "Oncology Care Model," Foley Hoag LLP, July 1, 2016, http://www.
foleyhoag.com/publications/alerts-and-updates/2016/june/oncology-
care-model.

[27] "Comprehensive ESRD Care Initiative: Frequently Asked

Questions," CMS, accessed December 7, 2016, https://innovation.cms.gov/Files/x/cecfaq.pdf.

[28] "The Quality Payment Program Overview Fact Sheet," CMS.gov.

[29] "The Quality Payment Program Overview Fact Sheet," CMS.gov.

[30] "Quality Payment Program," CMS, accessed December 7, 2016, https://www.cms.gov/Medicare/Quality-Initiatives-Patient-Assessment-Instruments/Value-Based-Programs/MACRA-MIPS-and-APMs/Quality-Payment-Program-Long-Version-Executive-Deck.pdf.

[31] "Health Care Payment Learning and Action Network," CMS, October 11, 2016, https://innovation.cms.gov/initiatives/Health-Care-Payment-Learning-and-Action-Network/.

[32] "The Quality Payment Program Overview Fact Sheet," CMS.gov.

[33] "Organization Quotes," Brainy Quotes, accessed December 7, 2016, http://www.brainyquote.com/quotes/keywords/organization.html.

[34] "The Quality Payment Program Overview Fact Sheet," CMS.gov.

[35] "Are physicians ready for MACRA and its changes? Perspectives from the Deloitte Center for Health Solutions 2016 Survey of US Physicians," Deloitte, 2016, http://www2.deloitte.com/content/dam/Deloitte/us/Documents/life-sciences-health-care/us-lshc-are-physicians-ready-MACRA.pdf.

Chapter 4

[1] Quotter, s.v. "W Edwards Deming," accessed December 2, 2016, http://www.quotter.net/2_w-edwards-deming_better-life-quote-of-the-day.

[2] *Goodreads*, s.v. "H. James Harrington," accessed December 1, 2016, http://www.goodreads.com/quotes/632992-measurement-is-the-first-step-that-leads-to-control-and.

[3] "National Strategy for Quality Improvement in Health Care," Department of Health & Human Services, March 2011, http://www.ahrq.gov/workingforquality/nqs/nqs2011annlrpt.pdf.

[4] Ibid.

[5] Ibid.

6 "HHS Measure Policy Council," NASHP, accessed December 8, 2016, http://www.nashp.org/sites/default/files/files/HHS_Measure_Policy_Council.pdf.

7 "CMS Quality Strategy 2016," CMS, accessed December 8, 2016, https://www.cms.gov/medicare/quality-initiatives-patient-assessment-instruments/qualityinitiativesgeninfo/downloads/cms-quality-strategy.pdf.

8 "Overview of the CMS Quality Strategy," CMS, accessed December 8, 2016, https://www.cms.gov/Medicare/Quality-Initiatives-Patient-Assessment-Instruments/QualityInitiativesGenInfo/Downloads/CMS-Quality-Strategy-Overview.pdf.

9 Morris and Bailey, "Measuring Health Care Quality."

10 Ibid.

11 Ibid.

12 Ibid.

13 "Good for Health, Good for Business: The Case for Measuring Patient Experience of Care," Aligning Forces for Quality, accessed December 5, 2016, http://forces4quality.org/node/3215.html.

14 Morris and Bailey, "Measuring Health Care Quality."

15 "Science of Improvement: Establishing Measures," Institute for Healthcare Improvement, accessed December 5, 2016, http://www.ihi.org/resources/Pages/HowtoImprove/ScienceofImprovementEstablishingMeasures.aspx.

16 "Types of Measures | Quality 101 | Quality & Innovation | SHM | Society of Hospital Medicine," SHM, accessed December 5, 2016, http://www.hospitalmedicine.org/Web/Quality___Innovation/Quality_101/Establishing_Measures/Types_of_Measures.aspx.

17 Morris and Bailey, "Measuring Health Care Quality."

18 David Blumenthal, Elizabeth Malphrus, and J. Michael McGinnis, eds., *Vital Signs: Core Metrics for Health and Health Care Progress* (Washington, D.C., The National Academies Press: 2015), http://www.lsuhsc.edu/administration/academic/cipecp/docs/IOM%20Core%20Metric%20for%20Health%20and%20Health%20Care%20Progress.pdf.

19 D. Blumenthal, E. Malphrus, and J.M. McGinnis, eds., "Health and Health Care Measurement in America," chap. 2 in *Vital Signs:*

Core Metrics for Health and Health Care Progress (Washington, DC: National Academies Press, 2015) http://www.ncbi.nlm.nih.gov/books/NBK316114/.

[20] Ibid.

[21] The website of the NCQA, accessed December 2, 2016, https://www.ncqa.org/.

[22] Blumenthal, Malphrus, and McGinnis, eds., "Health and Health Care Measurement in America," chap. 2 in *Vital Signs: Core Metrics for Health and Health Care Progress.*

[23] Ibid.

[24]"Achieving Results with Outcome Measures," Vital Health Software, accessed December 3, 2016, http://www.vitalhealthsoftware.com/products/patient-health-questionnaires/ichom-outcome-measures#sthash.dUMZVoQ1.dpuf.

[25] "About Us," PCORI, October 6, 2014, http://www.pcori.org/about-us.

[26] "Mission and Vision," The Leapfrog Group, accessed December 3, 2016, http://www.leapfroggroup.org/about/mission-and-vision.

[27] "About WHO," WHO, accessed December 3, 2016, http://www.who.int/about/en/.

[28] "Who we are?" ISQua, accessed December 3, 2016, http://www.isqua.org/who-we-are/who-we-are.

[29] "PQA Performance Measures," PQA, accessed December 3, 2016, http://pqaalliance.org/measures/default.asp.

[30] "Introduction," HHS, accessed December 3, 2016, http://www.hhs.gov/about/strategic-plan/introduction/index.html#overview.

[31] Blumenthal, Malphrus, and McGinnis, eds., "Health and Health Care Measurement in America," chap. 2 in *Vital Signs: Core Metrics for Health and Health Care Progress.*

[32] Ibid.

[33] "First Release of the Overall Hospital Quality Star Rating on Hospital Compare," CMS, July 27, 2016, https://www.cms.gov/Newsroom/MediaReleaseDatabase/Fact-sheets/2016-Fact-sheets-items/2016-07-27.html.

[34] Blumenthal, Malphrus, and McGinnis, eds., "Health and Health Care

Measurement in America," chap. 2 in *Vital Signs: Core Metrics for Health and Health Care Progress.*

[35] "CMS Quality Measure Development Plan" CMS.

[36] Ibid.

[37] "Transitioning from Volume to Value: Consolidation and Alignment of Quality Measures," Bipartisan Policy Center, April 2015, http://bipartisanpolicy.org/wp-content/uploads/2015/04/BPC-Health-Quality-Measures.pdf.

[38] "2013 Annual Progress Report to Congress" AHRQ.

[39] Ibid.

[40] "Core Quality Measures Collaborative Release," CMS.gov, February 16, 2016, https://www.cms.gov/Newsroom/MediaReleaseDatabase/Fact-sheets/2016-Fact-sheets-items/2016-02-16.html.

[41] "Specifications Manual for National Hospital Inpatient Quality Measures," The Join Commission, https://www.jointcommission.org/specifications_manual_for_national_hospital_inpatient_quality_measures.aspx.

[42] "Committee on Core Metrics for Better Health at Lower Cost," The National Academies of Science, accessed December 5, 2016, https://www.nationalacademies.org/hmd/Activities/Quality/CoreMetricsForBetterHealth.aspx.

[43] "Post-Acute Care Quality Initiatives," CMS.gov, October 20, 2015, https://www.cms.gov/Medicare/Quality-Initiatives-Patient-Assessment-Instruments/Post-Acute-Care-Quality-Initiatives/IMPACT-Act-of-2014-and-Cross-Setting-Measures.html.

[44] National Quality Forum, "NQF Provides Guidance to Help Reduce Variation in Healthcare Quality Measures," press release, Jan. 5, 2017, http://www.qualityforum.org/News_And_Resources/Press_Releases/2017/NQF_Provides_Guidance_to_Help_Reduce_Variation_in_Healthcare_Quality_Measures.aspx.

[45] "Transitioning from Volume to Value," Bipartisan Policy Center.

Chapter 5

[1] Eduardo Sabaté, ed., "Adherence to Long-Term Therapies: Evidence for Action," WHO, 2003, http://apps.who.int/iris/bitstream/10665/42682/1/9241545992.pdf.

[2] "The Growing Crisis of Chronic Disease in the United States," Partnership to Fight Chronic Disease.

[3] "Poor Medicine Adherence in Americans with Multiple Chronic Conditions—Anticipating & Addressing a Looming Threat," *PR Newswire*, October 15, 2013, http://www.prnewswire.com/news-releases/poor-medicine-adherence-in-americans-with-multiple-chronic-conditions---anticipating--addressing-a-looming-threat-227809681.html.

[4] Glen Slettin, "Pharmacist Collaboration Closes Gaps in Care," Express Scripts, February 28, 2013, http://lab.express-scripts.com/lab/insights/specialized-care/pharmacist-collaboration-closes-gaps-in-care#sthash.atJ3zXdX.dpuf.

[5] "The Growing Crisis of Chronic Disease in the United States," Partnership to Fight Chronic Disease.

[6] George Van Antwerp, "Medco 2009 Drug Trend Report Part 2," Enabling Healthy Decisions (blog), May 25, 2009, https://georgevanantwerp.com/2009/05/.

[7] "Medication Error Reports," FDA, October 20, 2016 http://www.fda.gov/Drugs/DrugSafety/MedicationErrors/ucm080629.htm.

[8] Griffin R. Resar and Nolan C. Haraden, "Using Care Bundles to Improve Health Care Quality," IHI, 2012, http://www.ihi.org/resources/pages/ihiwhitepapers/usingcarebundles.aspx.

[9] Eduardo Sabaté, ed., "Adherence to long-term therapies: evidence for action."

[10] Aja B. Williams, "Issue Brief: Medication Adherence and Health IT," Health IT, January 9, 2014, https://www.healthit.gov/sites/default/files/medicationadherence_and_hit_issue_brief.pdf.

[11] David P. Nau, "Proportion of Days Covered (PDC) as a Preferred Method of Measuring Medication Adherence," PQA, accessed

December 7, 2016, http://www.pqaalliance.org/images/uploads/files/
PQA%20PDC%20vs%20%20MPR.pdf.

[12] Lars Osterberg and Terrence Blaschke, "Adherence to Medication,"
The New England Journal of Medicine, 353 (August 4, 2005): 487-
497. doi: 10.1056/NEJMra050100.

[13] Chris Crawford, "One in Three Patients Not Filling Prescriptions,
Study Finds Physicians Can Have Positive Impact on Primary
Nonadherence," AAFP, April 28, 2014, http://www.aafp.org/news/
health-of-the-public/20140428nonadherencestudy.html.

[14] Marie T. Brown and Jennifer K. Bussell, "Medication Adherence:
WHO Cares?" *Mayo Clinic Proceedings* 86, no. 4 (April 2011): 304-
314. doi: 10.4065/mcp.2010.0575.

[15] Carla K. Johnson, "Many Patients Quit Medicine Too Early,"
Washington Post, September 25, 2006, http://www.washingtonpost.
com/wp-dyn/content/article/2006/09/25/AR2006092500771_pf.html.

[16] Ed Lamb, "Top 200 Prescription Drugs of 2007," Pharmacy
Times, May 1, 2008, http://www.pharmacytimes.com/publications/
issue/2008/2008-05/2008-05-8520.

[17] "Medication Adherence," Pharmacy Solution, LLC, accessed
December 7, 2016, http://www.pharmsolutions.org/Pages/
MedicationAdherence.aspx.

[18] "Medication Adherence," Pharmacy Solution, LLC, accessed
December 7, 2016, http://www.pharmsolutions.org/Pages/
MedicationAdherence.aspx.

[19] Kavita V. Nair, Daniel A. Belletti, Joseph J. Doyle, Richard R. Allen,
Robert B. McQueen, Joseph J. Saseen, Joseph Vande Griend, Jay V.
Patel, Angela McQueen, and Saira Jan, "Understanding barriers to
medication adherence in the hypertensive population by evaluating
responses to a telephone survey." *Patient Prefer Adherence* 5 (April
29, 2011): 195-206. doi: 10.2147/PPA.S18481.

[20] "Noncompliance with Medications: An Economic Tragedy with
Important Implications for Health Care Reform," NPC, April
1994, http://www.npcnow.org/system/files/research/download/

Noncompliance-with-Medications-An-Economic-Tragedy-with-Important-Implications-for-Health-Care-Reform-1994.pdf.

[21] E. Vermeire, H. Hearnshaw, P. Van Royen, and J. Denekens, "Patient adherence to treatment: three decades of research A comprehensive review." Abstract. *Journal of Clinical Pharmacy and Therapeutics* 26, no. 5 (October 2001): 331–342. https://www.ncbi.nlm.nih.gov/pubmed/11679023.

[22] F.H. Gwadry-Sridhar, E. Manias, Y. Zhang, A. Roy, K. Yu-Isenberg, D.A. Hughes, and M.B. Nichol, "A framework for planning and critiquing medication compliance and persistence using prospective study designs." Abstract. *Clinical Therapeutics* 31, no. 3 (February 2009): 421-435. doi: 10.1016/j.clinthera.2009.02.021.

[23] D.G. Pittman, W. Chen, S.J. Bowlin, and J.M. Foody, "Adherence to statins, subsequent healthcare costs, and cardiovascular hospitalizations." Abstract. American Journal of Cardiology 107, no. 11 (June 1, 2011): 1662-1666. doi: 10.1016/j.amjcard.2011.01.052.

[24] "A Tough Pill to Swallow: Medication Adherence and Cardiovascular Disease," American Heart Association, accessed December 7, 2016, https://www.heart.org/idc/groups/heart-public/@wcm/@adv/documents/downloadable/ucm_460769.pdf.

[25] C. McCowan, S. Wang, A.M. Thompson, B. Makubate, and D.J. Petrie, "The value of high adherence to tamoxifen in women with breast cancer: a community-based cohort study," *British Journal of Cancer* 109, no. 5 (September 3, 2013): 1172–1180. doi: 10.1038/bjc.2013.464.

[26] R.I. Horwitz, C.M. Viscoli, L. Berkman, R.M. Donaldson, S.M. Horwitz, C.J. Murray, D.F. Ransohoff, and J. Sindelar." Treatment adherence and risk of death after a myocardial infarction." Abstract. *Lancet* 336, no. 8,714 (September 1, 1990), 542-545. https://www.ncbi.nlm.nih.gov/pubmed/1975045.

[27] Jerry H. Gurwitz, Terry S. Field, Leslie R. Harrold, Jeffrey Rothschild, Kristin Debellis, Andrew C. Seger, Cynthia Cadoret, et al., "Incidence and Preventability of Adverse Drug Events Among Older

Persons in the Ambulatory Setting," *JAMA* 289, no. 9 (March 5, 2003): 1107-1116. doi:10.1001/jama.289.9.1107.

[28] J. Hong, C. Reed, D. Novick, J.M. Haro, and J. Aguado, "Clinical and economic consequences of medication non-adherence in the treatment of patients with a manic/mixed episode of bipolar disorder: results from the European Mania in Bipolar Longitudinal Evaluation of Medication (EMBLEM) study," Abstract. *Psychiatry Research* 190, no. 1 (November 30, 2011): 110-114. doi: 10.1016/j.psychres.2011.04.016.

[29] Regina M. Benjamin, "Medication Adherence: Helping Patients Take Their Medicines As Directed," Public Health Reports 127, no. 1 (January-February 2012): 2-3. https://www.ncbi.nlm.nih.gov/pmc/articles/PMC3234383/.

[30] Roy E. Hammarlund, Jana R. Ostrom, and Alice J. Kethley. "The Effects of Drug Counseling and Other Educational Strategies on Drug Utilization of the Elderly." Medical Care 23, no. 2 (Feb. 1985): 165-170. doi: http://dx.doi.org/10.1097/00005650-198502000-00007.

[31] Lisa Ward, "Take Your Heart Medicine—and Win a Prize! Researchers Test Ways to Motivate People to Take Their Medicine Consistently," The Wall Street Journal, June 8, 2014, http://www.wsj.com/articles/motivating-heart-patients-to-take-their-medicine-1402062220.

[32] "A Tough Pill to Swallow: Medication Adherence and Cardiovascular Disease," American Heart Association.

[33] Aurel O. Iuga, and Maura J McGuire, "Adherence and health care costs," *Journal of Risk Management and Healthcare Policy* 7 (February 20, 2014): 35-44. doi: 10.2147/RMHP.S19801.

[34] D. Esposito, A.D. Bagchi, J.M. Verdier, D.S. Bencio, and M.S. Kim, "Medicaid beneficiaries with congestive heart failure: association of medication adherence with healthcare use and costs," Abstract. *American Journal of Managed Care* 15, no. 7 (2009): 437–45 https://www.ncbi.nlm.nih.gov/pubmed/19589011.

[35] "Medication Adherence," Pharmacy Solution, LLC, accessed

December 7, 2016, http://www.pharmsolutions.org/Pages/
MedicationAdherence.aspx.

[36] Christina Sochacki, "Medication Adherence 101," California
Partnership for Access to Treatment, April 2013, http://www.caaccess.
org/pdf/medicationadherence_cahc.pdf.

[37] Gloria Nichols-English and Sylvie Poirier, "Optimizing Adherence
to Pharmaceutical Care Plans," JAPhA 40, no. 4 (July-August 2000):
475-485. doi: http://dx.doi.org/10.1016/S1086-5802(15)30405-8.

[38] P. Sleight, "The HOPE Study (Heart Outcomes Prevention
Evaluation)." Abstract. *Journal of the Renin-Angiotensin-Aldosterone
System* 1, no. 1 (March 2000): 18-20. doi: 10.3317/jraas.2000.002.

[39] "Randomised trial of cholesterol lowering in 4444 patients with
coronary heart disease: the Scandinavian Simvastatin Survival Study
(4S)," Abstract. *The Lancet* 344, no. 8934 (November 19, 1994):
1,383-1,389. doi: http://dx.doi.org/10.1016/S0140-6736(94)90566-5.

[40] M. Christopher Roebuck, Joshua N. Liberman, Marin Gemmill-
Toyama, and Troyen A. Brennan, "Medication Adherence Leads To
Lower Health Care Use And Costs Despite Increased Drug Spending,"
Health Affairs 30, no. 1 (January 2001): 91-99. doi: 10.1377/
hlthaff.2009.1087.

[41] R. James Dudl, Margaret C. Wang, Michelle Wong, and Jim
Bellows, "Preventing Myocardial Infarction and Stroke With
a Simplified Bundle of Cardioprotective Medications," *The
American Journal of Manged Care* 15, no. 10 (October 2009):
88-94, https://www.dmhc.ca.gov/Portals/0/AbouttheDMHC/RCI/
PromisingBestPractices/allphase.pdf.

[42] Michael C. Sokol, Kimberly A. McGuigan, Robert R. Verbrugge,
and Robert S. Epstein, "Impact of Medication Adherence on
Hospitalization Risk and Healthcare Cost," Vitality, 2005, http://www.
vitality.net/docs/managedcare_article.pdf.

[43] David Steeb and Lisa Webster, "Improving Care Transitions:
Optimizing Medication Reconciliation," Pharmacist.com, March 2012,
https://www.pharmacist.com/sites/default/files/files/2012_improving_
care_transitions.pdf.

[44] "The High 5s Project Standard Operating Protocol," WHO, September 2014, http://www.who.int/patientsafety/implementation/solutions/high5s/h5s-sop.pdf.

[45] "Patient Safety Systems Chapter, Sentinel Event Policy and RCA2," The Joint Commission, accessed December 7, 2016, http://www.jointcommission.org/SentinelEvents/SentinelEventAlert/sea_35.htm.

[46] "About Medication Errors," NCC MERP, accessed December 7, 2016, http://www.nccmerp.org/about-medication-errors.

[47] Jane H. Barnsteiner, "Medication Reconciliation," chap. 38 in *Patient Safety and Quality: An Evidence-Based Handbook for Nurses* (Rockville: Agency for Healthcare Research and Quality, 2008) http://www.ncbi.nlm.nih.gov/books/NBK2648/.

[48] Lisha Lo, Janice Kwan, Olavo A Fernandes, and Kaveh G Shojania, "Medication Reconciliation Supported by Clinical Pharmacists (NEW)," chap. 25 in *Making Health Care Safer II: An Updated Critical Analysis of the Evidence for Patient Safety Practices* (Rockville: Agency for Healthcare Research and Quality, 2013) http://www.ncbi.nlm.nih.gov/books/NBK133408/.

[49] "Sentinel Event Alert," The Joint Commission, January 25, 2006, http://www.jointcommission.org/assets/1/18/SEA_35.pdf.

[50] Bishr H. AbuYassin, Hisham Aljadhey, Mohammed Al-Sultan, Sulaiman Al-Rashed, Mansour Adam, and David W. Bates, "Accuracy of the medication history at admission to hospital in Saudi Arabia," *Saudi Pharmaceutical Journal* 19, no. 4 (October 19, 2011): 263-267. doi: 10.1016/j.jsps.2011.04.006.

[51] Ellen Nolte and Martin McKee, eds., "Caring for people with chronic conditions: A health system perspective," WHO Europe, 2008, http://www.euro.who.int/__data/assets/pdf_file/0006/96468/E91878.pdf.

[52] Steeb and Webster, "Improving Care Transitions: Optimizing Medication Reconciliation."

[53] "About The Partnership: Patient and family engagement," CMS, accessed December 7, 2016, https://partnershipforpatients.cms.gov/about-the-partnership/patient-and-family-engagement/the-patient-and-family-engagement.html.

[54] "Patient and Family Engagement: A Partnership for Culture Change" North Carolina Institute of Medicine.

[55] "Symposium on Patient Engagement (District of Columbia)," Health IT, accessed December 7, 2016, https://healthit.ahrq.gov/ahrq-funded-projects/symposium-patient-engagement.

[56] Ibid.

[57] "The U.S. Health Care Market: A Strategic View of Consumer Segmentation Deloitte Center for Health Solutions," Deloitte, 2012, http://www2.deloitte.com/content/dam/Deloitte/us/Documents/life-sciences-health-care/us-lshc-health-care-market-consumer-segmentation.pdf.

[58] Brian W. Jack, Veerappa K. Chetty, David Anthony, Jeffrey L. Greenwald, Gail M. Sanchez, Anna E. Johnson, Shaula R. Forsyth, et al, "A Reengineered Hospital Discharge Program to Decrease Rehospitalization," Abstract. *Annals of Internal Medicine* 150, no. 3 (February 3, 2009): 178-187, http://www.annals.org/content/150/3/178.

[59] "Patient and Family Engagement: A Partnership for Culture Change" North Carolina Institute of Medicine.

[60] Ibid.

[61] "Patient and Family Engagement: A Partnership for Culture Change" North Carolina Institute of Medicine.

[62] Ibid.

[63] "The U.S. Health Care Market," Deloitte.

[64] "National Health Expenditures 2015 Highlights," CMS, accessed December 7, 2016, https://www.cms.gov/research-statistics-data-and-systems/statistics-trends-and-reports/nationalhealthexpenddata/downloads/highlights.pdf.

[65] "U.S. prescription drug spending jumps to record $374 billion," Chicago Tribune, April 14, 2015, http://www.chicagotribune.com/business/ct-drug-spending-0415-biz-20150414-story.html.

[66] "U.S. health agency estimates 2015 prescription drug spend rose to $457 billion," Reuters, March 8, 2016, http://www.reuters.com/article/us-usa-healthcare-pricing-idUSKCN0WA2O0.

[67] "Generic Drugs: Questions and Answers," FDA, November 29,

2016, http://www.fda.gov/Drugs/ResourcesForYou/Consumers/QuestionsAnswers/ucm100100.htm

[68] *Vocabulary.com*, s.v. "brand-name drug," accessed December 7, 2016, https://www.vocabulary.com/dictionary/brand-name%20drug.

[69] "Specialty Drugs and Health Care Costs," The PEW Charitable Trusts, November 16, 2015, http://www.pewtrusts.org/en/research-and-analysis/fact-sheets/2015/11/specialty-drugs-and-health-care-costs.

[70] John Powter, "Prescription Trends—How and Why Costs Are Increasing," GDP Advisors, October 10, 2015, http://info.gdpadvisors.com/blog/prescription-trends-how-and-why-costs-are-increasing.

[71] "Budget-Busters: The Shift to High-Priced Innovator Drugs in the USA," Evaluate, accessed December 7, 2016, http://www.evaluategroup.com/public/Reports/EvaluatePharma-Budget-Busters-the-Shift-to-High-Priced-Innovator-Drugs.aspx.

[72] "Specialty at Retail: Considerations and Opportunities for Independent Pharmacies," Health Mart Pharmacies, accessed December 7, 2016, http://becomeahealthmart.com/Websites/becomeapharmacy/images/White_Paper_Specialty_at_Retail_-_Considerations_and_Opportunities_for_Independent_Pharmacies.pdf.

[73] Ibid.

[74] Suzanne Delbanco and Andréa Elizabeth Caballero, "The Payment Reform Landscape: Specialty Pharmacy — Can Payment Reform Offer Relief?" Health Affairs Blog, November 19, 2015, http://healthaffairs.org/blog/2015/11/19/the-payment-reform-landscape-specialty-pharmacy-can-payment-reform-offer-relief/.

[75] "2011 Drug Trend Report," Express Scripts, April 2012, https://lab.express-scripts.com/lab/drug-trend-report/~/media/b2d069aa4a2b4b188879a81ab0bab8aa.ashx.

[76] "Specialty Drugs: Issues and Challenges: Advancing Effective Strategies to Address Soaring Drug Costs While Ensuring Access to Effective Treatments and Promoting Continued Medical Innovation," AHIP, July 2015, https://www.ahip.org/wp-content/uploads/2015/07/IssueBrief_SpecialtyDrugs_7.9.15.pdf.

[77] John Graham, "Crisis In Pharma R&D: It Costs $2.6 Billion To Develop A New Medicine; 2.5 Times More Than In 2003," *Forbes*, November 26, 2014, http://www.forbes.com/ sites/theapothecary/2014/11/26/crisis-in-pharma-rd-it-costs-2-6-billion-to-develop-a-new-medicine-2-5-times-more-than-in-2003/#4218f02c1641.

[78] Topher Spiro, Maura Calsyn, and Thomas Huelskoetter, "Enough Is Enough: The Time Has Come to Address Sky-High Drug Prices," Center for American Progress, September 2015, https:// cdn.americanprogress.org/wp-content/uploads/2015/09/15131852/ DrugPricingReforms-report1.pdf.

[79] Sreedhar Potarazu, "Rising cost of prescription drugs threatens health care gains," CNN, August 26, 2015, http://www.cnn. com/2015/08/26/opinions/potarazu-drug-price-hikes/.

[80] Ibid.

[81] Ibid.

[82] Lee Graczyk, "Americans can't afford U.S. medication, need a safe alternative," The Hill (blog), November 12, 2014, http://thehill.com/blogs/congress-blog/ healthcare/223650-americans-cant-afford-us-medication-need-a-safe-alternative.

[83] "IFHP publishes 2013 Price Report," International Federation of Health Plans, accessed December 7, 2016, http://www.ifhp. com/1404121/.

[84] "2013 Comparative Price Report Variation in Medical and Hospital Prices by Country," International Federation of Health Plans, accessed December 7, 2016, https://static1.squarespace.com/static/518a3cfee4b0a77d03a62c98/t/ 534fc9ebe4b05a88e5fbab70/1397737963288/2013+iFHP+FIN AL+4+14+14.pdf.

[85] Don Wright, Paul D. Hughes, and Wanda K. Jones, "ADE Prevention: 2014 Action Plan Conference," Health.gov, October 30, 2014, https://health.gov/hcq/pdfs/2014-ADE-Action-Plan-Conference-Slides.pdf.

[86] Ronda G. Hughes and Mary A. Blegen, "Medication Administration Safety," chap. 37 in *Patient Safety and Quality: An Evidence-Based Handbook for Nurses* (Rockville: Agency for Healthcare Research and Quality, 2008) http://www.ncbi.nlm.nih.gov/books/NBK2656/.

[87] Ibid.

[88] K.H. Yu, R.L. Nation, and M.J. Dooley, "Multiplicity of medication safety terms, definitions and functional meanings: when is enough enough?" *Quality & Safety in Health Care* 4 (July 30, 2005): 358-363, https://www.ncbi.nlm.nih.gov/pmc/articles/PMC1744082/pdf/v014p00358.pdf.

[89] L. La Pietra, L. Calligaris, L. Molendini, R. Quattrin, and S. Brusaferro, "Medical errors and clinical risk management: state of the art," *Acta Otorhinolaryngol Italica* 25, no. 6 (December 2005): 339-346, http://www.ncbi.nlm.nih.gov/pmc/articles/PMC2639900/.

[90] Rachel M. Kruer, Andrew S. Jarrell, and Asad Latif, "Reducing medication errors in critical care: a multimodal approach," The *Journal of Clinical Pharmacology* 6 (September 1, 2014): 117-126. doi: 10.2147/CPAA.S48530.

[91] Ibid.

[92] Ronald A. Nosek, Jr., Judy McMeekin, and Geoffrey W. Rake, *Advances in Patient Safety: From Research to Implementation (Volume 4: Programs, Tools, and Products)* (Rockville: Agency for Healthcare Research and Quality, 2005), http://www.ncbi.nlm.nih.gov/books/NBK20623/.

[93] Ibid.

[94] G.M. Kuo, R.L. Phillips, D. Graham, J.M. Hickner, "Medication errors reported by US family physicians and their office staff." Abstract. *Quality & Safety in Health Care* 17, no. 4 (August 2008): 286-290. doi: 10.1136/qshc.2007.024869.

[95] James Reason, "Human error: models and management," BMJ 320, no. 7,237 (March 18, 2000): 768-770, https://www.ncbi.nlm.nih.gov/pmc/articles/PMC1117770/.

[96] Ibid.

[97] Ibid.

[98] James Reason, "Human error models and management," The Western Journal of Medicine 172, no. 6 (June 2000): 393-396 http://www.ncbi.nlm.nih.gov/pmc/articles/PMC1070929/.

[99] Ronda G. Hughes and Mary A. Blegen, "Medication Administration Safety," chap. 37 in *Patient Safety and Quality: An Evidence-Based Handbook for Nurses.*

[100] Ibid.

[101] Ibid.

[102] "National Action Plan for Adverse Drug Event Prevention," U.S. Department of Health and Human Services, 2014, https://health.gov/hcq/pdfs/ade-action-plan-508c.pdf.

[103] "Antibiotic Resistance Threats in the US," CDC, September 16, 2013, http://www.cdc.gov/features/antibioticresistancethreats/.

[104] National Action Plan for Adverse Drug Event Prevention," U.S. Department of Health and Human Services.

[105] Rose A. Rudd, Noah Aleshire, Jon E. Zibbell, and R. Matthew Gladden, "Increases in Drug and Opioid Overdose Deaths—United States, 2000–2014 Weekly," CDC, January 1, 2016, http://www.cdc.gov/mmwr/preview/mmwrhtml/mm6450a3.htm.

[106] "Understanding the Epidemic," CDC, June 21, 2016, http://www.cdc.gov/drugoverdose/epidemic/index.html.

[107] H.Y. Chang, M. Daubresse, S.P. Kruszewski, and G.C. Alexander, "Prevalence and treatment of pain in EDs in the United States, 2000 to 2010." Abstract. American Journal of Emergency Medicine 32, no. 5 (May 2014): 421-431. doi: 10.1016/j.ajem.2014.01.015.

[108] Nora D. Volkow, "America's Addiction to Opioids: Heroin and Prescription Drug Abuse," National Institute on Drug Abuse, May 14, 2014, https://www.drugabuse.gov/about-nida/legislative-activities/testimony-to-congress/2016/americas-addiction-to-opioids-heroin-prescription-drug-abuse.

[109] Theodore J. Cicero, Matthew S. Ellis, Hilary L. Surratt, and Steven P. Kurtz, "The Changing Face of Heroin Use in the United States: A Retrospective Analysis of the Past 50 Years," *JAMA Psychiatry* 71, no. 7 (2014): 821-826. doi:10.1001/jamapsychiatry.2014.366.

[110] Volkow, "America's Addiction to Opioids."

[111] Elizabeth R. Seaquist, John Anderson, Belinda Childs, Philip Cryer, Samuel Dagogo-Jack, Lisa Fish, Simon R. Heller, Henry Rodriguez, MD; James Rosenzweig, and Robert Vigersky, "Hypoglycemia and Diabetes," Diabetes Care 36, no. 5 (2013): 1,384-1395. http://www.medscape.com/viewarticle/803608_3.

[112] K.J. Lipska, J.S. Ross, Y. Wang, S.E. Inzucchi, K. Minges, A.J. Karter, E.S. Huang, M.M. Desai, T.M. Gill, and H.M. Krumholz, "National trends in US hospital admissions for hyperglycemia and hypoglycemia among Medicare beneficiaries, 1999 to 2011," Abstract. *JAMA Internal Medicine* 174, no. 7 (July 2014): 1,116-1,124. doi: 10.1001/jamainternmed.2014.1824.

[113] "Effects of Intensive Glucose Lowering in Type 2 Diabetes," *The New England Journal of Medicine* 358 (June 12, 2008): 2,545-2,559. doi: 10.1056/NEJMoa0802743.

[114] Gregory Piazza, Thanh Nha Nguyen, Deborah Cios, Matthew Labreche, Benjamin Hohlfelder, John Fanikos, Karen Fiumara, and Samuel Z. Goldhaber, "Anticoagulation-Associated Adverse Drug Events," *The American Journal of Medicine* 124, no. 12 (December 2011): 1,136-1,142. doi: 10.1016/j.amjmed.2011.06.009.

[115] "Warfarin, diabetes drugs cause emergency hospitalization among the elderly," Patient Education Center, accessed December 7, 2016, http://www.patienteducationcenter.org/articles/warfarin-diabetes-drugs-cause-emergency-hospitalization-among-the-elderly/#sthash.0ZxCnJeh.dpuf.

[116] "2014 Summary Report on Antimicrobials Sold or Distributed for Use in Food-Producing Animals," FDA, December 2015, http://www.fda.gov/downloads/ForIndustry/UserFees/AnimalDrugUserFeeActADUFA/UCM476258.pdf.

[117] "Antibiotic/Antimicrobial Resistance," CDC, October 25, 2016, https://www.cdc.gov/drugresistance/.

[118] Fleming-Dutra, Hersh, Shapiro, Bartoces, Enns, File, Finkelstein, et al., "Prevalence of Inappropriate Antibiotic Prescriptions."

[119] James Baggs, Scott K. Fridkin, Lori A. Pollack, Arjun Srinivasan,

[128] Michel Elie, Martin G. Cole, François J. Primeau, and François Bellavance, "Delirium Risk Factors in Elderly Hospitalized Patients," Journal of General Internal Medicine 13, no. 3 (March 1998): 204-212. doi: 10.1046/j.1525-1497.1998.00047.x.

[129] Maher, Hanlon, and Hajjar, "Clinical Consequences of Polypharmacy in Elderly."

[130] "Drug Research and Children," FDA, May 4, 2016, http://www.fda.gov/Drugs/ResourcesForYou/Consumers/ucm143565.htm.

[131] "Sentinel Event Alert," The Joint Commission, April 11, 2008, https://www.jointcommission.org/assets/1/18/SEA_39.PDF.

[132] "Promoting Safety of Medications for Children," WHO, accessed December 7, 2016, http://www.who.int/medicines/publications/essentialmedicines/Promotion_safe_med_childrens.pdf.

[133] Ibid.

Chapter 6

[1] Sven Stegemann, ed., Developing Drug Products in an Aging Society, (AG Switzerland: Springer International Publishing, 2016), 490, https://books.google.com/books?id=NPJNDQAAQBAJ.

[2] "Overview of Medication Adherence Where Are We Today?" Adult Meducation, 2006, http://www.adultmeducation.com/overviewofmedicationadherence_4.html.

[3] "ISMP Safe Practice Guidelines for Adult IV Push Medications," ISMP, 2015, http://www.ismp.org/Tools/guidelines/ivsummitpush/ivpushmedguidelines.pdf.

[4] "Use, Abuse, Misuse & Disposal of Prescription Pain Medication Clinical Reference," ACPM, 2011, http://www.acpm.org/?UseAbuseRxClinRef.

[5] Donald E. Morisky, Alfonso Ang, Marie Krousel-Wood, and Harry J. Ward, "Predictive Validity of A Medication Adherence Measure in an Outpatient Setting," The Journal of Clinical Hypertension 10, no. 5 (May 2008): 348-354. http://www.ncbi.nlm.nih.gov/pmc/articles/PMC2562622/.

[6] Lisa D. Chew, Katharine A. Bradley, and Edward J. Boyko, "Brief Questions to Identify Patients With Inadequate Health Literacy," STFM, September 2004, https://www.stfm.org/fmhub/fm2004/September/Lisa588.pdf.

[7] Elizabeth Oyekan, Ananda Nimalasuriya, John Martin, Ron Scott, R. James Dudl, and Kelley Green, "The B-SMART Appropriate Medication-Use Process: A Guide for Clinicians to Help Patients— Part 1: Barriers, Solutions, and Motivation," *The Permanente Journal* 13, no. 1 (2009): 62-69. https://www.ncbi.nlm.nih.gov/pmc/articles/PMC3034468/.

[8] Ibid.

[9] A.J. Forster, H. J. Murff, J.F. Peterson, T.K. Gandhi, and D.W. Bates, "The incidence and severity of adverse events affecting patients after discharge from the hospital," *Annals of Internal Medicine* 138, no. 3 (2003): 161–167. http://www.ncbi.nlm.nih.gov/pubmed/12558354.

[10] Osterberg and Blaschke, "Adherence to Medication," 487–497.

[11] "2017 National Patient Safety Goals," The Joint Commission, accessed December 7, 2016, https://www.jointcommission.org/standards_information/npsgs.aspx.

[12] Mark D. Levitz, "Medication Reconciliation: The Role of the Pharmacy Technician," *Pharmacy Times*, August 9, 2013, http://www.pharmacytimes.com/publications/directions-in-pharmacy/2013/august2013/medication-reconciliation-the-role-of-the-pharmacy-technician.

[13] "Guide to Patient and Family Engagement in Hospital Quality and Safety," AHRQ, June 2013, http://www.ahrq.gov/professionals/systems/hospital/engagingfamilies/index.html.

[14] Stephanie Rennke, Marwa H Shoeb, Oanh K Nguyen, Yimdriuska Magan, Robert M Wachter, and Sumant R Ranji, "Interventions To Improve Care Transitions at Hospital Discharge (NEW)," chap. 37 in *Making Health Care Safer II: An Updated Critical Analysis of the Evidence for Patient Safety Practices* (Rockville: Agency for Healthcare Research and Quality, 2013), http://www.ncbi.nlm.nih.gov/books/NBK133366/.

[15] "Educating Patients About Safe Medication Use," Davis's Drug Guide.com, http://www.drugguide.com/ddo/view/Davis-Drug-Guide/110092/all/Educating_Patients_About_Safe_Medication_Use.

[16] "Patient and Family Engagement: A Partnership for Culture Change A Report of the NCIOM Task Force on Patient and Family Engagement." North Carolina Institute of Medicine.

[17] "Overspending driven by oversized single dose vials of cancer drugs," *BMJ*, March 1, 2016, doi: http://dx.doi.org/10.1136/bmj.i788.

[18] Ron Shinkman, "Hospitals throw away $3 billion worth of cancer drugs annually," *FierceHealthcare*, March 3, 2016, http://www.fiercehealthcare.com/finance/hospitals-throw-away-3-billion-worth-cancer-drugs-annually.

[19] Gigi Y.C. Wong, "Cost Impact of Using Patients' Own Multidose Medications in Hospital," Abstract. *The Canadian Journal of Hospital Pharmacy* 67, no. 1 (January-February, 2014): 9-16. https://www.ncbi.nlm.nih.gov/pmc/articles/PMC3952918/.

[20] Ibid.

[21] "Improving Medication Safety," AHA, accessed December 7, 2016, http://www.aha.org/advocacy-issues/tools-resources/advisory/96-06/991207-quality-adv.shtml.

[22] "2016-2017 Targeted Medication Safety Best Practices for Hospitals," ISMP, accessed December 7, 2016, http://www.ismp.org/Tools/BestPractices/TMSBP-for-Hospitals.pdf.

[23] Abha Agrawal, "Medication errors: prevention using information technology systems," *British Journal of Clinical Pharmacology* 67, no. 6 (June 2009): 681-686, https://www.ncbi.nlm.nih.gov/pmc/articles/PMC2723209/.

[24] R. Amarasingham, L. Plantinga, M. Diener-West, D.J. Gaskin, and N.R. Powe NR, "Clinical information technologies and inpatient outcomes: a multiple hospital study," Abstract. Archives of Internal Medicine 169, no. 2 (January 2009): 108–114. doi: 10.1001/archinternmed.2008.520.

[25] R.C. Boothman, A.C. Blackwell, D.A. Campbell Jr., E. Commiskey,

and S. Anderson, "A better approach to medical malpractice claims? The University of Michigan experience." *Abstract. Journal of Health & Life Science Law 2*, no. 2 (January 2009): 125-159. https://www. ncbi.nlm.nih.gov/pubmed/19288891.

[26] Neil Chesanow, "5 Easy Ways to Improve Compliance That Many Doctors Don't Do," Medscape, February 11, 2015, http://www. medscape.com/viewarticle/837428_3.

[27] Vera Gruessner, "Patient Engagement Expands with Telehealth, Mobile Devices," mHealth Intelligence, November 2, 2015, http:// mhealthintelligence.com/news/patient-engagement-expands-with-telehealth-mobile-devices.

[28] Rachel Zimmerman, "Health Boost: Story-Sharing Kiosk For Hospital Patients Coping With Illness Set To Launch," *WBUR*, October 29, 2015, http://www.wbur.org/commonhealth/2015/10/29/ patients-sharing-stories.

[29] "Mobile Technology Fact Sheet," Pew Research Center, December 27, 2013, http://www.pewinternet.org/fact-sheets/mobile-technology-fact-sheet/.

[30] Vera Gruessner, "Top Four Patient Engagement Trends to Follow from October," mHealth Intelligence, November 2, 2015, http:// mhealthintelligence.com/news/top-four-patient-engagement-trends-to-follow-from-october.

[31] Miriam Chan, "Reducing Cost-Related Medication Nonadherence in Patients With Diabetes," Physician's Practice, April 15, 2010, http://www.physicianspractice.com/articles/reducing-cost-related-medication-nonadherence-patients-diabetes.

[32] "10 Ways to reduce your drug costs," *Consumer Reports*, March 2009, http://www.consumerreports.org/cro/2012/04/10-ways-to-reduce-your-drug-costs/index.htm.

[33] "PREVENTING ERRORS IN YOUR PRACTICE Prescription Writing to Maximize Patient Safety," AAFP, 2002, http://www.aafp. org/fpm/2002/0700/p27.html.

[34] Jeff E. Freund, Beth A. Martin, Mara A. Kieser, Staci M. Williams, and Susan L. Sutter, "Transitions in Care: Medication Reconciliation

in the Community Pharmacy Setting After Discharge," *Innovations in Pharmacy* 4, no. 2 (2013): 1-6. http://pubs.lib.umn.edu/cgi/ viewcontent.cgi?article=1119&context=innovations.

[35] Ibid.

[36] "CVS/pharmacy Encourages Consumers to Consult With Pharmacists: CARE 1on1™ program offers dedicated time with pharmacists to review savings, safety and side effects when transferring or filling a new ongoing medication," *PR Newswire*, June 20, 2011, http://www.prnewswire.com/news-releases/cvspharmacy-encourages-consumers-to-consult-with-pharmacists-124182029.html.

[37] "CVS Caremark Study Finds Integrated Pharmacy-Based Program Improved Diabetes Medication Initiation and Adherence Rates," CVS Health, January 9, 2012, https://cvshealth.com/newsroom/press-releases/cvs-caremark-study-finds-integrated-pharmacy-based-program-improved-diabetes.

[38] Allison Gilchrist, "5 Tips to Help Patients Save Money on Prescriptions," *Pharmacy Times*, February 28, 2016, http://www. pharmacytimes.com/news/5-tips-to-help-patients-save-money-on-prescriptions#sthash.DEqrmmtY.dpuf.

[39] Rama P. Nair, Daya Kappil, and Tonja M. Woods, "10 Strategies for Minimizing Dispensing Errors," *Pharmacy Times*, January 19, 2010, http://www.pharmacytimes.com/publications/issue/2010/january2010/ p2pdispensingerrors-0110.

[40] Ibid.

[41] "Reducing Hospital Readmissions With Enhanced Patient Education," Boston University, accessed December 7, 2016, https://www.bu.edu/ fammed/projectred/publications/news/krames_dec_final.pdf.

[42] "Consumer Reports AdWatch," *Consumer Reports*, April 2012, http://www.consumerreports.org/cro/2012/04/consumer-reports-adwatch/index.htm.

[43] "One way to reduce the cost of specialty drugs: Find the right place to get them," Aetna, 2015, https://news.aetna.com/2015/08/one-way-reduce-cost-specialty-drugs-find-right-place-get/.

[44] "Adverse Drug Events (ADE)," CMS.gov, accessed December 7, 2016, https://partnershipforpatients.cms.gov/p4p_resources/tsp-adversedrugevents/tooladversedrugeventsade.html.

[45] Catherine M. Mullahy and Michael G. Goldstein, "Dancing, not wrestling: Motivational interviewing helps case managers cultivate relationships and elicit change," CCMC, 2012, https://ccmcertification.org/sites/default/files/downloads/2012/10%20-%20Dancing,%20not%20wrestling.%20Motivational%20interviewing%20helps%20case%20managers%20cultivate%20relationships%20and%20e-licit%20change.pdf.

[46] Richard Scott, ed., "Motivational Interviewing: An Emerging Trend in Medical Management," Professional Patient Advocate Institute, accessed December 7, 2016, http://www.patientadvocatetraining.com/wp-content/themes/patientadvocate/static/pdf/ppai_specialreport_mi.pdf.

[47] Mullahy and Goldstein, "Dancing, not wrestling."

[48] Ibid.

[49] Garry Welch, Gary Rose, and Dennis Ernst, "Motivational Interviewing and Diabetes: What Is It, How Is It Used, and Does It Work?" *Diabetes Spectrum* 19, no. 1 (January 2006): 5-11. doi: http://dx.doi.org/10.2337/diaspect.19.1.5.

[50] Albert Bandura and Daniel Cervone, "Self-Evaluative and Self-Efficacy Mechanisms Governing the Motivational Effects of Goal Systems," *Journal of Personality and Social Psychology* 45, no. 5 (1983): 1,017-1,028. https://web.stanford.edu/dept/psychology/bandura/pajares/Bandura1983JPSP.pdf.

[51] Tommy Newberry, *Success Is Not an Accident: Change Your Choices; Change Your Life* (Carol Stream: Tyndall House Publishers, Inc., 2007), 68, https://books.google.com/books?id=Fe7wfvw2SHQC.

[52] Vermeire, Hearnshaw, Royen, and Denekens, "Patient adherence to treatment: three decades of research. A comprehensive review." 331–342.

[53] Joe Carlson, "Doc communication, medication adherence tied: study," *Modern Healthcare*, December 31, 2012, http://www.modernhealthcare.com/article/20121231/NEWS/312319981.

[54] Elizabeth Oyekan, Ananda Nimalasuriya, John Martin, Ron Scott, R. James Dudl, and Kelley Green, "The B-SMART Appropriate Medication-Use Process: A Guide for Clinicians to Help Patients-Part 2: Adherence, Relationships, and Triage," *The Permanente Journal* 13, no. 4 (2009): 50-54, https://www.ncbi.nlm.nih.gov/pmc/articles/PMC2911835/.

Chapter 7

[1] "What is Integrative Medicine?" AIHM, accessed December 8, 2016, https://www.aihm.org/about/what-is-integrative-medicine/.
[2] Brown and Bussell, "Medication Adherence: WHO Cares?" 304-314.
[3] Mullahy and Goldstein, "Dancing, not wrestling."
[4] "AHA 2017 Environmental Scan," *H&HN Magazine*, September 12, 2016, http://www.hhnmag.com/articles/7616-aha-2017-environmental-scan.
[5] Rick Pollack, "A Road Map to What Will Be Trending in Health Care in 2017: The AHA Environmental Scan," *H&HN Magazine*, September 7, 2016, http://www.hhnmag.com/articles/7601-road-map-to-health-care-in-2017-aha-environmental-scan.
[6] "2017 AHA Environmental Scan," B.E. Smith, accessed December 8, 2016, https://www.besmith.com/thought-leadership/articles/2017-aha-environmental-scan.
[7] "Trends in Chronic Care and Wellness for Patients and Consumers," *H&HN Magazine*, September 7, 2016, http://www.hhnmag.com/articles/7602-consumers-and-patients-trends-in-chronic-care-andwellness.
[8] Rick Pollack, "A Road Map to What Will Be Trending in Health Care in 2017."
[9] "Edward A. Chow, Henry Foster, Victor Gonzalez, and LaShawn McIver, "The Disparate Impact of Diabetes on Racial/Ethnic Minority Populations," Clinical Diabetes 30, no. 3 (July 2012): 130-133. doi: http://dx.doi.org/10.2337/diaclin.30.3.130.
[10] "Health Statistics," The National Institute of Diabetes and Digestive

and Kidney Diseases, accessed March 7, 2012, http://www.diabetes. niddk.nih.gov/dm/pubs/statistics.

[11] "The Growing Crisis of Chronic Disease in the United States," Partnership to Fight Chronic Disease.

[12] "The Great Healthcare Debates: Prescriptions for meaningful reform," AMCP, accessed December 8, 2016, http://www.amcp.org/ WorkArea/DownloadAsset.aspx?id=12182.

[13] *Goodreads*, s.v. "Steve Jobs," accessed December 8, 2016, http:// www.goodreads.com/quotes/861193-deciding-what-not-to-do-is-as-important-as-deciding.

[14] Lou Diorio and Dave Thomas, "Lean Concepts & Pharmacy," LDT, 2011, http://ldthealthsolutions.com/_articles/ LeanConceptsAndPharmacy.pdf.

[15] "Clinical Guidelines and Standardization of Practice to Improve Outcomes," ACOG, April 2015, http://www.acog.org/Resources-And-Publications/Committee-Opinions/Committee-on-Patient-Safety-and-Quality-Improvement/Clinical-Guidelines-and-Standardization-of-Practice-to-Improve-Outcomes.

[16] S. Lawrence Kocot, "Realigning Medicare Part D Incentives: A New Model For Medication Therapy Management," Health Affairs Blog, September 28, 2015, http://healthaffairs.org/blog/2015/09/28/ realigning-medicare-part-d-incentives-a-new-model-for-medication-therapy-management/.

[17] Ibid.

Chapter 8

[1] Michael E. Porter, "What Is Value in Health Care?" *The New England Journal of Medicine* 363 (December 23, 2010): 2,477-2,482. doi: 10.1056/NEJMp1011024.

[2] Ninon Lewis, "A Primer on Defining the Triple Aim," IHI (blog), October 17, 2014, http://www.ihi.org/communities/blogs/_layouts/ ihi/community/blog/itemview.aspx?List=81ca4a47-4ccd-4e9e-89d9-14d88ec59e8d&ID=63.

[3] "Part C and D Performance Data," CMS.gov, November 16, 2016, https://www.cms.gov/Medicare/Prescription-Drug-Coverage/PrescriptionDrugCovGenIn/PerformanceData.html.

[4] Ibid.

[5] Ibid.

[6] Ibid.

[7] "Quality Measures," Quality Payment Program, accessed December 7, 2016, https://qpp.cms.gov/measures/quality.

[8] "Accountable Care Organization 2015 Program Analysis Quality Performance Standards Narrative Measure Specifications," CMS.gov, January 9, 2015, https://www.cms.gov/Medicare/Medicare-Fee-for-Service-Payment/sharedsavingsprogram/Downloads/ACO-NarrativeMeasures-Specs.pdf.

[9] "Physician Quality Reporting System," CMS.gov, October 11, 2016, https://www.cms.gov/Medicare/Quality-Initiatives-Patient-Assessment-Instruments/PQRS/index.html.

[10] "The Hospital Readmissions Reduction (HRR) Program," CMS.gov, accessed December 7, 2016, https://www.cms.gov/Medicare/Quality-Initiatives-Patient-Assessment-Instruments/Value-Based-Programs/HRRP/Hospital-Readmission-Reduction-Program.html.

[11] "Health Care Provider Patient Safety," NCSL, March 2011, http://www.ncsl.org/research/health/health-care-provider-patient-safety.aspx.

[12] "Patient Safety," National Quality Forum, accessed December 7, 2016, http://www.qualityforum.org/Topics/Patient_Safety.aspx.

[13] "Consumer Assessment of Healthcare Providers & Systems (CAHPS)," CMS.gov, November 4, 2016, https://www.cms.gov/Research-Statistics-Data-and-Systems/Research/CAHPS/.

[14] "ACO CAHPS Frequently Asked Questions," Press Ganey, 2016, http://www.pressganey.com/docs/default-source/default-document-library/aco-cahps-faq_010416.pdf?sfvrsn=0.

[15] "The National Quality Strategy: Fact Sheet," AHRQ, September 2014, http://www.ahrq.gov/workingforquality/nqs/nqsfactsheet.htm.

[16] Ibid.

[17] "2011 Report to Congress: National Strategy for Quality Improvement in Health Care," AHRQ, March 2011, http://www.ahrq. gov/workingforquality/nqs/nqs2011annlrpt.htm.

[18] Chris Morran, "CDC Reports "Worrisome" News On Antibiotic Use In Hospitals," *Consumerist*, September 19, 2016, https://consumerist. com/2016/09/19/cdc-reports-worrisome-news-on-antibiotic-use-in-hospitals/.

[19] Paige Minemyer, "Antibiotic stewardship programs reduce unneeded prescriptions, infections," *FierceHealthcare*, June 9, 2016, http://www. fiercehealthcare.com/healthcare/antibiotic-stewardship-programs-reduce-unneeded-prescriptions-bacterial-infections.

[20] "Prescription Drug Monitoring Programs (PDMPs)," CDC, March 23, 2016, http://www.cdc.gov/drugoverdose/pdmp/.

[21] "PHARMACOGENOMICS PROGRAM," Mayo Clinic, accessed December 7, 2016, http://mayoresearch.mayo.edu/center-for-individualized-medicine/pharmacogenomics.asp.

[22] "Pharmacist Interactions Can Improve Outcomes," CVS Health, accessed December 7, 2016, https://cvshealth.com/thought-leadership/pharmacist-interactions-can-improve-outcomes.

[23] M.M. Spence, A.F. Makarem, S.L. Reyes, L.L. Rosa, C. Nguyen, E.A. Oyekan, and A.T. Kiyohara, "Evaluation of an outpatient pharmacy clinical services program on adherence and clinical outcomes among patients with diabetes and/or coronary artery disease." Abstract. *Journal of Managed Care & Specialty Pharmacy* 20, no. 10 (October 2014): 1,036-1,045. https://www.ncbi.nlm.nih.gov/pubmed/25278326.

[24] "Medication Management Center," UF Medication Management Center College of Pharmacy, accessed December 5, 2016, http://mmc. pharmacy.ufl.edu/.

[25] Ibid.

[26] Roebuck, Liberman, Gemmill-Toyama, and Brennan, "Medication Adherence Leads to Lower Health Care Use and Costs Despite Increased Drug Spending," 91-99.

[27] Payal Kohli, Seamus P. Whelton, Steven Hsu, Clyde W. Yancy, Neil J. Stone, Jonathan Chrispin, Nisha A. Gilotra, et al., "Clinician's Guide to the Updated ABCs of Cardiovascular Disease Prevention," *Journal of the American Health Association* 3, no. 5 (September 22, 2014). doi: http://dx.doi.org/10.1161/JAHA.114.001098.

[28] "Walgreens Addresses Growing Need for Mental Health Resources with New Platform, Campaign and Access to Expanded Services," Walgreens Newsroom, May 10, 2016, http://news.walgreens.com/press-releases/general-news/walgreens-addresses-growing-need-for-mental-health-resources-with-new-platform-campaign-and-access-to-expanded-services.htm.

[29] *Goodreads*, s.v. "Peter F. Drucker," accessed December 5, 2016, http://www.goodreads.com/quotes/172730-what-s-measured-improves.

[30] "Performance Management & Measurement," HRSA, accessed December 7, 2016, http://www.hrsa.gov/quality/toolbox/methodology/performancemanagement/index.html.

[31] "People Play Differently When They Are Keeping Score," The 4DX Blog, November 27, 2012, http://www.4dxbook.com/blog/category/the-4dx-book/.

[32] Lucian L. Leape, "Transparency and Public Reporting Are Essential for a Safe Health Care System," accessed December 7, 2016, IPRO, http://www.whynotthebest.org/contents/view/142.

[33] Ibid.

[34] M. E. Porter and E. O. Teisberg, "How Physicians Can Change the Future of Health Care," Abstract. *Journal of the American Medical Association* 297, no. 10 (March 14, 2007): 1,103–1,011. doi: 10.1001/jama.297.10.1103.

[35] Leape, "Transparency and Public Reporting Are Essential."

Chapter 9

[1] *QuoteHD*, s.v. "Mike Parker Quotes," accessed December 5, 2016, http://www.quotehd.com/quotes/mike-parker-quote-when-you-dont-invest-in-infrastructure-you-are-going-to-pay.

[2] Andrew Kingery, "The Basics of Pharmacy Benefits Management (PBM) 2009," Anthem, 2009, https://www11.anthem.com/shared/va/f5/s1/t0/pw_b135247.pdf.

[3] Craig Schilling and John Mbagwu, "Breakout III: Drug Reconciliation and Medication Adherence–Two Sides of the Same Coin," EHCCA, October 7, 2014, http://www.ehcca.com/presentations/capgma1/schilling_b3.pdf.

[4] RxAnte website, accessed December 7, 2016, https://www.rxante.com.

[5] Allazo Health website, accessed December 7, 2016, http://allazohealth.com.

[6] Briova Rx website, accessed December 7, 2016, https://www.briovarx.com/index.html.

[7] "Pharmacy On the Go," CVS, accessed December 7, 2016, http://www.cvs.com/mobile/mobile-cvs-pharmacy/.

[8] Abbe Steel, "Engaging Patients for Healthier Outcomes," Express Scripts, June 26, 2013, http://lab.express-scripts.com/lab/insights/adherence/engaging-patients-for-healthier-outcomes.

[9] "Maintaining the Affordability of the Prescription Drug Benefit" AMCP.

[10] Thomas Reuters, "Express Scripts releases list of costly drugs it won't cover for 2017," *Business Insurance*, August 2, 2016, http://www.businessinsurance.com/article/20160802/NEWS03/160809963/express-scripts-releases-list-of-costly-drugs-it-wont-cover-for-2017.

[11] "2015 Global health care outlook Common goals, competing priorities," Deloitte.

[12] "Pharmacy Benefit Managers (PBMs): Generating Savings for Plan Sponsors and Consumers," That's What PBMS Do, February 2016, http://thatswhatpbmsdo.com/wp-content/uploads/2016/02/visante-pbm-savings-study-Feb-2016.pdf.

[13] "Maintaining the Affordability of the Prescription Drug Benefit" AMCP.

[14] "Pharmacy Benefit Managers (PBMs)" That's What PBMS Do.

[15] "Follow The Pill: Understanding the U.S. Commercial Pharmaceutical Supply Chain," Kaiser Family, March 2005, https://kaiserfamilyfoundation.files.wordpress.com/2013/01/follow-the-pill-

understanding-the-u-s-commercial-pharmaceutical-supply-chain-report.pdf.

[16] Ibid.

[17] "The Challenges, Solutions, and Strategies Driving Pharmaceutical Supply Chain Innovation," LogiPharma, 2015, https://cdn2.hubspot.net/hubfs/476052/offers/whitepapers/LogiPharma_White_Paper/Challenges_Solutions_Strategies_Pharma-Supply_Chain_Innovation_Report.pdf.

[18] "Drug Shortages & Supply Chain Info," Pharma, accessed December 7, 2016, http://www.phrma.org/advocacy/safety/drug-shortages-supply-chain.

[19] "Medication Adherence," Omnicell, accessed December 7, 2016, http://www.omnicell.com/Products/Medication_Adherence.aspx.

[20] Walt Berghahn, "Medication Adherence Efforts In D.C. Show Upsurge: Should Smarter Pharmaceutical Packaging Follow?" *BNP Media*, February 2016, http://digital.bnpmedia.com/article/Medication+Adherence+Efforts+In+D.C.+Show+Upsurge%3AShould+Smarter+Pharmaceutical+Packaging+Follow%3F/2380595/0/article.html.

[21] Thomas Grant, "Medication adherence," Team Consulting, accessed December 7, 2016, https://www.team-consulting.com/insights/medication-adherence/.

[22] Andy Fry and Julian Dixon, "Device Usability and Compliance: The Implications, Opportunities and Requirements," Slide Share.net, June 21, 2011, http://www.slideshare.net/team_medical/device-usability-and-compliance-the-implications-opportunities-and-requirements.

[23] "Pharma 2020: Supplying the future Which path will you take?" PWC, accessed December 7, 2016, http://www.pwc.com/gx/en/pharma-life-sciences/pharma-2020/assets/pharma-2020-supplying-the-future.pdf.

[24] Ibid.

[25] Ebel, Larsen, and Shah, "Strengthening health care's supply chain."

[26] Ibid.

[27] "Save Time and Money With a Mail-Order Pharmacy," *News USA*, accessed December 7, 2016, http://www.newsusa.com/articles/article/save-time-and-money-with-a-mail-order-pharmacy.aspx.

[28] "Drug Supply Chain Integrity," FDA.

[29] Ebel, Larsen, and Shah, "Strengthening health care's supply chain."

[30] Ibid.

[31] "Drug Shortages & Supply Chain Info," Pharma.

[32] Walter Berghahn, "Packaging, serialization and medication adherence: the coming connection," *Pharmaceutical Commerce*, July 18, 2012, http://pharmaceuticalcommerce.com/opinion/packaging-serialization-and-medication-adherence-the-coming-connection/.

[33] Brian Johnson, "A Pharmaceutical Company's View on Supply-Chain Security: A Perspective from Pfizer," *Pharmaceutical Technology*, September 2, 2011, http://www.pharmtech.com/pharmaceutical-companys-view-supply-chain-security-perspective-pfizer?id=&sk=&date=&%0A%09%09%09&pageID=2.

[34] "Clinical and Business Analytics," H&HN, June 15, 2016, http://www.hhnmag.com/articles/7369-clinical-and-business-analytics.

[35] Ed Burns, "descriptive analytics," WhatIs.com, December 2015, http://whatis.techtarget.com/definition/descriptive-analytics.

[36] Ibid.

[37] John Pagliuca, "Leveraging Data to Improve Medication Compliance," *Scio Health Analytics* (blog), September 29, 2016, http://www.sciohealthanalytics.com/blog/leveraging-data-improve-medication-compliance.

[38] "OptumRx and Walgreens Partner to Improve Consumer Convenience, Cost Savings and Outcomes," Walgreens Newsroom, March 17, 2016, http://news.walgreens.com/press-releases/general-news/optumrx-and-walgreens-partner-to-improve-consumer-convenience-cost-savings-and-outcomes.htm.

[39] "Accountable Care Coalition of Greater New York and AllazoHealth Receive 2014 Pilot Health Tech NYC Grant: Medication adherence pilot program targets Medicare beneficiaries with developmental disabilities and intellectual challenges," *Business Wire*, July 9, 2014, http://www.businesswire.com/news/home/20140709005319/en/Accountable-Care-Coalition-Greater-York-AllazoHealth-Receive.

[40] "EnvisionInsurance Partnership with RxAnte Uses Predictive

Technologies to Improve Care and Costs for Patients with Chronic Conditions," RxAnte, July 19, 2016, https://www.rxante.com/1256/envisioninsurance-partnership-with-rxante-uses-predictive-technologies-to-improve-care-and-costs-for-patients-with-chronic-conditions/.

[41] "OptumRx and Walgreens Partner" Walgreens Newsroom.

[42] Dominique Comer, Joseph Couto, Ruth Aguiar, and Daniel J. Elliott, "Usefulness of Pharmacy Claims for Medication Reconciliation in Primary Care | Page 2," *American Journal of Managed Care* 21, no. 7 (July 16, 2015). http://www.ajmc.com/journals/issue/2015/2015-vol21-n7/usefulness-of-pharmacy-claims-for-medication-reconciliation-in-primary-care/p-2.

[43] Harry Totonis, Paul L. Uhrig, May Ann Chaffee, David Yakimischak, Seth Joseph, and Ajit A. Dhavle, "An Rx for America's Healthcare Health IT & E-Prescribing," Surescripts, accessed December 7, 2016, http://surescripts.com/docs/default-source/PressRelease-Library/ebookanrxforamerica'shealthcare.pdf.

[44] Jennifer Bresnick, "Surescripts Ups Patient Safety, Savings with Interoperability," *HealthITAnalytics*, May 21, 2015, http://healthitanalytics.com/news/surescripts-ups-patient-safety-savings-with-interoperability.

[45] Scott Mace, "Data Analytics Takes on Medication Management," *Health Leaders Media*, February 11, 2014, http://www.healthleadersmedia.com/technology/data-analytics-takes-medication-management?page=0%2C2.

[46] Ibid.

[47] "Patient Engagement & Satisfaction," MedeAnalytics, accessed December 7, 2016, http://medeanalytics.com/business-issues/patient-experience-satisfaction

[48] "IBM Watson Health Cloud Capabilities Expand," *FierceMarkets*, September 10, 2015, http://assets.fiercemarkets.net/public/004-Healthcare/internal/watsonhealthcloud.pdf.

[49] "Big data gives new insight into blood pressure reduction role of

commonly prescribed drug," *EurekAlert!* July 28, 2015, https://www.eurekalert.org/pub_releases/2015-07/iu-bdg072815.php.

[50] "Drug Cost Opportunity Analytics: Rapidly identify top medication drivers and benchmark performance, and track antibiotic usage and susceptibility." CaridnalHealth, accessed December 7, 2016, http://www.cardinalhealth.com/en/services/acute/business-solutions/financial-consulting/drug-cost-control-and-analytics/drug-cost-opportunity-analytics.html.

[51] Ibid.

[52] Patti Romeril, "How to Use Data to Improve Hospital Drug Distribution: Memorial Hermann reduced readmissions, improved patient safety and lowered the costs of patient care with adverse drug events analytics." *H&HN*, September 3, 2015, http://www.hhnmag.com/articles/3237-how-to-use-data-to-improve-hospital-drug-distribution.

[53] Ibid.

[54] "Health IT: Advancing America's Health Care," HealthIT.gov, accessed December 7, 2016, https://www.healthit.gov/sites/default/files/pdf/health-information-technology-fact-sheet.pdf.

[55] "What is an electronic health record (EHR)?" HealthIT.gov, March 16, 2013, https://www.healthit.gov/providers-professionals/faqs/what-electronic-health-record-ehr. .

[56] Ibid.

[57] "FDASIA Health IT Report: Proposed Strategy and Recommendations for a Risk-Based Framework," FDA, April 2014, http://www.fda.gov/downloads/AboutFDA/CentersOffices/OfficeofMedicalProductsandTobacco/CDRH/CDRHReports/UCM391521.pdf.

[58] Ibid.

[59] "Improved Diagnostics & Patient Outcomes," HealthIT.gov, March 19, 2014, https://www.healthit.gov/providers-professionals/improved-diagnostics-patient-outcomes.

[60] Aja B. Williams, "Issue Brief: Medication Adherence and Health IT."

[61] S.B. Joseph, M.J. Sow, M.F. Furukawa, S. Posnack, and J.G. Daniel. "E-prescribing adoption and use increased substantially following the

start of a federal incentive program." Abstract. *Health Affairs* 32, no. 7 (July 2013): 1,221-1,227. doi: 10.1377/hlthaff.2012.1197.

[62] H.B. Bosworth, B.B. Granger, P. Mendys, R. Brindis, R. Burkholder, S.M. Czajkowski, J.G. Daniel, et al., "Medication adherence: a call for action." Abstract. American Heart Journal 162, no. 3 (September 2011): 412-424. doi: 10.1016/j.ahj.2011.06.007.

[63] Aja B. Williams, "Issue Brief: Medication Adherence and Health IT."

[64] Ibid.

[65] "Patient Participation," HealthIT.gov, March 19, 2014, https://www.healthit.gov/providers-professionals/patient-participation.

[66] "Improved Diagnostics & Patient Outcomes," HealthIt.gov.

[67] "Pharmacy Management Systems," McKesson, accessed December 7, 2016, http://betterpharmacytech.com/about-us/pms/.

[68] "Fully Integrated Pharmacy Information Management System," VersaSuite, accessed December 7, 2016, http://versasuite.com/pharmacy-information-management-system/.

[69] "Enterprise Pharmacy System," PDX Inc., accessed December 7, 2016, https://www.pdxinc.com/software/enterprise_pharmacy.asp

[70] "Evaluating Hospital Pharmacy Inventory Management and Revenue Cycle Processes," AHIA, 2015, https://www.ahia.org/assets/Uploads/pdfUpload/WhitePapers/HospitalPharmacyInventory ManagementandRevenueCycleProcesses.pdf.

[71] "Medication Adherence and Clinical Performance for Pharmacies," McKesson, accessed December 7, 2016, http://www.mckesson.com/pharmacies/medication-adherence-and-clinical-performance/.

[72] Bev Johnson, Marie Abraham, Jim Conway, Laurel Simmons, Susan Edgman-Levitan, Pat Sodomka, Juliette Schlucter, and Dan Ford, "Partnering with Patients and Families to Design a Patientand Family-Centered Health Care System," IPFCC, April 2008, http://www.ipfcc.org/pdf/PartneringwithPatientsandFamilies.pdf.

[73] Zachary A. Marcum, Julia Driessen, Carolyn T. Thorpe, Walid F. Gellad, and Julie M. Donohue, "Impact of Multiple Pharmacy Use on Medication Adherence and Drug-drug Interactions in Older Adults

with Medicare Part D," *Journal of the American Geriatrics Society* 62, no. 2 (January 21, 2014): 244-252. doi: 10.1111/jgs.12645.

74 Zach Schladetzky, "Trend: What is Pharmacy Load Balancing?" TELEPHRAM (blog), May 16, 2016, http://blog.telepharm.com/trend-what-is-pharmacy-load-balancing.

75 "Office of Justice Programs Announces Grant Awards of More Than $8.8 Million to Help Reduce Prescription Drug Abuse, Misuse, Diversion," The United States Department of Justice, September 23, 2016, https://www.justice.gov/opa/pr/office-justice-programs-announces-grant-awards-more-88-million-help-reduce-prescription-drug.

76 "The consumer's guide to finding good medication management apps," Script Your Future, accessed December 7, 2016, http://www.scriptyourfuture.org/home/the-consumers-guide-to-finding-good-medication-management-apps/.

77 "O BAR," Ochsner, accessed December 7, 2016, https://www.ochsner.org/shop/o-bar/.

78 *Goodreads*, s.v. "Benjamin Franklin," accessed December 7, 2016, http://www.goodreads.com/quotes/21262-tell-me-and-i-forget-teach-me-and-i-may.

79 David Ollier Weber, "Health System's 'Genius Bar' Links Patients' Devices for Better Engagement Outcomes: Ochsner makes patient engagement easy through mobile and wearable technology," *H&HN,* August 2, 2016, http://www.hhnmag.com/articles/7502-health-systems-genius-bar-links-patients-devices-for-better-engagement-outcomes.

80 Charles L. Hooper, "Pharmaceuticals: Economics and Regulation," Library of Economics and Liberty, 2008, http://www.econlib.org/library/Enc/PharmaceuticalsEconomicsandRegulation.html.

81 "Pharmacy Auditing and Dispensing: The Self-Audit Control Practices to Improve Medicaid Program Integrity and Quality Patient Care Checklist," CMS.gov, accessed December 7, 2016, https://www.cms.gov/Medicare-Medicaid-Coordination/Fraud-Prevention/Medicaid-Integrity-Education/Downloads/pharmacy-selfaudit-checklist.pdf.

[82] Bob Miller, "Pharmacy Compliance Audits - Are You Prepared?" Healthcare Consultants, July 28, 2015, http://www.pharmacy-staffing. com/blog/posts/pharmacy-compliance-audits-are-you-prepared.html.
[83] "FDA Gives Pharmacies Another Four Months to Comply With Track and Trace Requirements," RAPS, June 30, 2015, http://www. raps.org/Regulatory-Focus/News/2015/06/30/22804/FDA-Gives-Pharmacies-Another-Four-Months-to-Comply-With-Track-and-Trace-Requirements/.
[84] "Fact Sheet–FDA Opioids Action Plan," FDA, September 13, 2016, http://www.fda.gov/NewsEvents/Newsroom/FactSheets/ucm484714.htm.
[85] "CDC Releases Guideline for Prescribing Opioids for Chronic Pain: Recommendations to improve patient care, safety, and help prevent opioid misuse and overdose," CDC, March 15, 2016, http://www.cdc.gov/media/releases/2016/p0315-prescribing-opioids-guidelines.html.
[86] "Injury Prevention & Control: Opioid Overdose," CDC.
[87] Mark Lowery, ed., "Protect your pharmacy against cyber and physical attacks," *Drug Topics Voice of the Pharmacist*, December 10, 2015, http://drugtopics.modernmedicine.com/drug-topics/news/protect-your-pharmacy-against-cyber-and-physical-attacks?page=0,0.

Chapter 10

[1] *BrainyQuote*, s.v. "Simon Mainwaring Quotes," accessed December 7, 2016, https://www.brainyquote.com/quotes/quotes/s/simonmainw493933.html.
[2] Daniela Molnau, "High-performance Teams: Understanding Team Cohesiveness," iSixSigma, accessed December 7, 2016, https://www.isixsigma.com/implementation/teams/high-performance-teams-understanding-team-cohesiveness/.
[3] Chris Musselwhite, "Building and Leading High Performance Teams: You don't have to be Michael Jordan or Mia Hamm to have the skills you need to build and lead high performing teams." Inc. January 1, 2007, http://www.inc.com/resources/leadership/articles/20070101/musselwhite.html.

[4] *Goodreads*, s.v. "Mark Twain," accessed December 7, 2016, http://www.goodreads.com/quotes/505050-the-two-most-important-days-in-your-life-are-the.

[5] "Alice in Wonderland quotes," Alice-in-wonderland.net, accessed December 7, 2016, http://www.alice-in-wonderland.net/resources/chapters-script/alice-in-wonderland-quotes/.

[6] "PRESS KIT," 4dxbook.com, accessed December 7, 2016, http://www.4dxbook.com/pdf/press_kit.pdf.

[7] Josh Bersin, "New Research Unlocks the Secret of Employee Recognition," Forbes, June 13, 2013, http://www.forbes.com/sites/joshbersin/2012/06/13/new-research-unlocks-the-secret-of-employee-recognition/#2515ad7e2d94.

[8] "The Positive Impact of Employee Recognition," TriNet Group, accessed December 7, 2016, http://www.trinet.com/hr-insights/articles/the-positive-impact-of-employee-recognition.

[9] "Guiding You Toward Success: Meet the Leadership behind Integrated Healthcare Strategies," Integrated Healthcare Strategies, Kathy Hall," Integrated Healthcare Strategies, accessed December 7, 2016, http://www.integratedhealthcarestrategies.com/knowledgecenter_bio.aspx?l=y&id=2274.

[10] "Guiding You Toward Success: Meet the Leadership behind Integrated Healthcare Strategies, James R. Rice," Integrated Healthcare Strategies, accessed December 7, 2016, http://www.integratedhealthcarestrategies.com/knowledgecenter_bio.aspx?l=y&id=2267.

[11] Ibid.

[12] Ibid.

[13] Cynthia D. McCauley, Charles J. Palus, Wilfred H. Drath, Richard L. Hughes, John B. McGuire, Patricia M.G. O'Connor, and Ellen Van Velsor, "INTERDEPENDENT LEADERSHIP IN ORGANIZATIONS EVIDENCE FROM SIX CASE STUDIES," CCL, 2008, http://www.ccl.org/wp-content/uploads/2015/04/interdependentLeadership.pdf.

[14] Wilfred H. Drath, Charles J. Palus, and John B. McGuire, "Developing Interdependent Leadership," chap. 14 from *The Center*

for Creatve Leadership Handbook of Leadership Development, (San Francisco: Jossey-Bass, 2010), http://www.academia.edu/7034290/ Developing_an_interdependent_leadership_culture.

[15] McCauley, Palus, Drath, Hughes, McGuire, O'Connor, and Van Velsor, "INTERDEPENDENT LEADERSHIP."

[16] Ellen Van Velsor, Cynthia D. McCauley, and Marian N. Ruderman, eds., "Developing Interdependent Leadership," chap. 14 from *The Center for Creative Leadership Handbook of Leadership Development* (San Francisco: Jossey-Bass, 2010), http://solutions.ccl.org/ The_Center_for_Creative_Leadership_Handbook_of_Leadership_ Development_3rd_Edition.

[17] Bruce W. Tuckman, "Developmental Sequence in Small Groups'" *Psychological Bulletin* 63, no. 6 (1965): 384–399, http://openvce.net/ sites/default/files/Tuckman1965DevelopmentalSequence.pdf.

[18] "Pharmacist Collaboration Closes Gaps in Care," Express Scripts, February 13, 2013, http://lab.express-scripts.com/lab/insights/specialized-care/pharmacist-collaboration-closes-gaps-in-care#sthash.atJ3zXdX.dpuf.

[19] "The Growing Crisis of Chronic Disease in the United States," Partnership to Fight Chronic Disease.

[20] "Development and Implementation of Curricula Strategies in Medication Therapy Management by Colleges and Schools of Pharmacy," AACP, December 2011, http://www.aacp.org/ resources/education/Documents/DevelopmentandImplementation ofCurriculaStrategiesinMTMbyCollegesandSchoolsofPharmacy-SummaryReportofSubmissions.pdf.

[21] "Integrating Medication Therapy Management (MTM) Into the Curricula of Schools and Colleges of Pharmacy: Recommendations and Strategies from an American Pharmacists Association MTM in the Curricula Expert Panel," APha, March 2012, http://www.pharmacist. com/sites/default/files/files/mtm_integrating_curricula_032012.pdf.

Chapter 11

[1] "ADHERENCE TO LONG-TERM THERAPIES Evidence for action," WHO, 2003, http://www.who.int/chp/knowledge/publications/adherence_introduction.pdf.

[2] "2017 AHA Environmental Scan," *H&HN*, accessed December 7, 2016, http://www.hhnmag.com/ext/resources/inc-hhn/pdfs/PartnerArticles/2016/EnviroScan_2017.pdf.

[3] "New Kaiser/New York Times Survey Finds One in Five Working-Age Americans With Health Insurance Report Problems Paying Medical Bills," Kaiser Family Foundation, January 05, 2016, http://kff.org/health-costs/press-release/new-kaisernew-york-times-survey-finds-one-in-five-working-age-americans-with-health-insurance-report-problems-paying-medical-bills/.

[4] "Better Care. Smarter Spending. Healthier People" CMS.gov.

[5] Susan DeVore, "Six Big Trends To Watch In Health Care For 2016," *Health Affairs Blog*, December 30, 2015, http://healthaffairs.org/blog/2015/12/30/six-big-trends-to-watch-in-health-care-for-2016/.

[6] "Prescription Opioid Overdose Data," CDC, June 21, 2016, http://www.cdc.gov/drugoverdose/data/overdose.html.

[7] "Precision Medicine Initiative," FDA, October 3, 2016, http://www.fda.gov/ScienceResearch/SpecialTopics/PrecisionMedicine/default.htm.

[8] Zachary Brennan, "Regulatory Explainer: 21st Century Cures Redux and What It will Mean for FDA," November 28, 2016, http://www.raps.org/Regulatory-Focus/News/2016/11/28/26242/Regulatory-Explainer-21st-Century-Cures-Redux-and-What-it-Will-Mean-for-FDA/

[9] "Important Role for Pharmacy in House-Passed 21st Century Cures Bill," NACDS, July 7, 2015, http://www.nacds.org/Article/2432/2015-07-10/important-role-for-pharmacy-in-house-passed-21st-century-cures-bill

[10] Michael E. Porter, "What Is Value in Health Care?" 2,477-2,481.

[11] Ibid.

About the Author

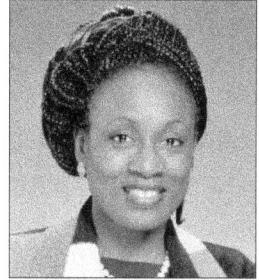

Elizabeth Oyekan, Pharm.D, FCSHP, CPHQ
Author . Executive . Senior Advisor . Faculty

Dr. Elizabeth Oyekan is the author of the following books:
- ***Medication A.R.E.A.S. Bundle***: *Prescription for Healthcare Value to Optimize Patient Health Outcomes, Reduce Total Costs, and Improve Organization Performance*
- ***The Ten Elements of L.E.A.D.E.R.S.H.I.P.*** *Intelligence: Behaviors & Skills to lead in uncertain & complex healthcare & business environments*
- ***The B-SMART Handbook with Pharmaceutical Pearls*** - *Helping your patients Be Smart about appropriate medication use*

She is also a senior advisor with a major organization and a faculty member at the Institute of Healthcare Improvement (IHI). Prior to these roles, Dr. Elizabeth Oyekan was the Vice President of Operations and Quality for Kaiser Permanente Colorado, Colorado's leading integrated health care provider and not-for-profit health plan. With oversight of more than $1.5 billion budget, the Operations and Quality aspects of Kaiser Permanente Colorado serves more than 650,000 members in 28 medical offices ranging from Fort Collins in the North to Denver / Boulder and to Pueblo in the South.

Oyekan assumed this role in 2013 and in her role, she oversees Behavioral Health, Call Center, Clintech, Lab, Labor Management Partnership, Medical Imaging, Medical Specialties, Nursing, Pharmacy, Population Care & Prevention Services, Primary Care, Quality & Risk

Management, Surgical Specialties, Women's Health, visions essentials, and Business Operations Support Services.

Her career at Kaiser Permanente has spanned more than 23 years, and she has successfully managed different aspects of the organization including Vice President of Operations, National Quality Leader for Pharmacy, Director of Pharmacy, Administrator for Perioperative Services, Director of Population Management, and various other Pharmacy leadership roles.

Under Oyekan's leadership, Kaiser Permanente Colorado has maintained its Medicare 5 star status, developed a solid leadership infrastructure to address the changing healthcare landscape, and worked interdependently to bring a new level of business acumen to Operations. In Kaiser Southern California, Oyekan co-led the development and implementation of the Outpatient Pharmacy Clinical Services, and developed the BSMART Strategy for all Kaiser Permanente Regions – provider tools used to optimize medication adherence and appropriate medication use in patients to improve their health outcomes. The BSMART Strategy won the CBI Strategic Patient Award in 2009. She has worked with IHI and the KP Adherence Team on strategies to improve Medication Adherence in our African American Population with Hypertension.

In all her roles, Oyekan has been dedicated to contributing to delivering on the Quad Aim – **better health** for members, patients, and the communities we serve, **better service and care** for each patient, **better and more effective costs** per capita, supported by the most effective team members.

In 2015, Dr. Oyekan was awarded the Most Powerful and Influential Women Award presented by the Colorado Diversity Council for her contributions.

A California & Colorado resident for over 30 years, Dr. Oyekan earned her Doctorate in Pharmacy Degree from the University of Southern California, completed her administrative and clinical residency at Kaiser Permanente Los Angeles Medical Center, and graduated from the executive leadership program at Harvard University.

Dr. Oyekan is a member of the National Association of Health Services Executives, Academy of Managed Care Pharmacy, National Association of Healthcare Quality, and the Care Management Society of America and currently serves on the Board of Directors for the Denver Hospice. She is an active member of the community, has served on many Boards, and is involved in medical missions locally and internationally as well as community youth orchestras.

She is married to Richard and they have 3 children who have travelled extensively and lived in various countries.

www.ingramcontent.com/pod-product-compliance
Lightning Source LLC
Chambersburg PA
CBHW071317210326
41597CB00015B/1258